PROXY MOM

ISBN 9781681123349
Library of Congress Control Number: 2024930523

Translation made in arrangement with Am-Book
(www.am-book.com)
Printed in Turkey by Elma Basim
First printed June 2024

This title is also available wherever e-books are sold (ISBN 9781681123356)

SOPHIE ADRIANSEN • MATHOU
TRANSLATION: MONTANA KANE

PROXY MOM

MY EXPERIENCE WITH POSTPARTUM DEPRESSION

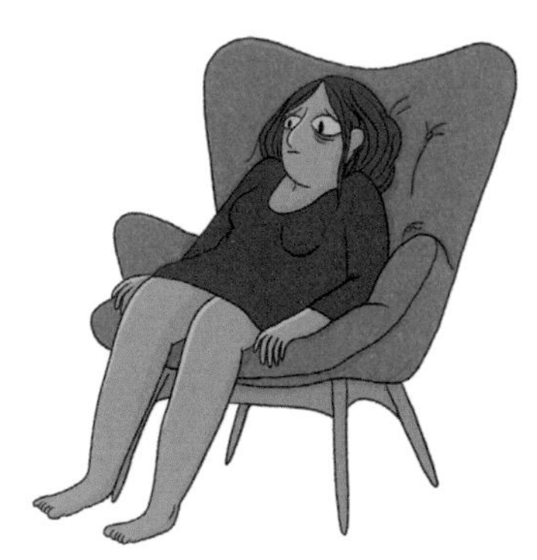

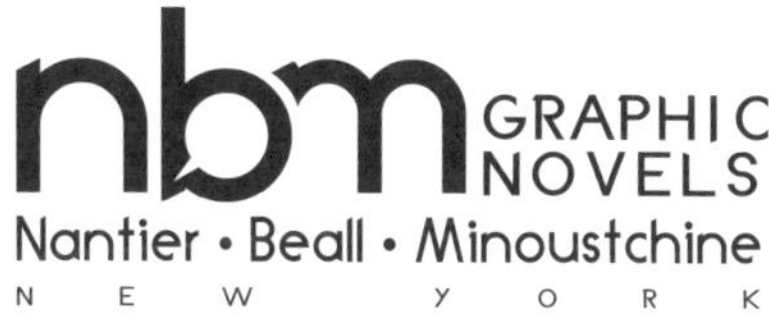

nbm GRAPHIC NOVELS
Nantier • Beall • Minoustchine
NEW YORK

One sees things better with eyes that have cried.

Ivoirian proverb

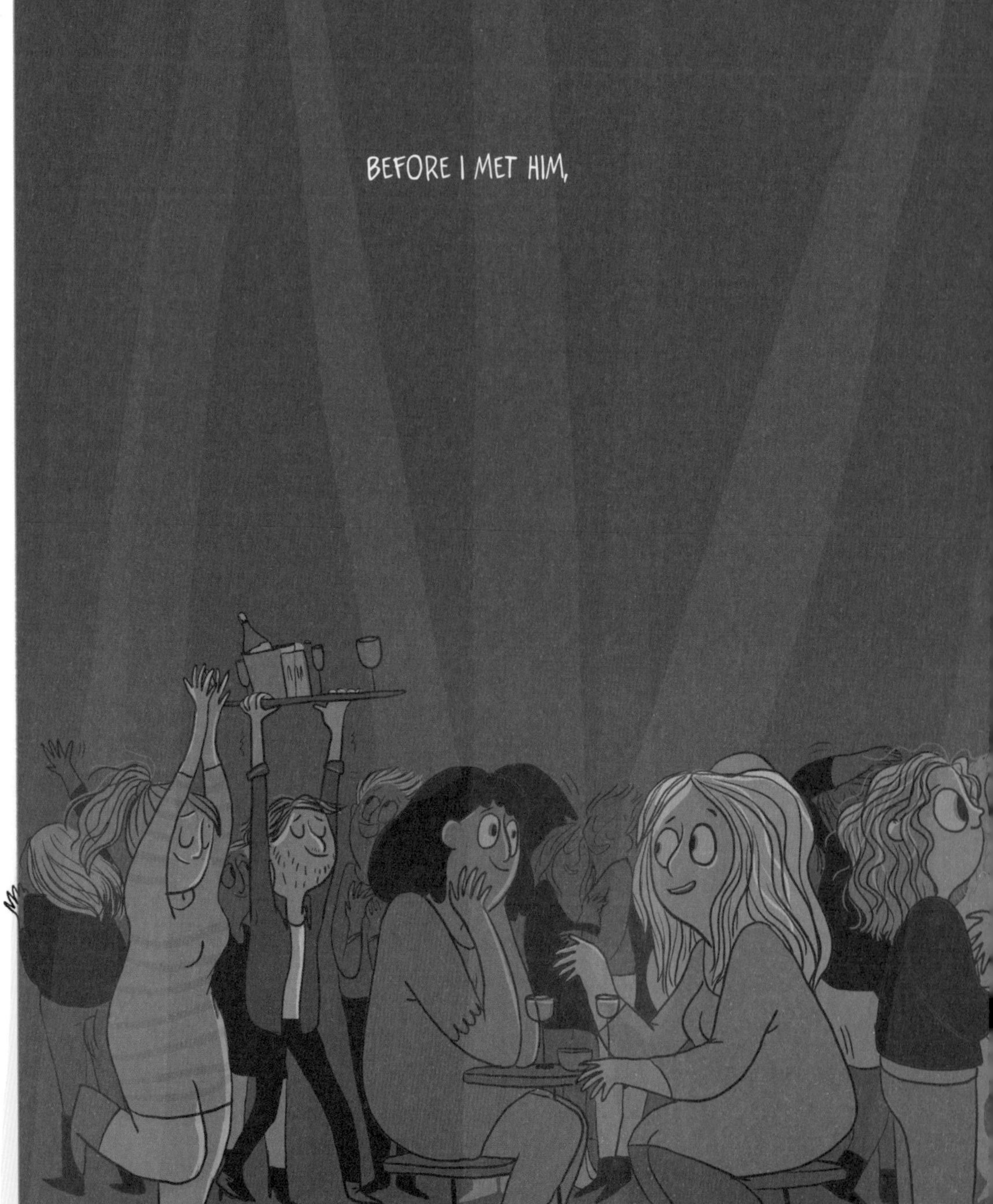
BEFORE I MET HIM,

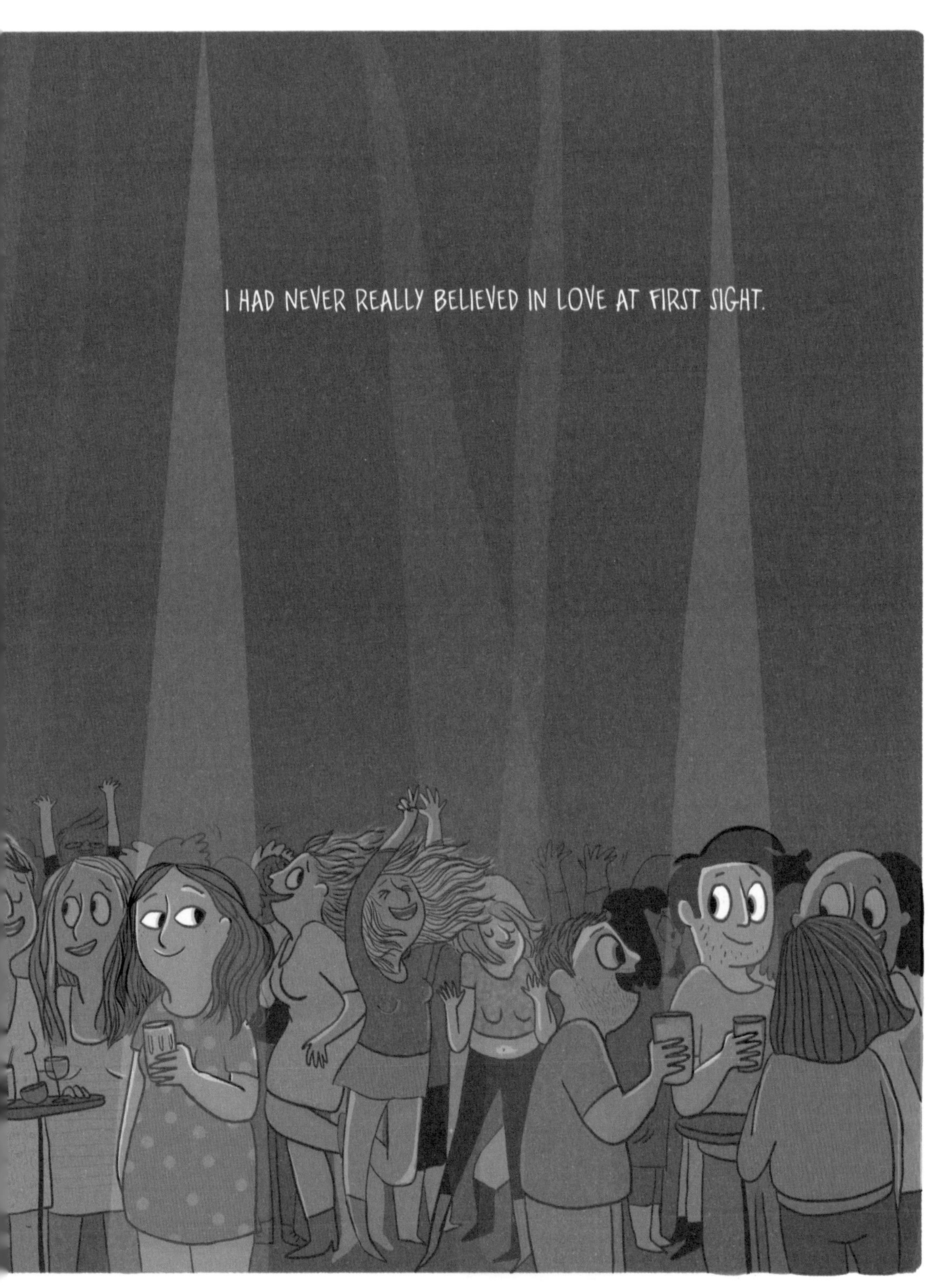
I HAD NEVER REALLY BELIEVED IN LOVE AT FIRST SIGHT.

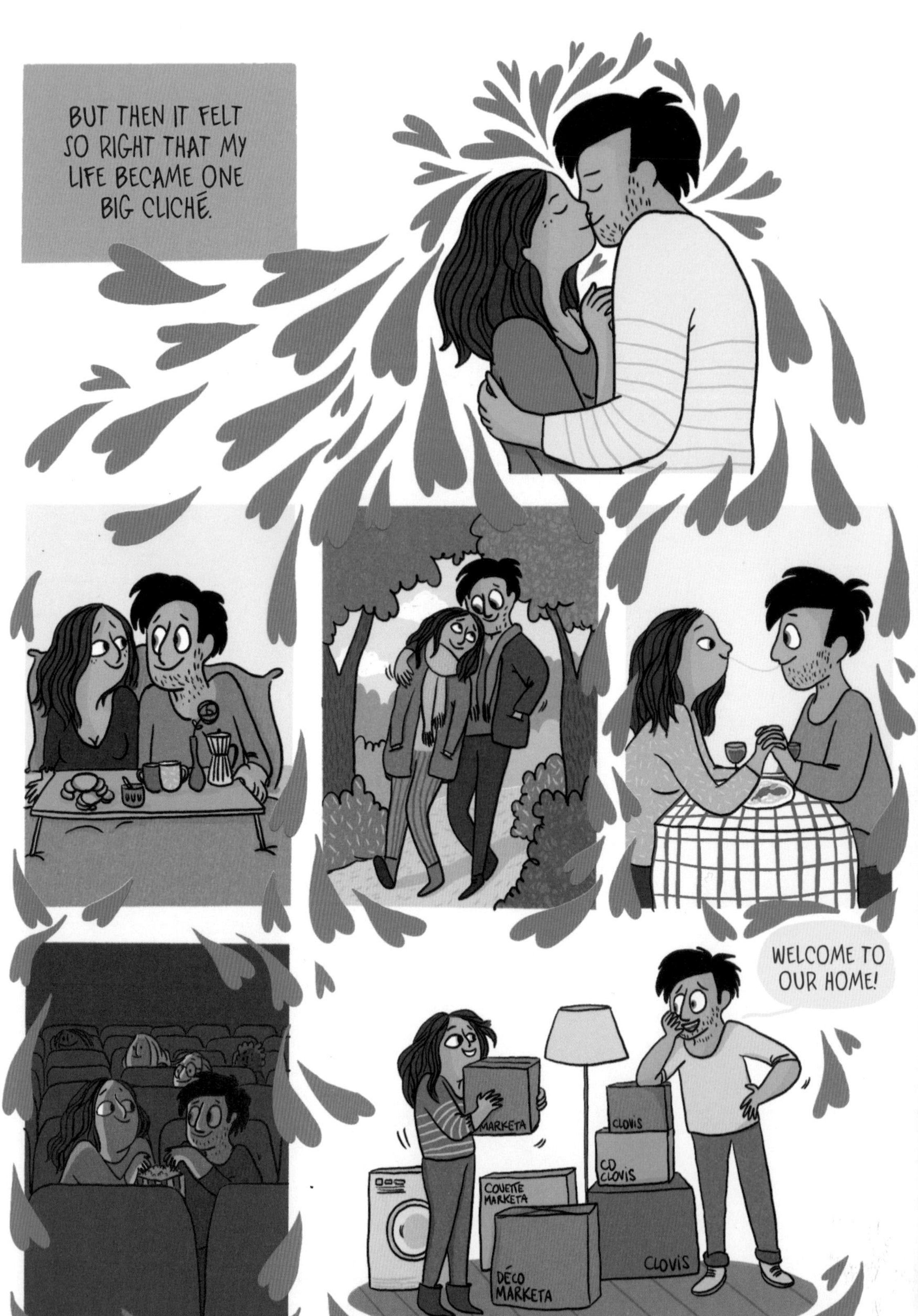

BUT THEN IT FELT SO RIGHT THAT MY LIFE BECAME ONE BIG CLICHÉ.

WELCOME TO OUR HOME!

MARKETA

CLOVIS

CD CLOVIS

COUETTE MARKETA

DÉCO MARKETA

CLOVIS

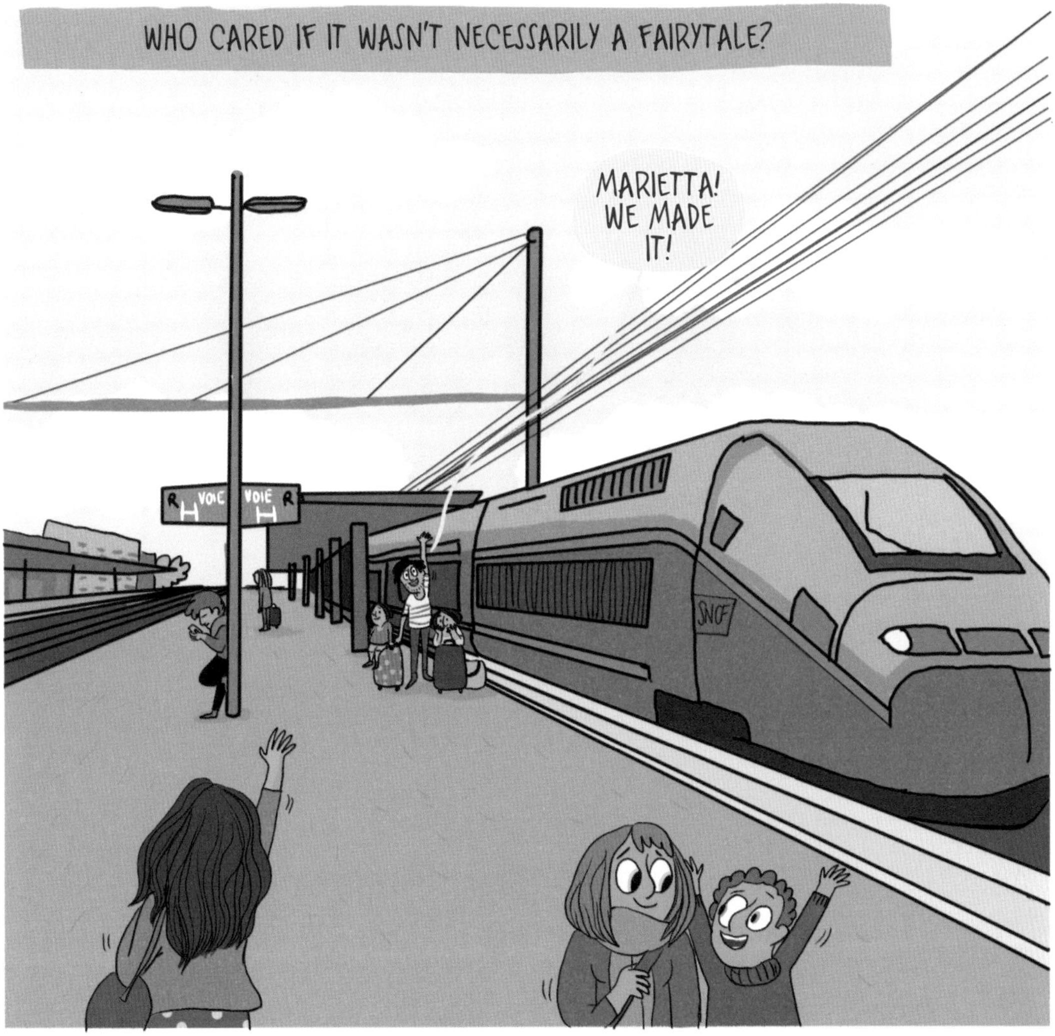

WHO CARED IF IT WASN'T NECESSARILY A FAIRYTALE?

MARIETTA! WE MADE IT!

AS SOMEONE WHO'D ALWAYS FELT A LITTLE LEFT OUT,
IT WAS AS IF I WERE STARRING IN MY OWN LIFE FOR THE FIRST TIME.

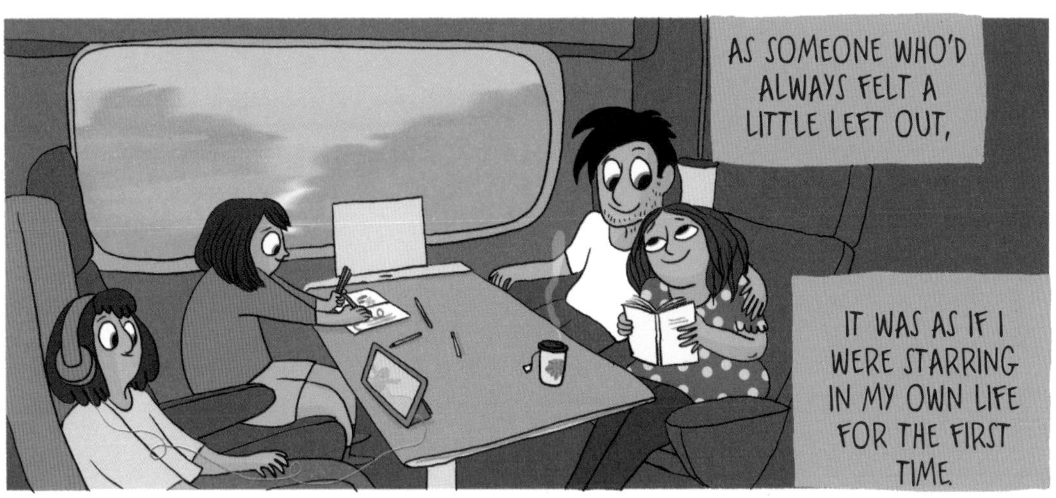

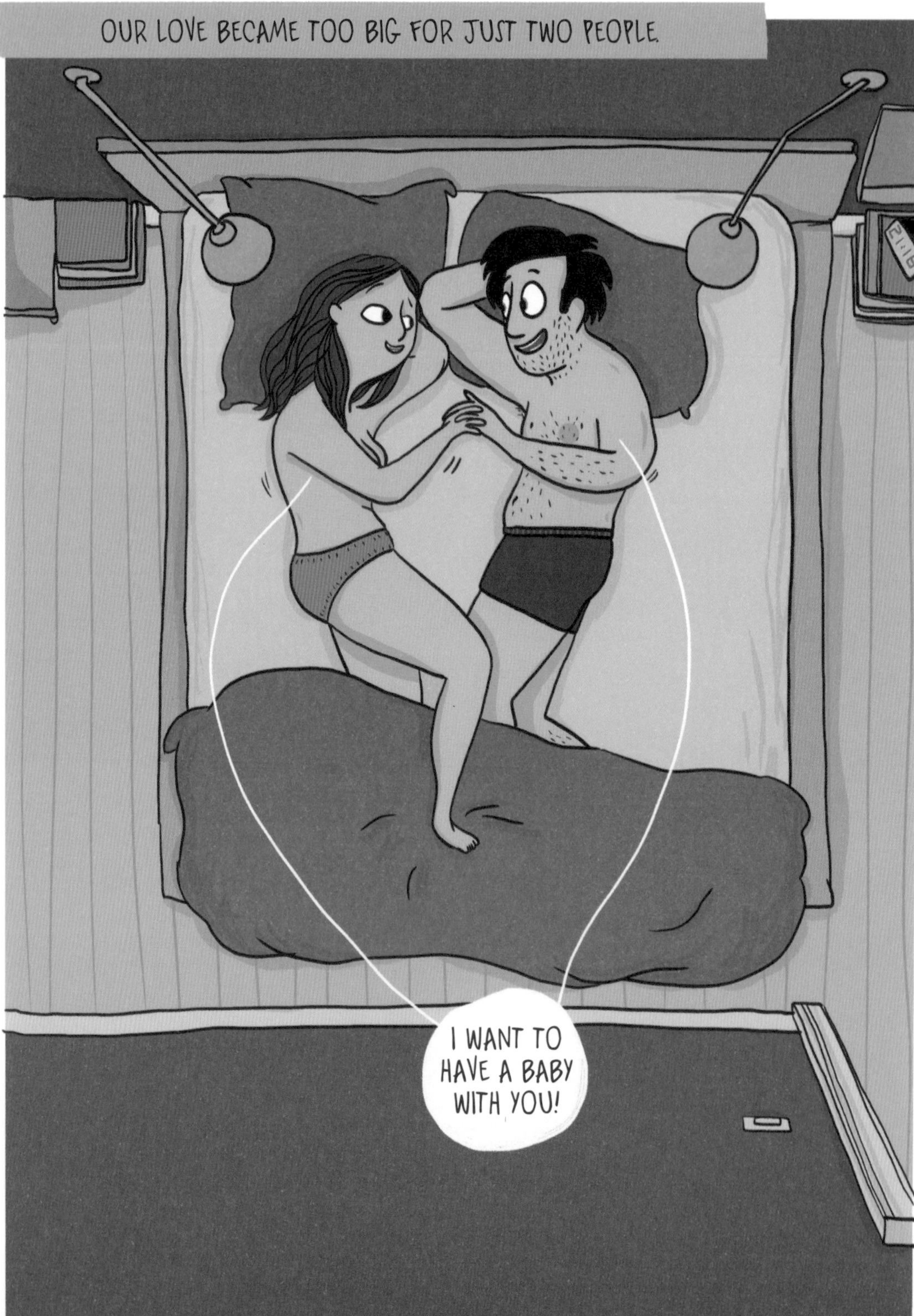
OUR LOVE BECAME TOO BIG FOR JUST TWO PEOPLE.
I WANT TO HAVE A BABY WITH YOU!

AND IT FELT AWESOME.

IT'S POSITIVE!!!
WE'RE HAVING A BABY!
OH MY GOD!

IT'S A GIRL!
LAMPE
I'LL NURSE HER IN THIS CHAIR AT NIGHT!

CHECK OUT MY NEW TRAY!

AS BIG AS A HOUSE? NO, A PAINT STORE!

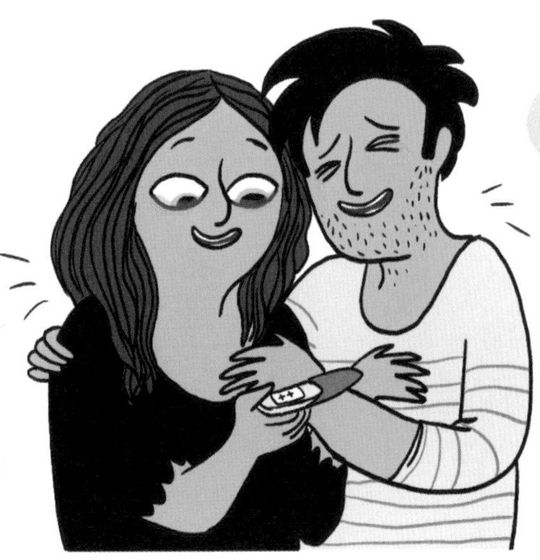

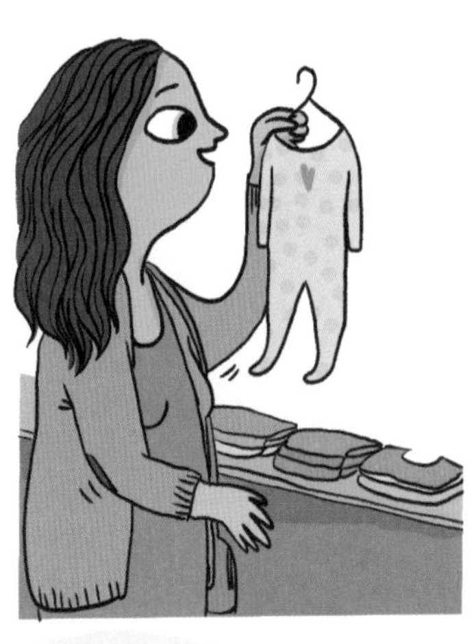

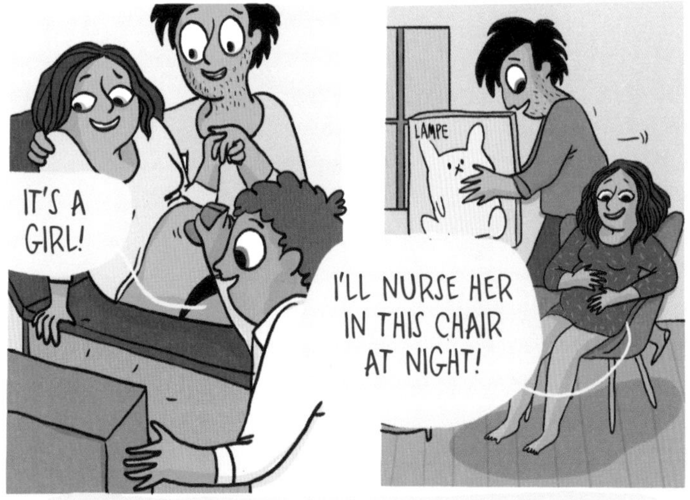

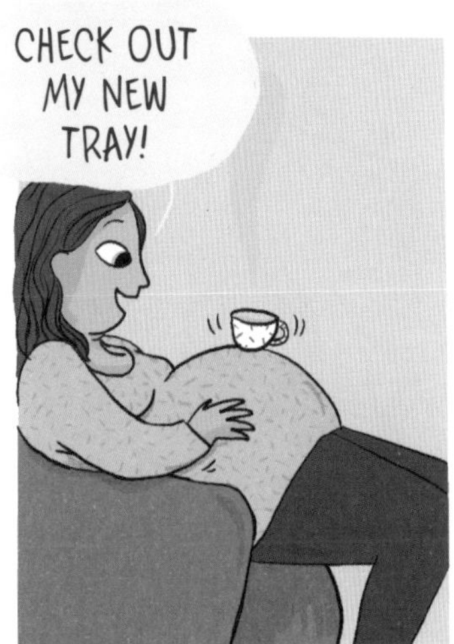

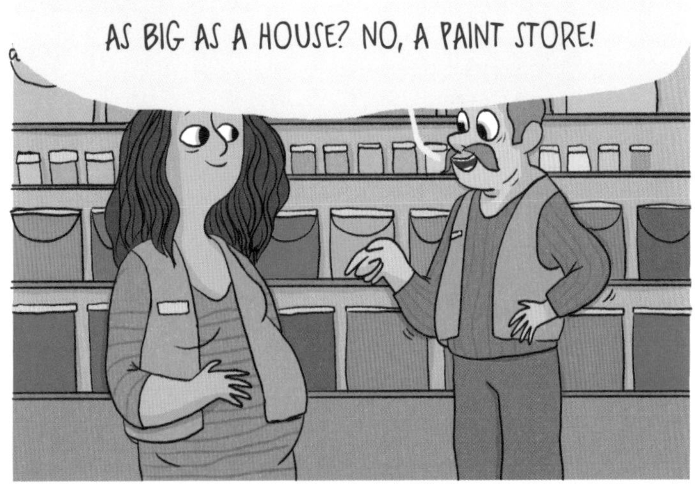

AND THEN ONE DAY I CAME CRASHING DOWN FROM MY CLOUD.

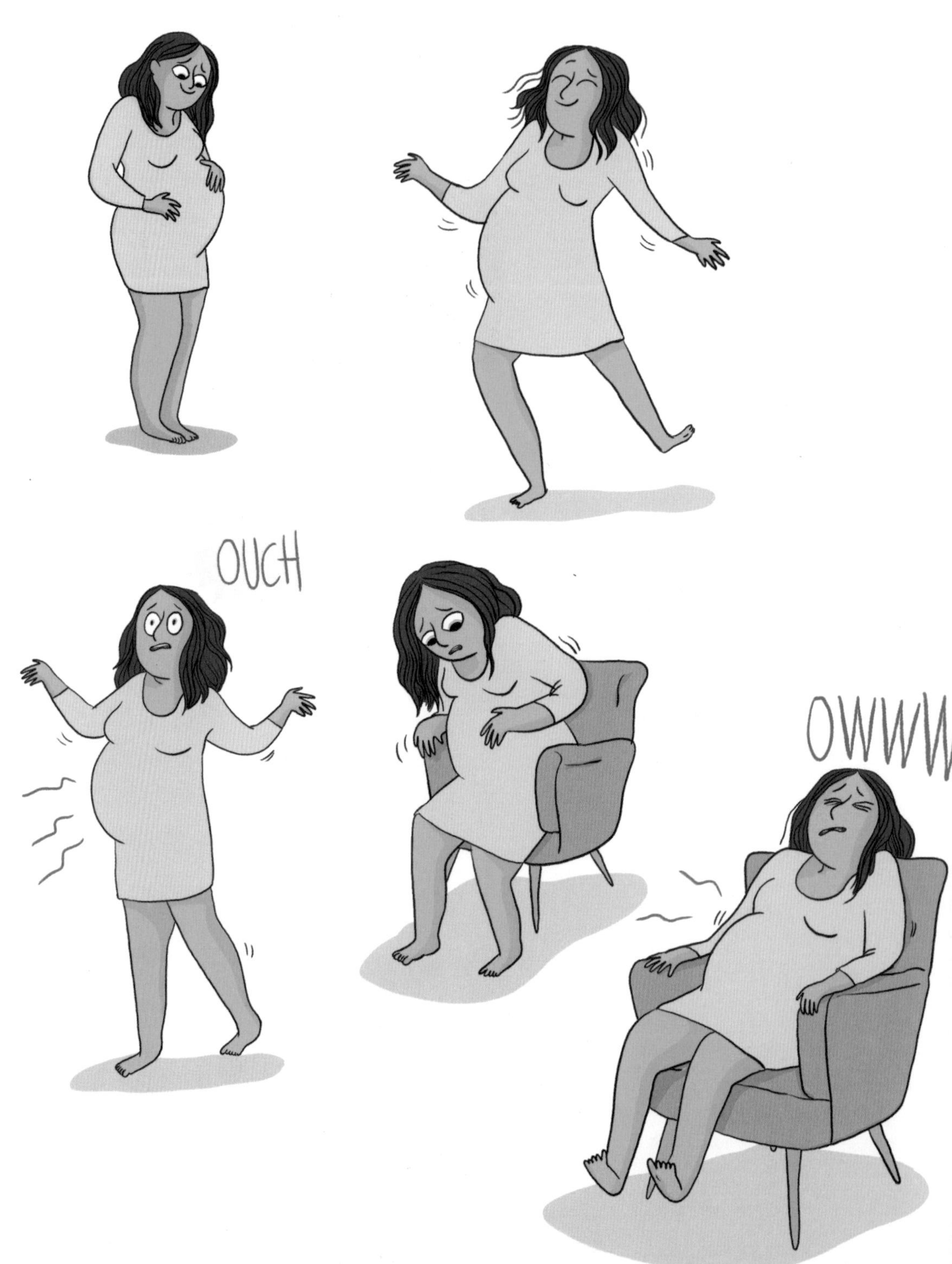

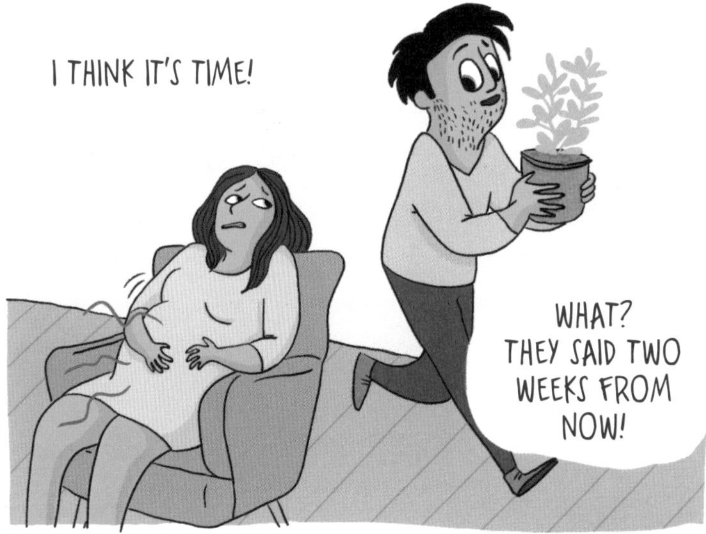
I THINK IT'S TIME!
WHAT? THEY SAID TWO WEEKS FROM NOW!
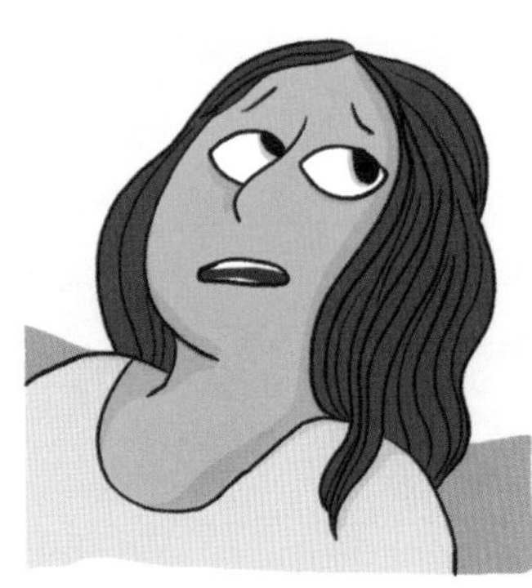
YEAH, WELL, SHE SEEMS INTENT ON COMING OUT NOW!
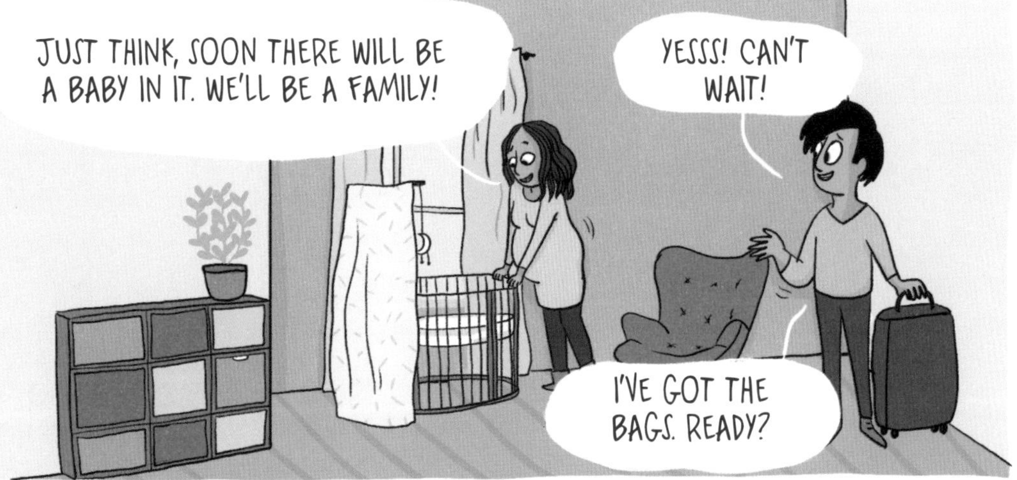
JUST THINK, SOON THERE WILL BE A BABY IN IT. WE'LL BE A FAMILY!
YESSS! CAN'T WAIT!
I'VE GOT THE BAGS. READY?
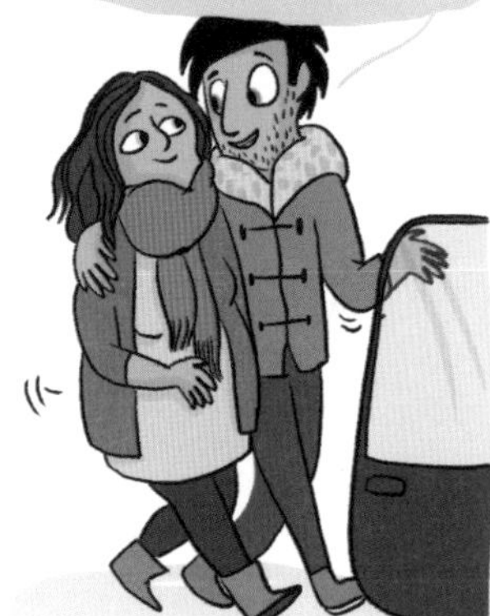
YOUR CHARIOT AWAITS, MILADY!
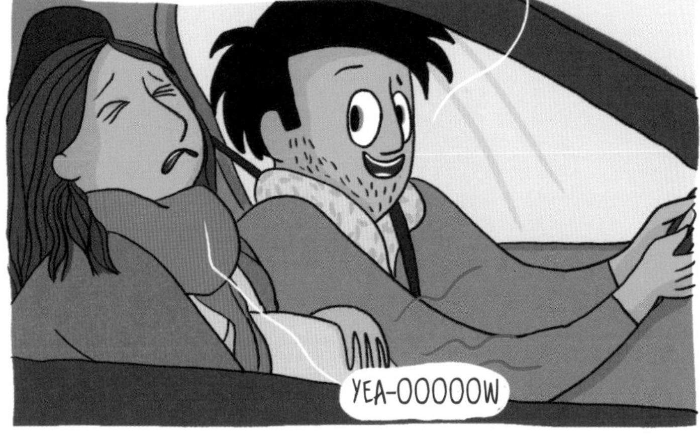
WE'RE ABOUT TO MEET HER! CAN YOU BELIEVE IT?
YEA-OOOOOW

YOU'RE HAVING BRAXTON-HICKS CONTRACTIONS, I.E. WHAT WE CALL FALSE LABOR
GET SOME REST, TAKE BATHS, AND DON'T LIFT HEAVY OBJECTS.
DRINK LOTS OF WATER AND LIE DOWN AS MUCH AS POSSIBLE.

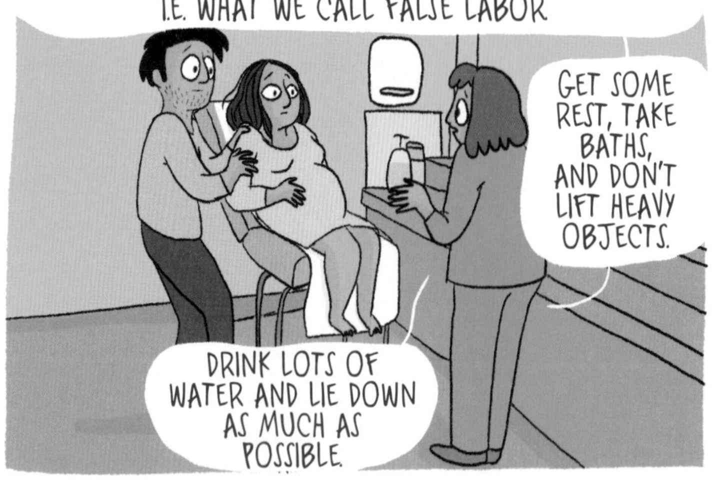

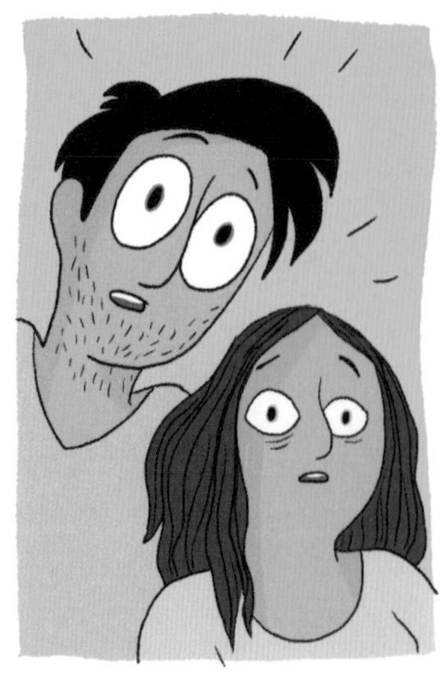

THE LAST WEEKS OF MY PREGNANCY WERE NOTHING LIKE I HAD IMAGINED.

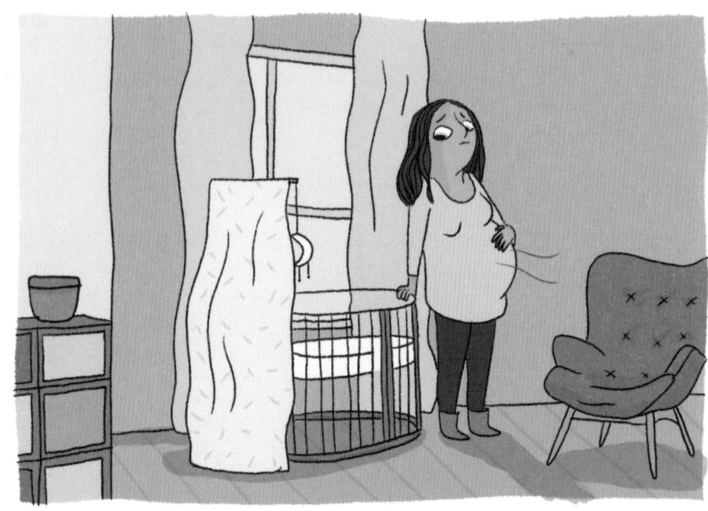

I ACCEPTED THE NOTION THAT IT WAS JUST A FALSE START.

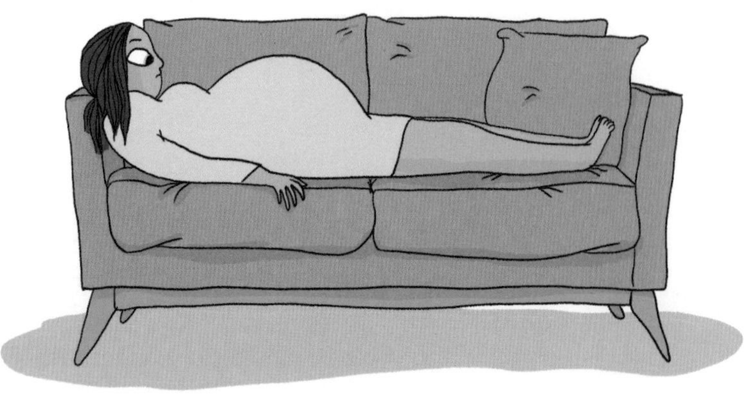

BUT COMING DOWN FROM MY CLOUD MEANT SAYING GOODBYE TO LIGHTNESS.

UGH
OWW

TIME FOR BED!
HANG IN THERE!

GNEEEE

MY POOR BABY...

ALL YOU CAN DO, MARIETTA, IS REST AND BE PATIENT.

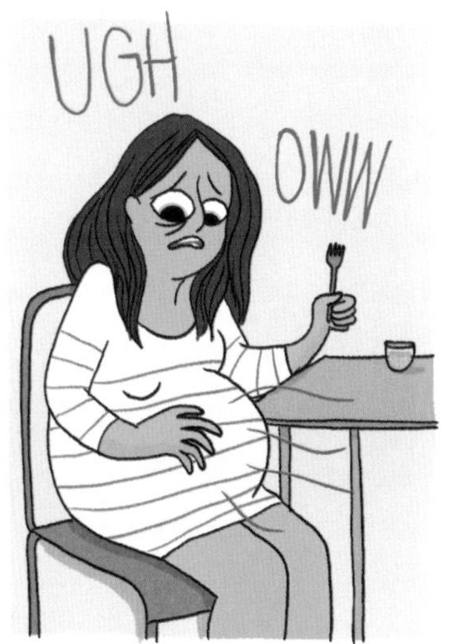

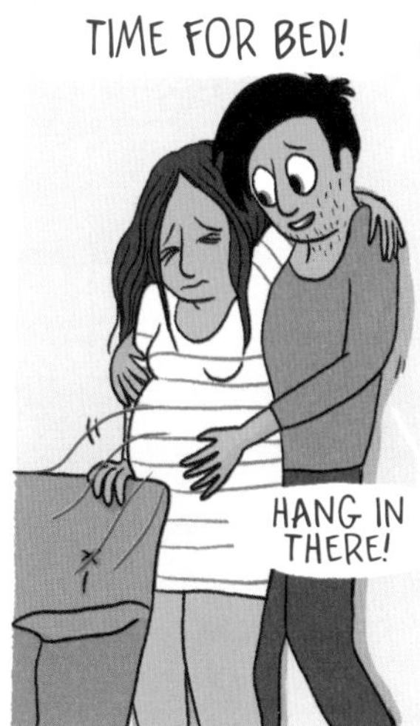

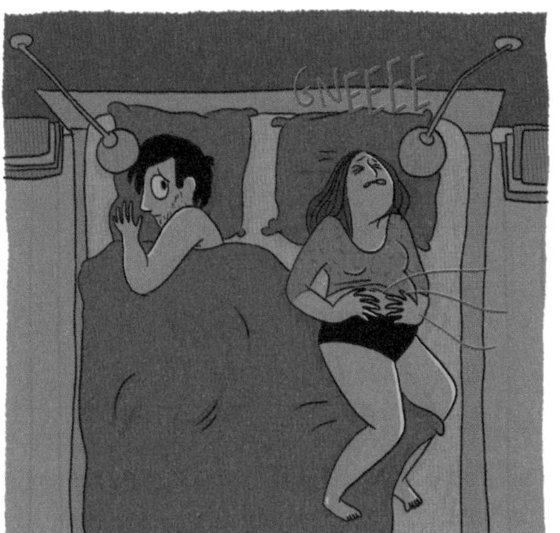

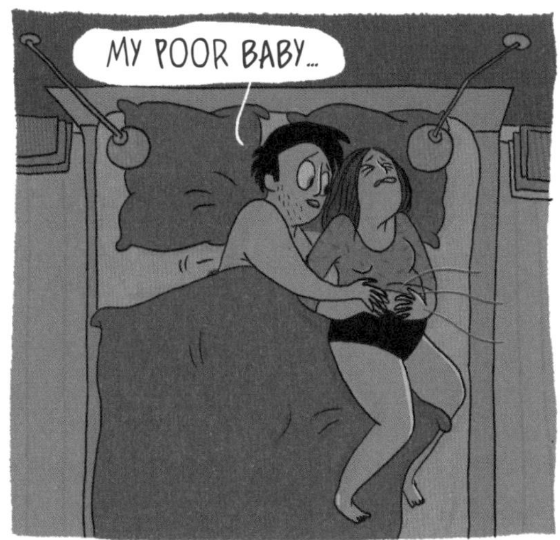

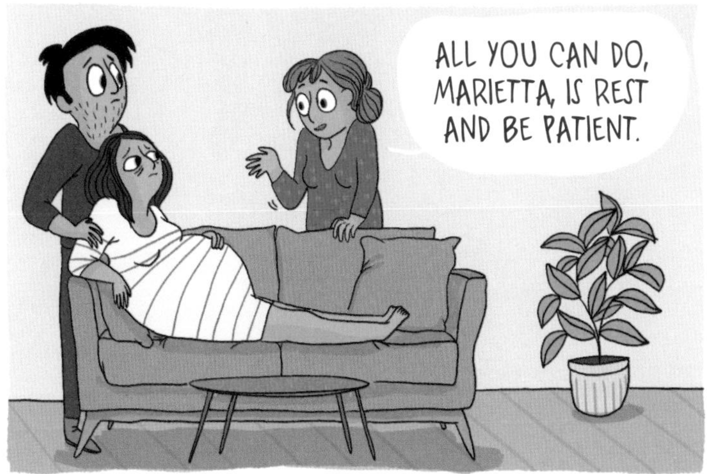

PATIENCE AND PAIN: MY NEW REALITY.

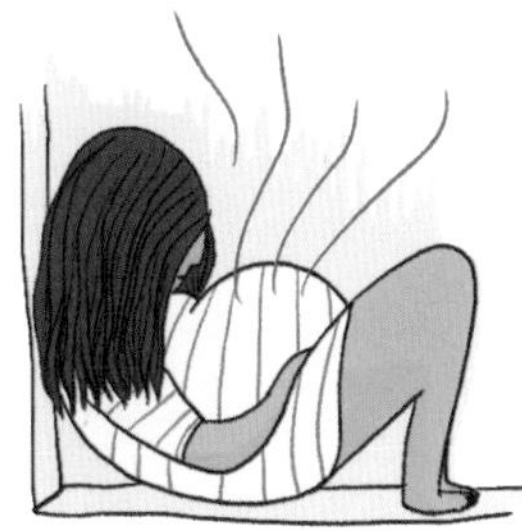

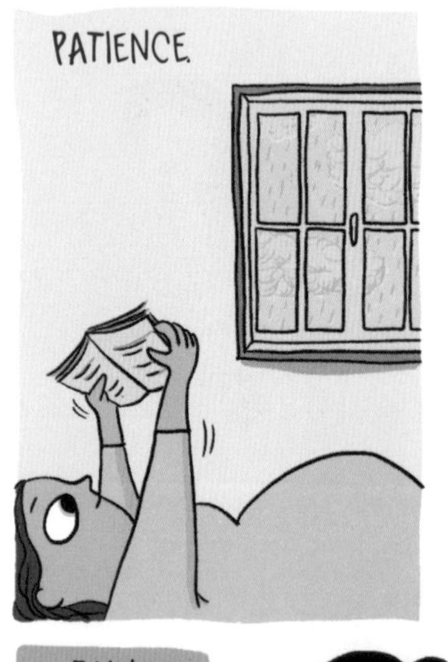
PATIENCE.

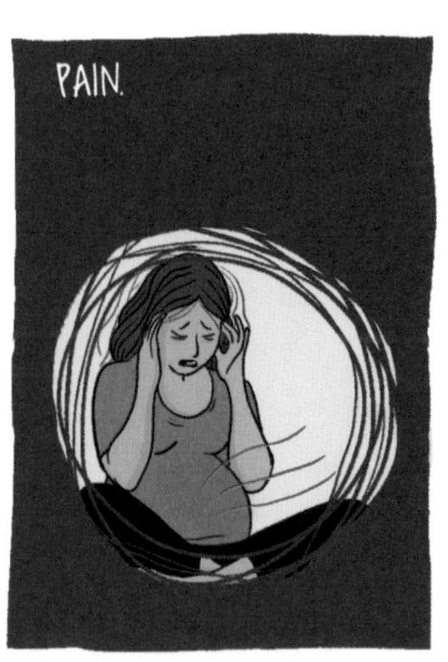
PAIN.

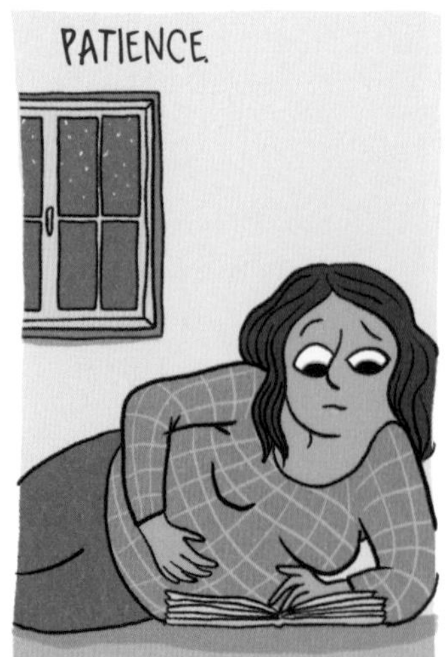
PATIENCE.

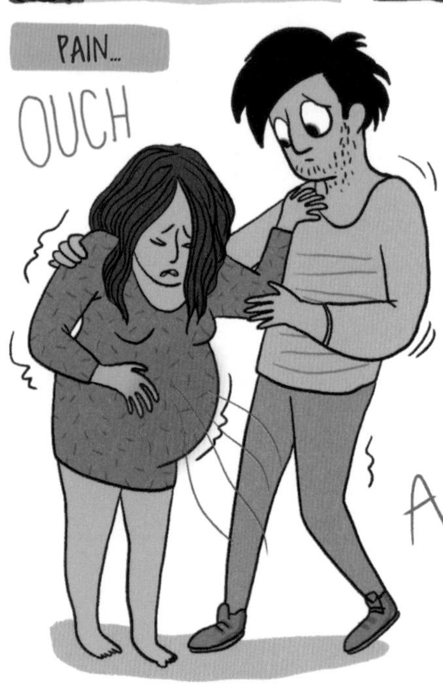
PAIN...
OUCH

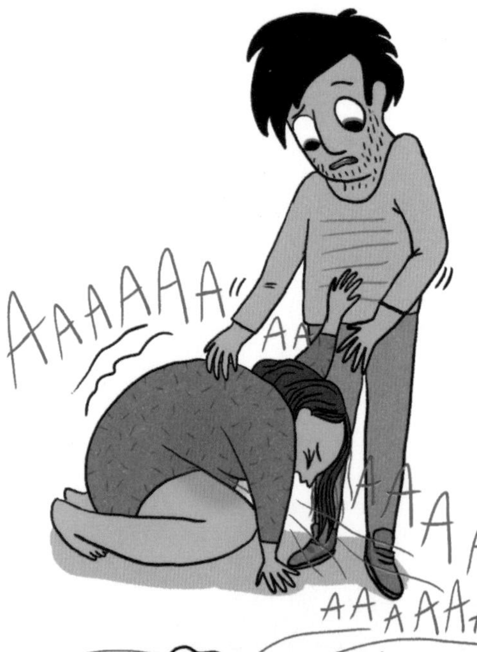
AAAAAAA
AA
AAAA

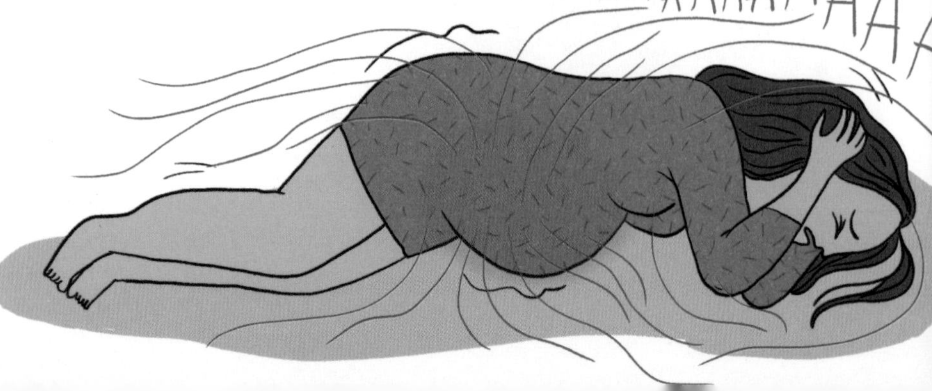
AAAAAAAAAAA

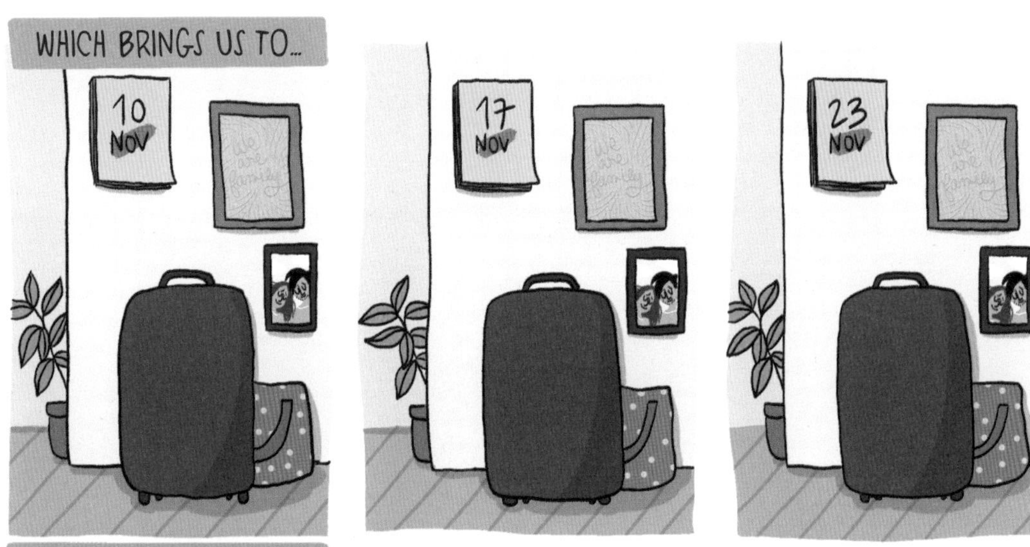
WHICH BRINGS US TO...
10 NOV
17 NOV
23 NOV

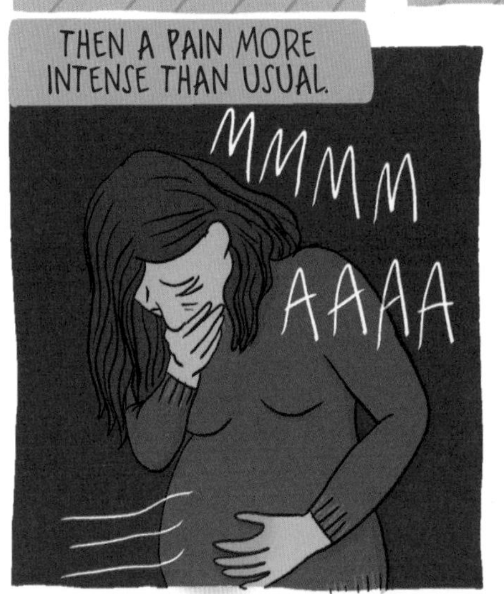
THEN A PAIN MORE INTENSE THAN USUAL.
MMMM
AAAA

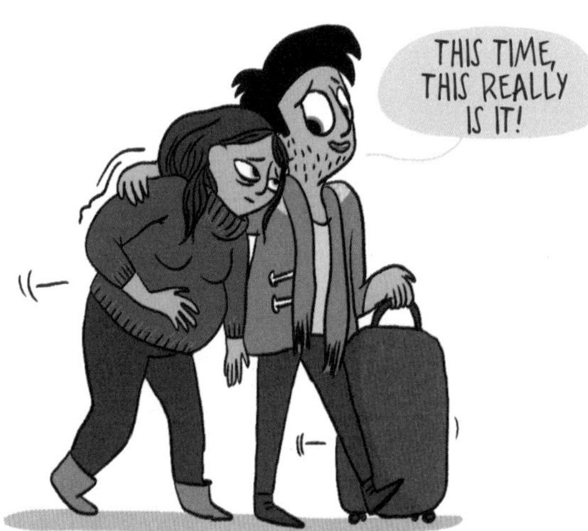
THIS TIME, THIS REALLY IS IT!

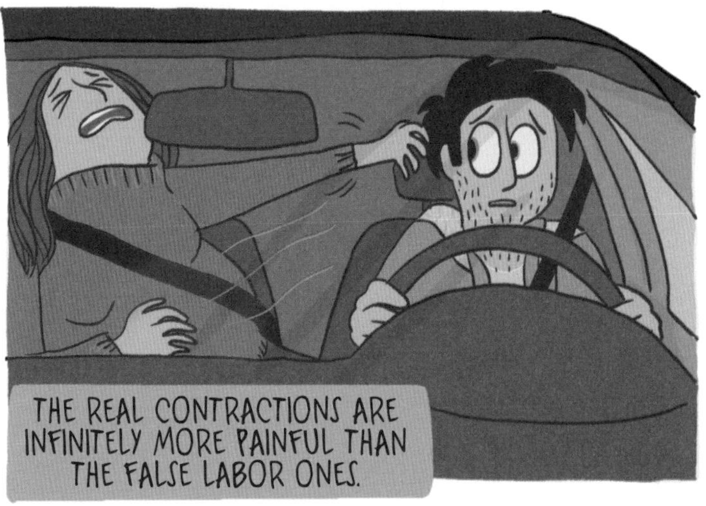
THE REAL CONTRACTIONS ARE INFINITELY MORE PAINFUL THAN THE FALSE LABOR ONES.

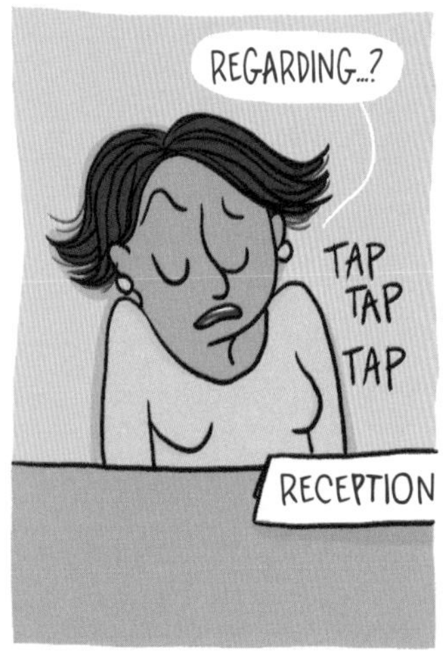
REGARDING...?
TAP
TAP
TAP
RECEPTION

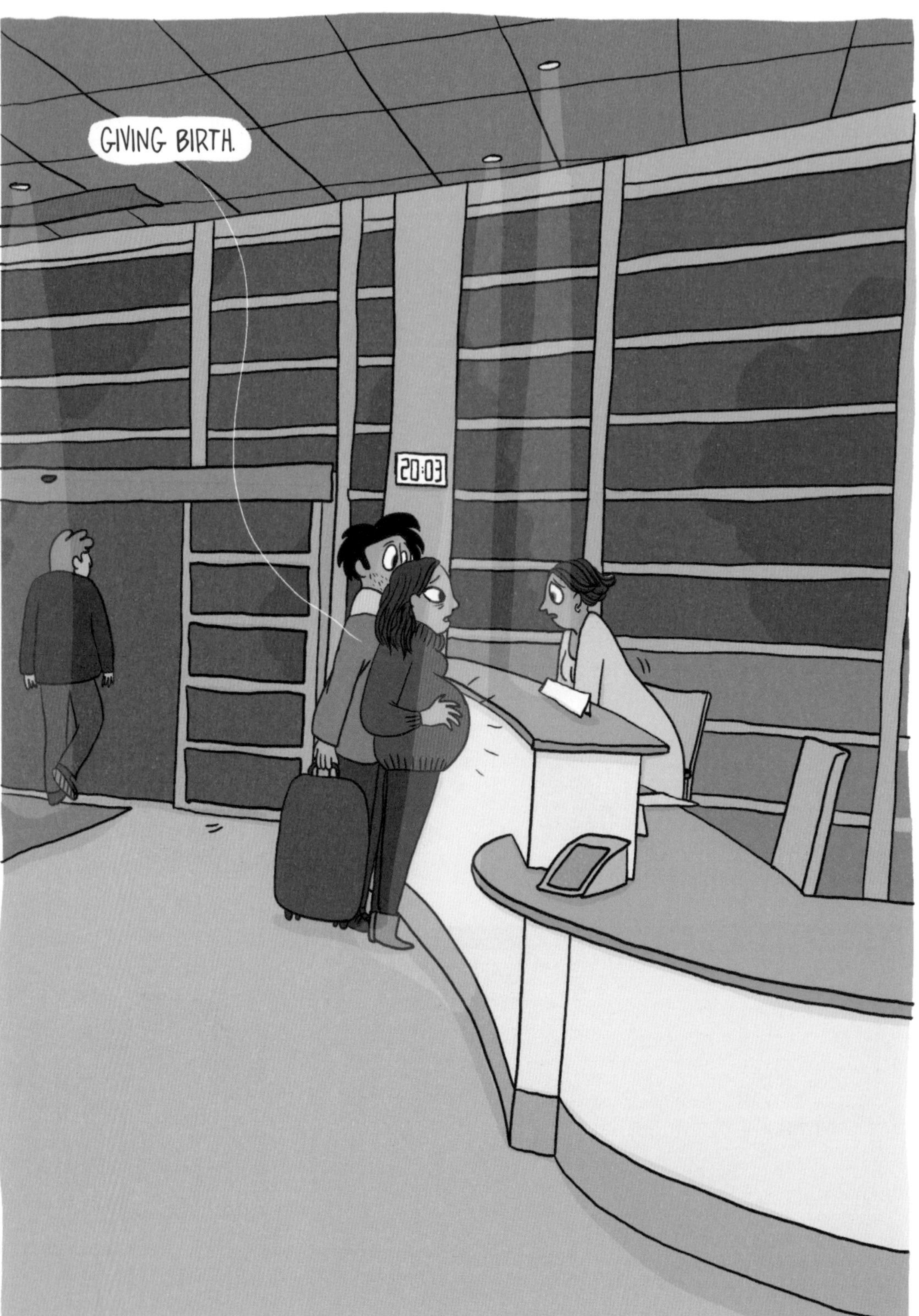
GIVING BIRTH.
20:03

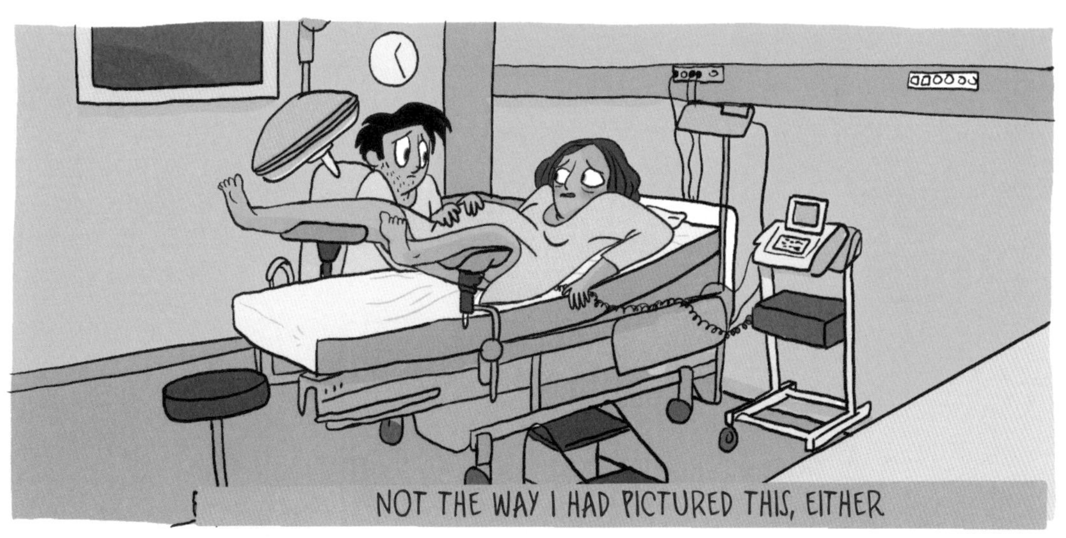
NOT THE WAY I HAD PICTURED THIS, EITHER

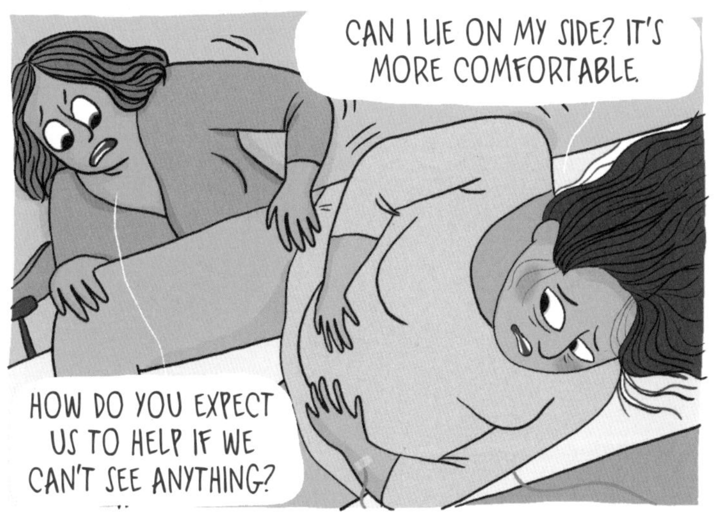
CAN I LIE ON MY SIDE? IT'S MORE COMFORTABLE.
HOW DO YOU EXPECT US TO HELP IF WE CAN'T SEE ANYTHING?

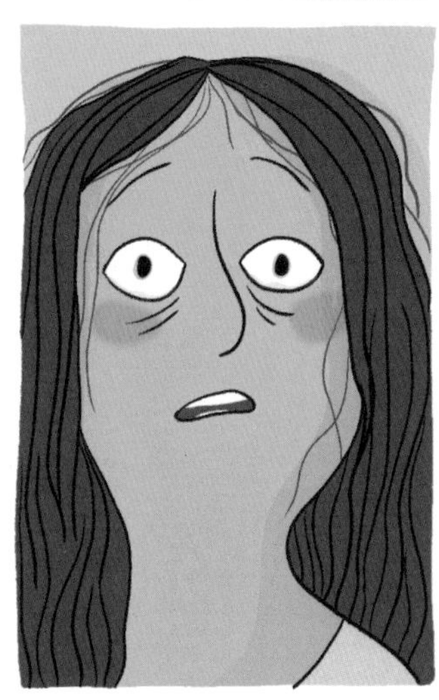

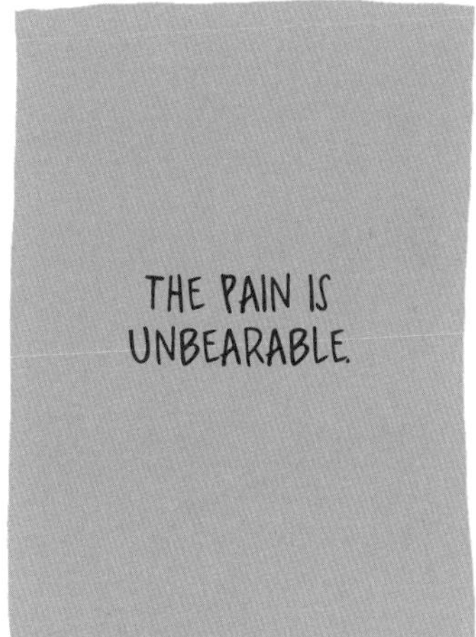
THE PAIN IS UNBEARABLE.

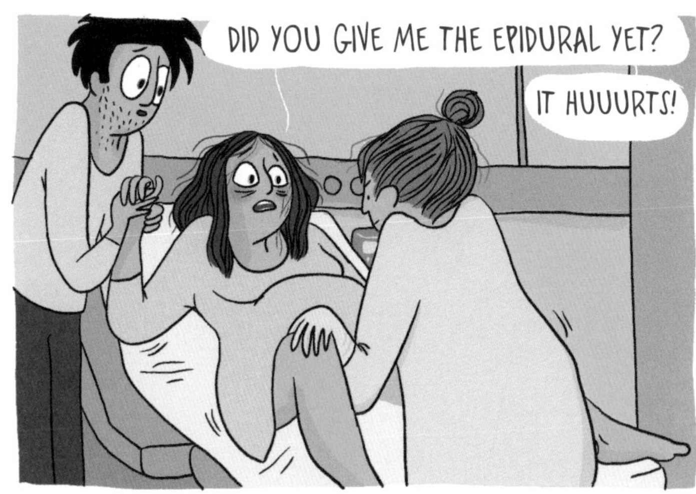
DID YOU GIVE ME THE EPIDURAL YET?
IT HUUURTS!

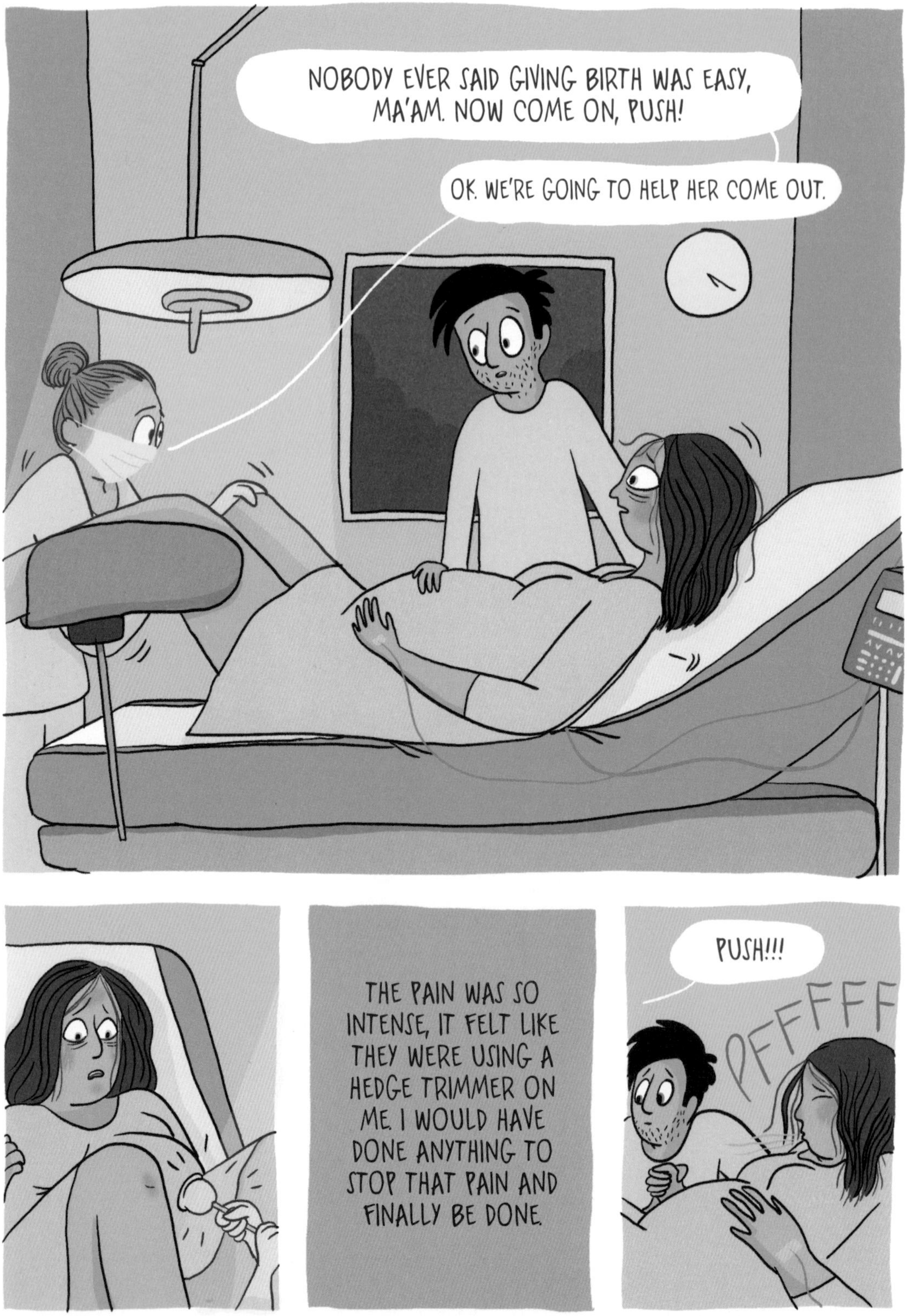

NOBODY EVER SAID GIVING BIRTH WAS EASY, MA'AM. NOW COME ON, PUSH!

OK. WE'RE GOING TO HELP HER COME OUT.

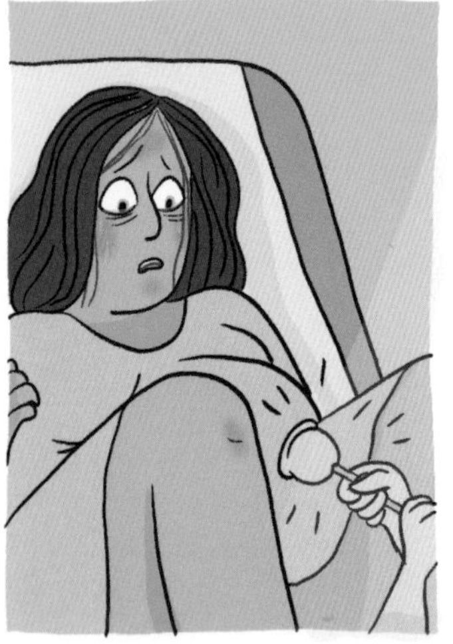

THE PAIN WAS SO INTENSE, IT FELT LIKE THEY WERE USING A HEDGE TRIMMER ON ME. I WOULD HAVE DONE ANYTHING TO STOP THAT PAIN AND FINALLY BE DONE.

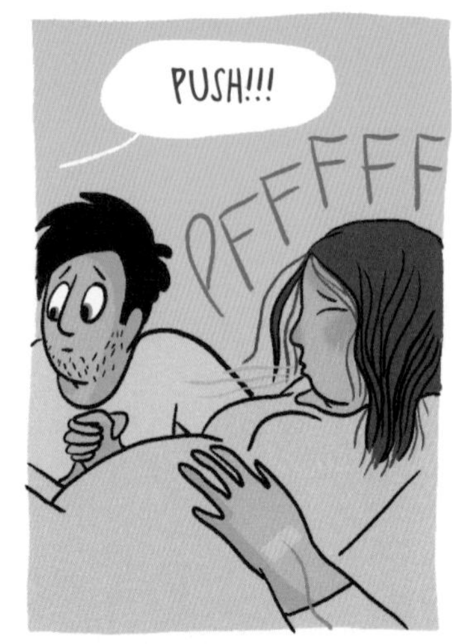

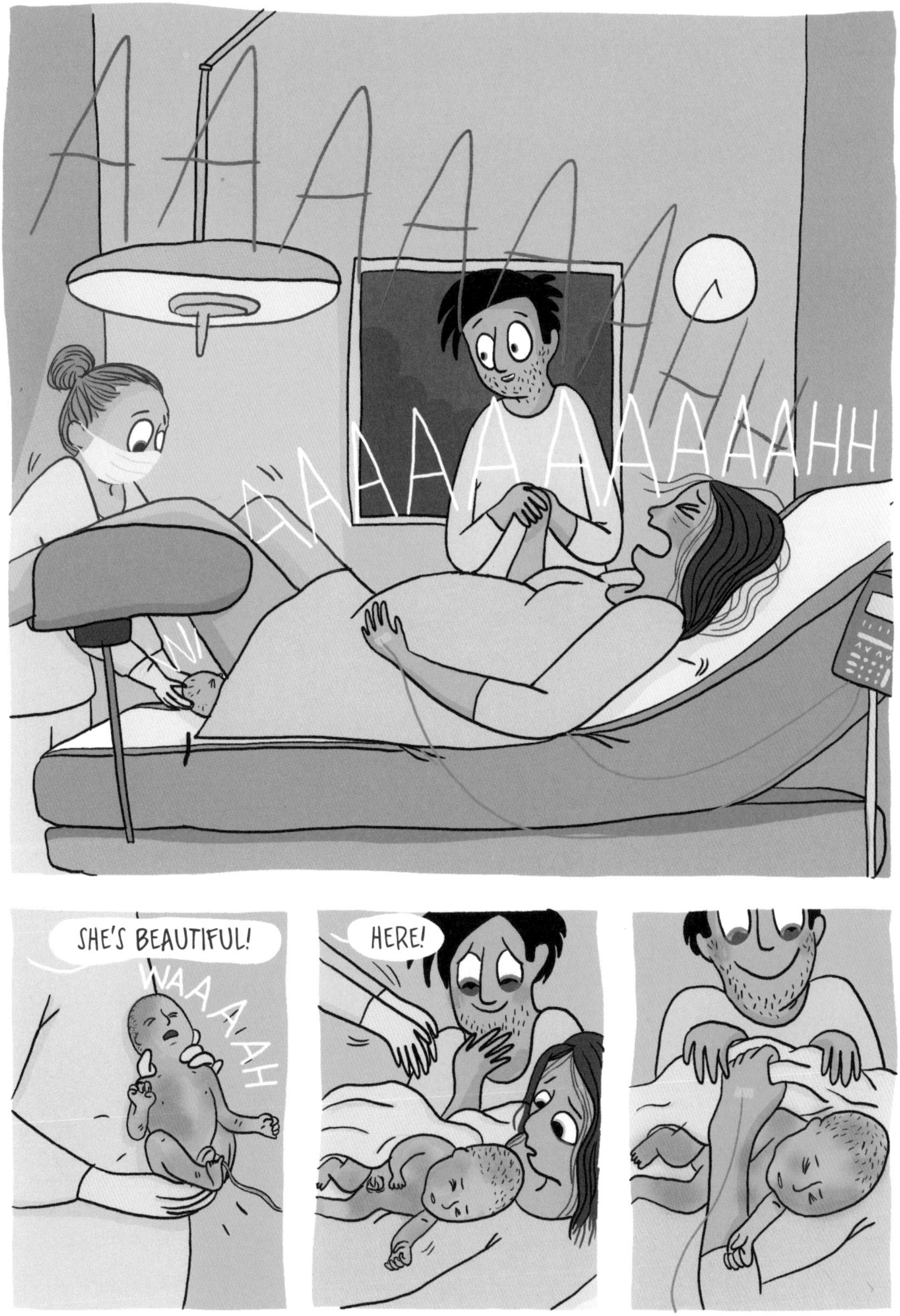

AAAAAAAAAHH

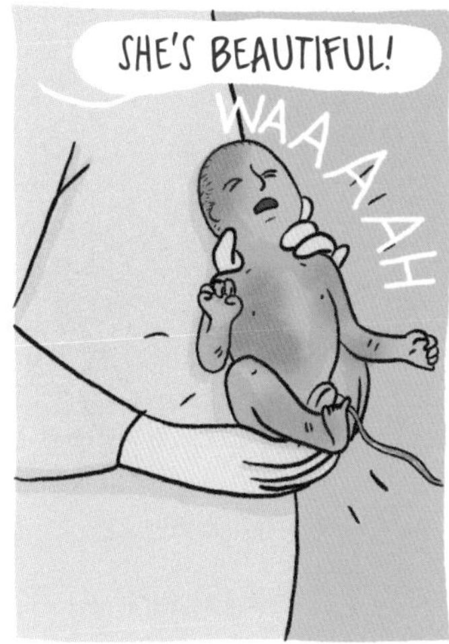
SHE'S BEAUTIFUL!
WAAAAH

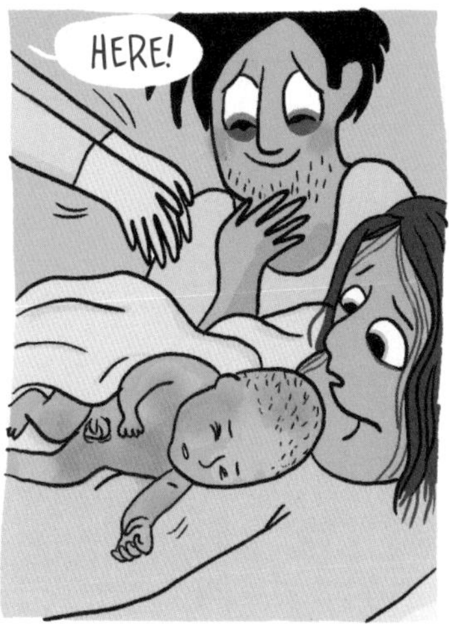
HERE!

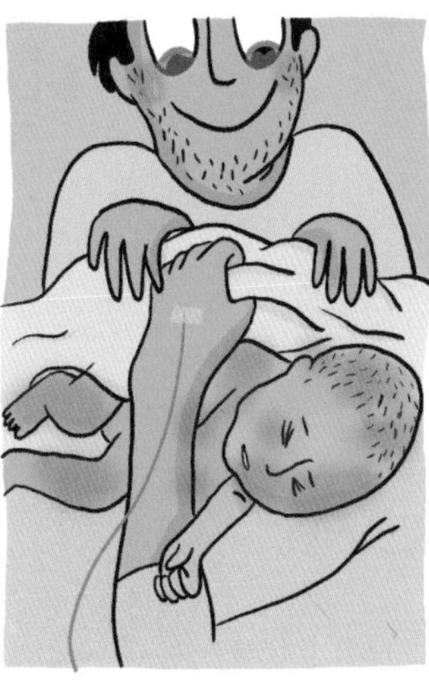

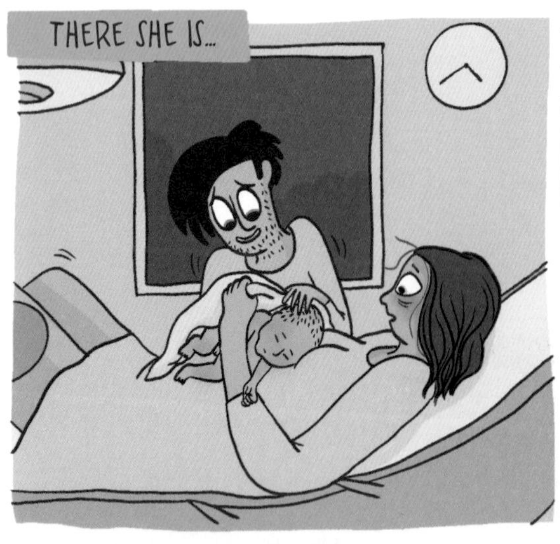
THERE SHE IS...

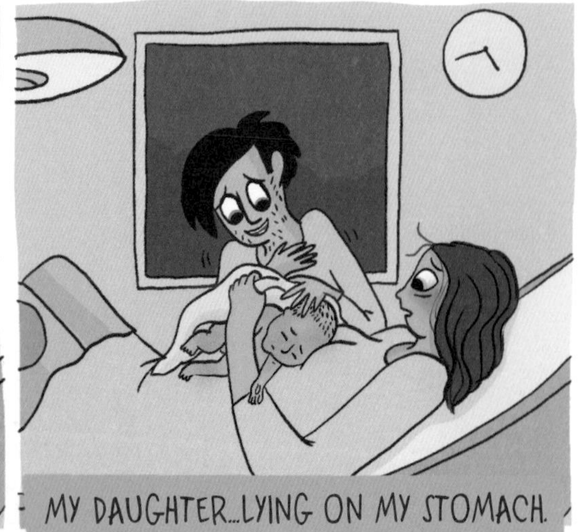
MY DAUGHTER...LYING ON MY STOMACH.

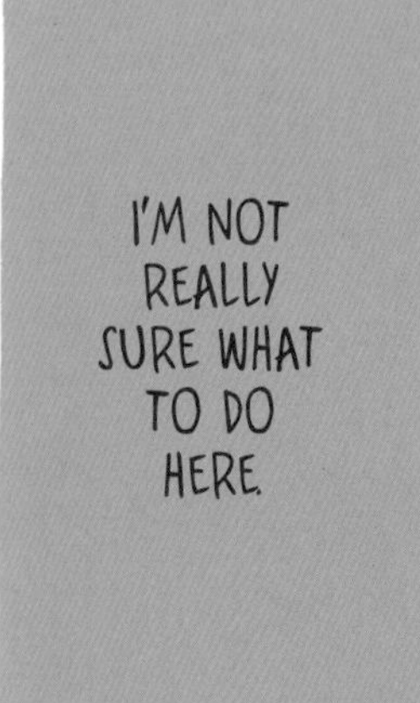
I'M NOT REALLY SURE WHAT TO DO HERE.

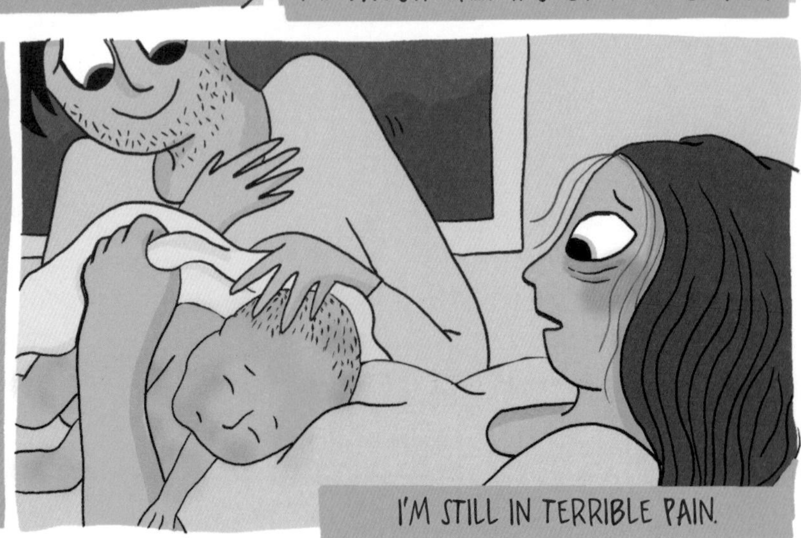
I'M STILL IN TERRIBLE PAIN.

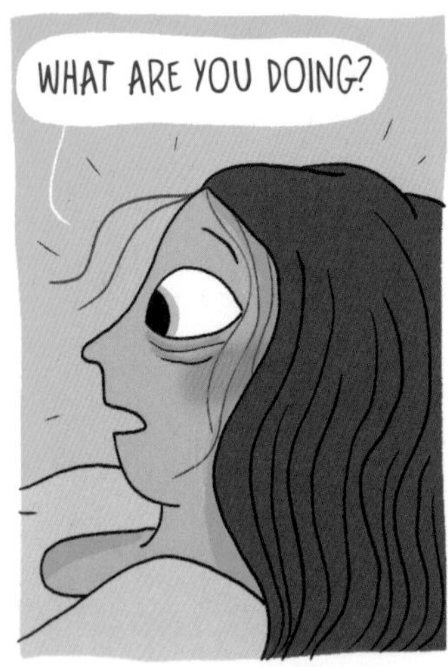
WHAT ARE YOU DOING?

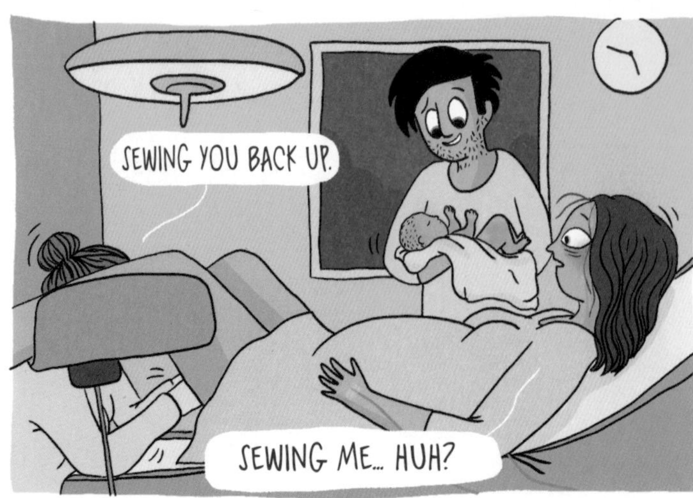
SEWING YOU BACK UP.
SEWING ME... HUH?

D+1

SHE'S SO PURE...

DID MY BODY REALLY MAKE THAT?

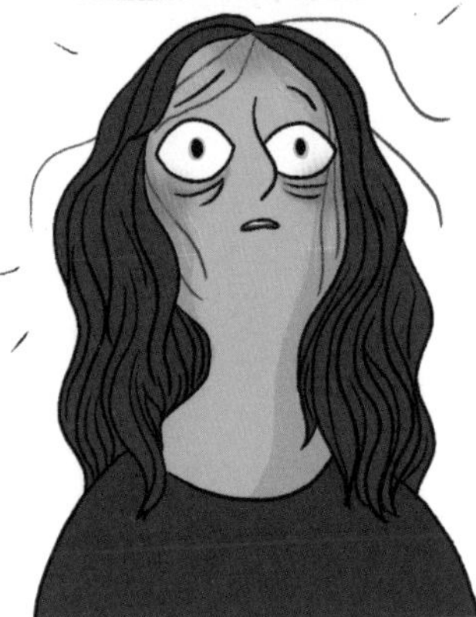

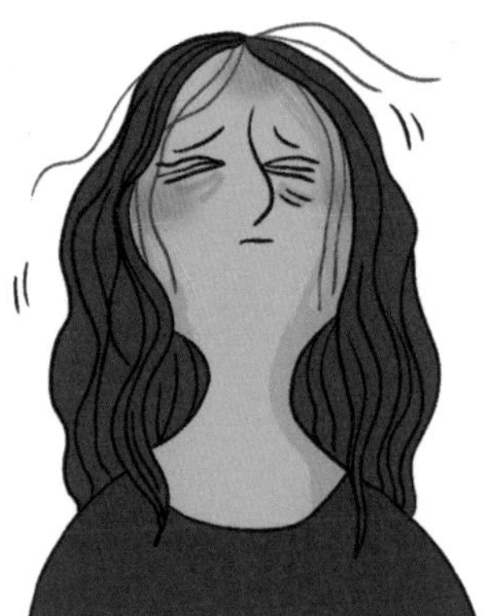

HOW IS THAT EVEN POSSIBLE?

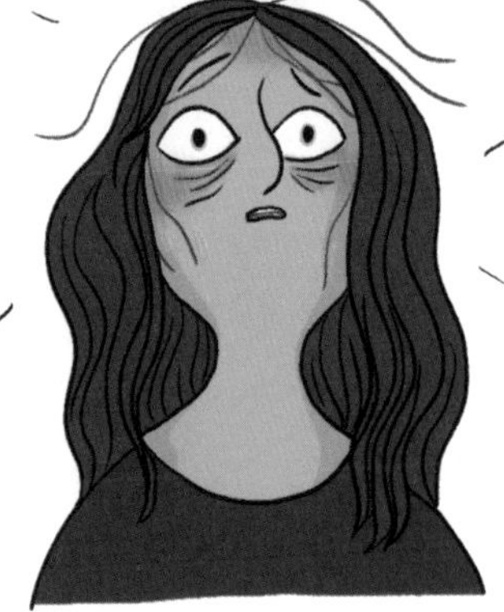

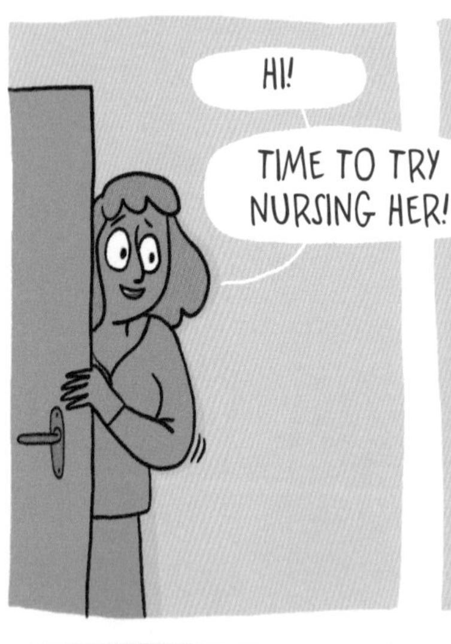
HI!
TIME TO TRY NURSING HER!

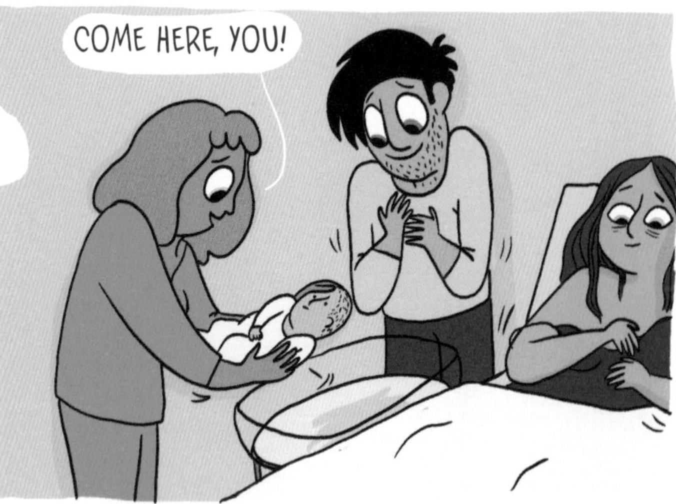
COME HERE, YOU!

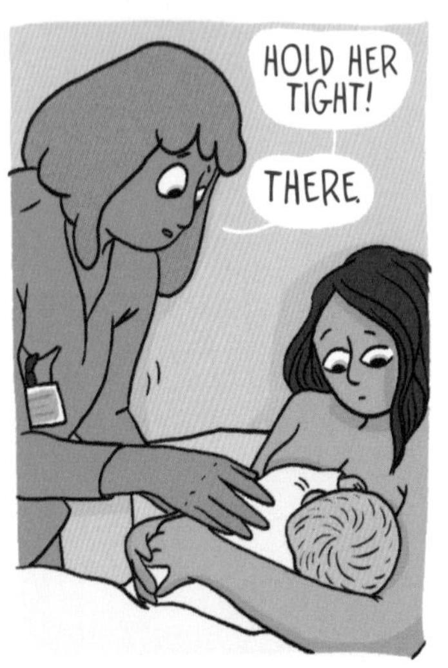
HOLD HER TIGHT!
THERE.

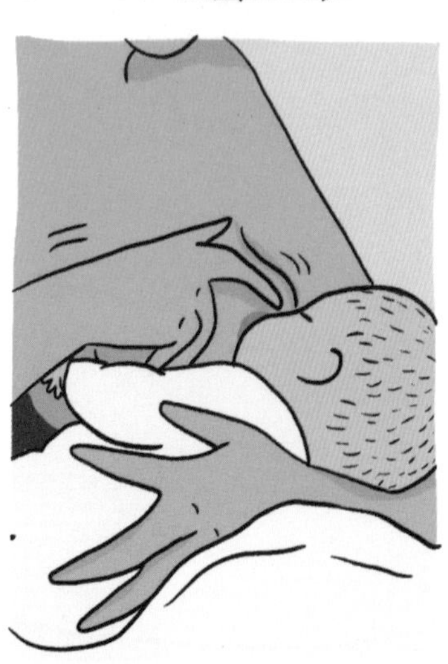

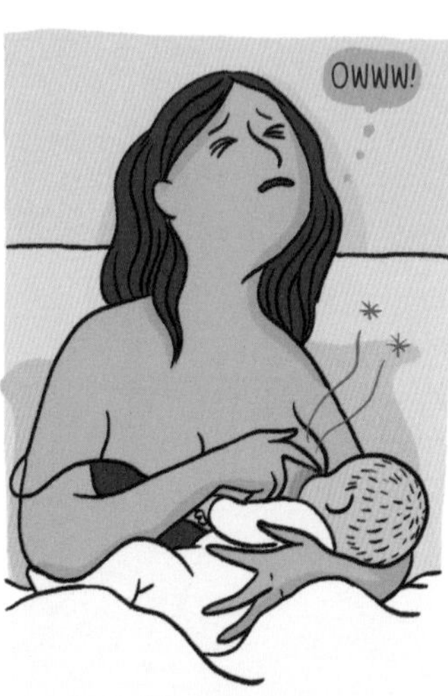
OWWW!

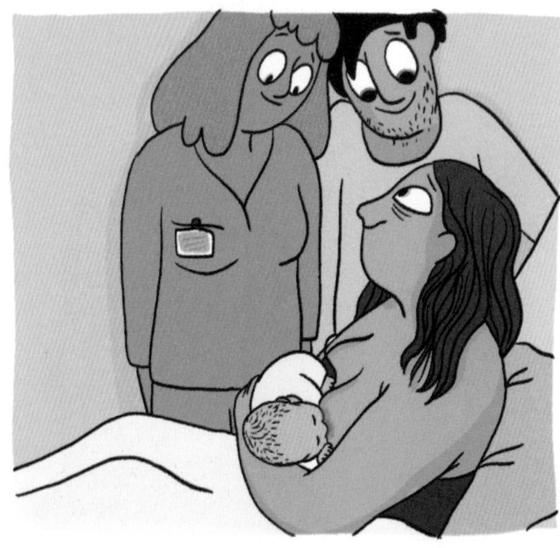

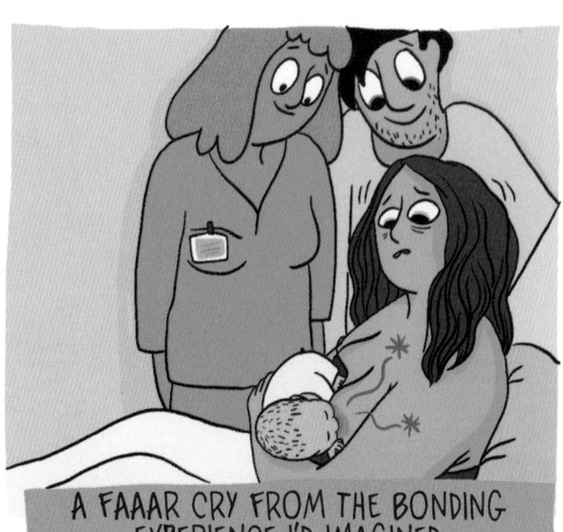
A FAAAR CRY FROM THE BONDING EXPERIENCE I'D IMAGINED.

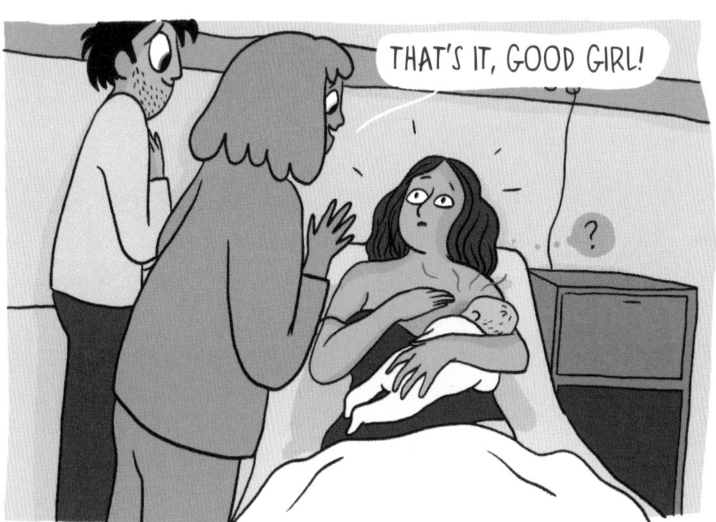
THAT'S IT, GOOD GIRL!
?

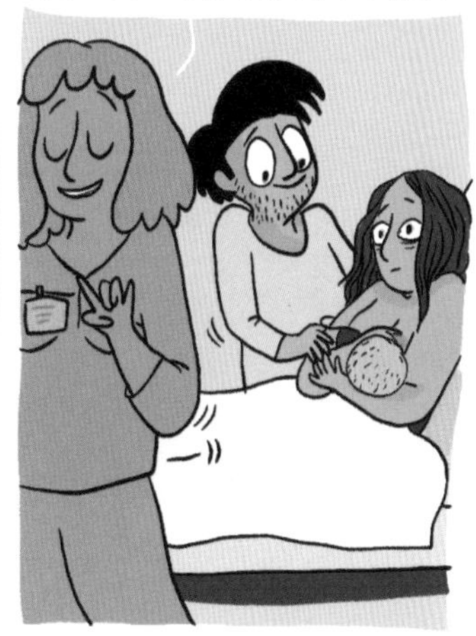
I'LL BE BACK IN TWO HOURS FOR ROUND TWO!

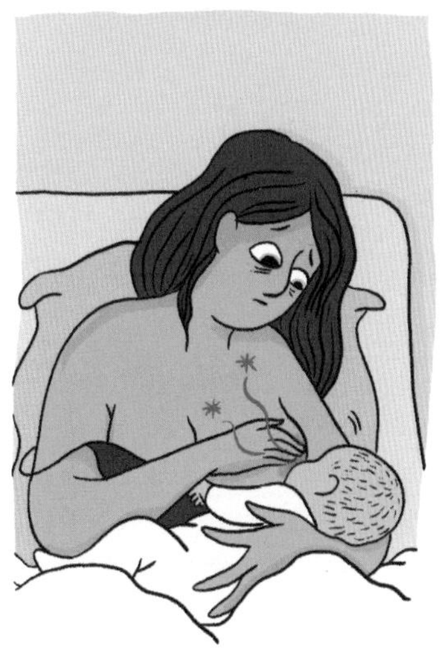

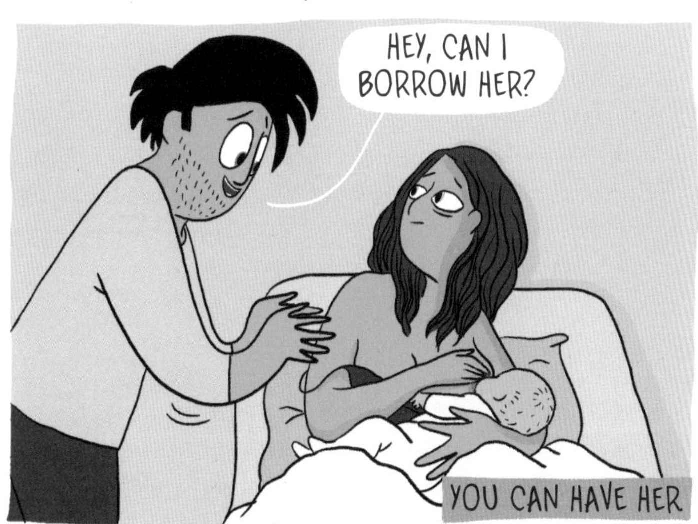
HEY, CAN I BORROW HER?
YOU CAN HAVE HER

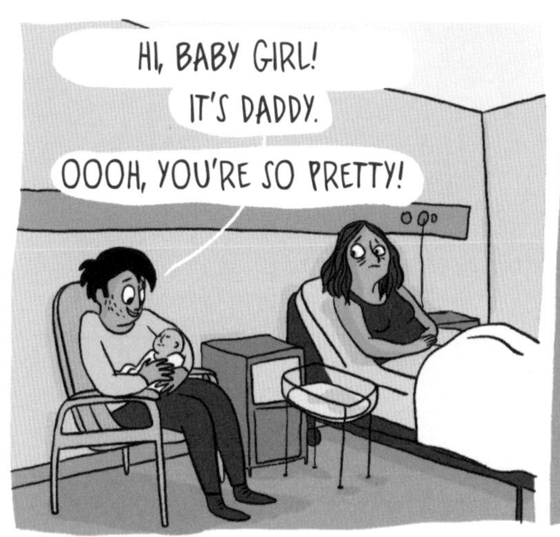
HI, BABY GIRL!
IT'S DADDY.
OOOH, YOU'RE SO PRETTY!

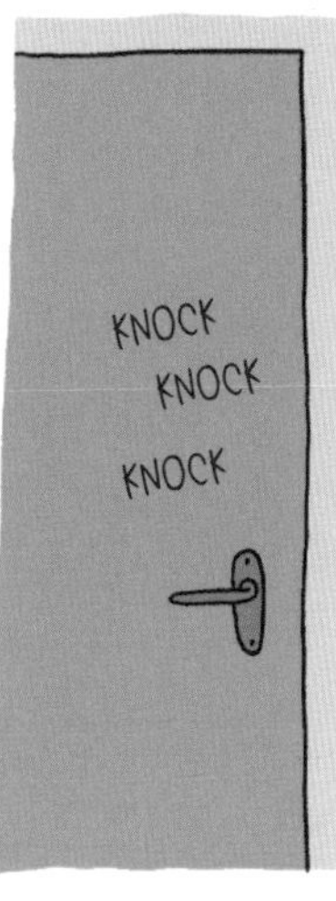
KNOCK
KNOCK
KNOCK

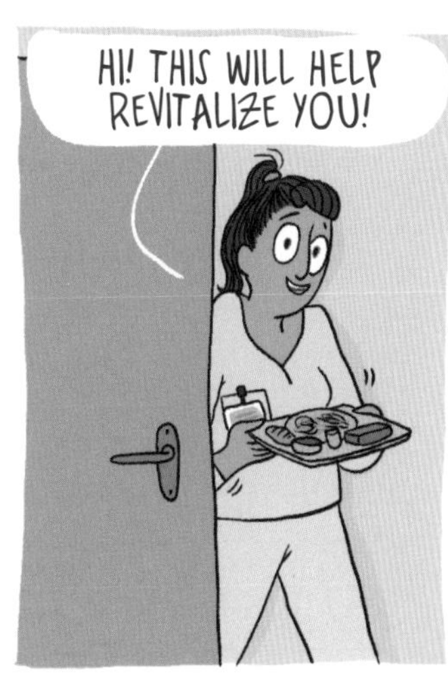
HI! THIS WILL HELP REVITALIZE YOU!

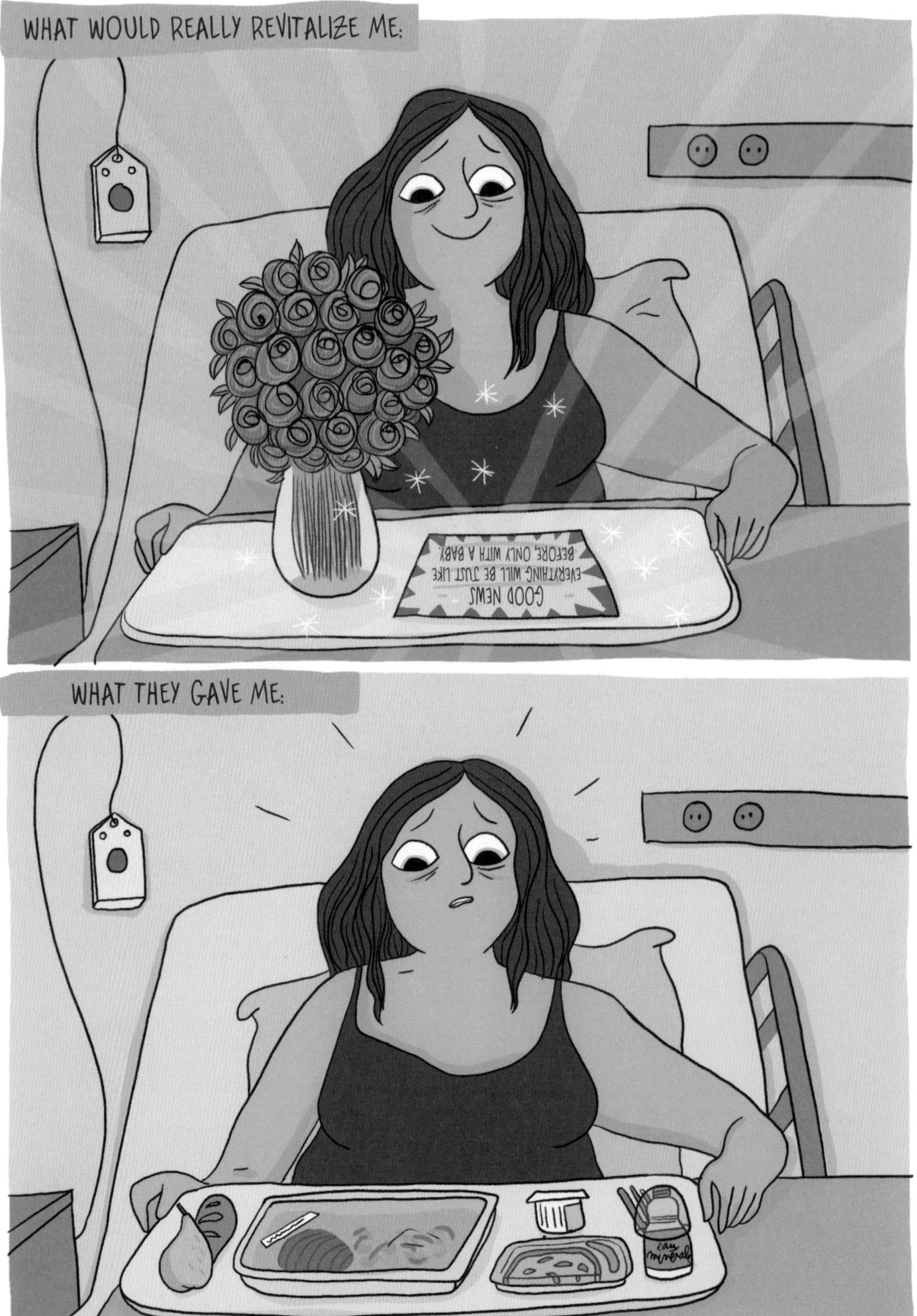
WHAT WOULD REALLY REVITALIZE ME:
GOOD NEWS!
EVERYTHING WILL BE JUST LIKE BEFORE, ONLY WITH A BABY.
WHAT THEY GAVE ME:
eau minérale

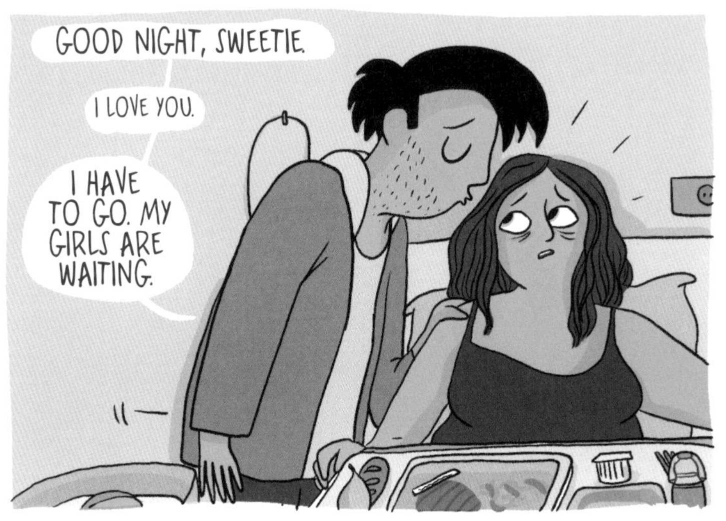
GOOD NIGHT, SWEETIE.
I LOVE YOU.
I HAVE TO GO. MY GIRLS ARE WAITING.

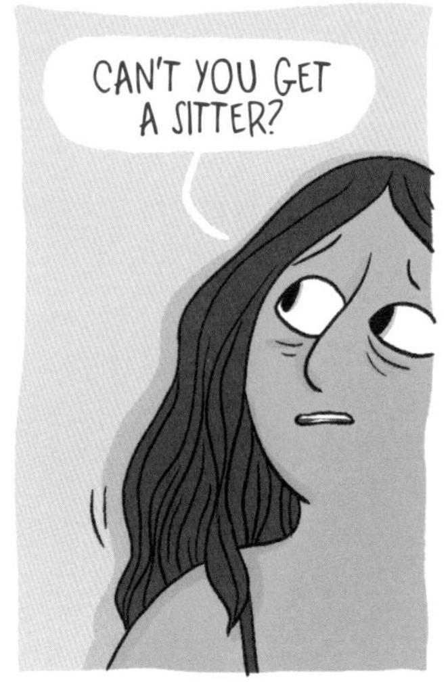
CAN'T YOU GET A SITTER?

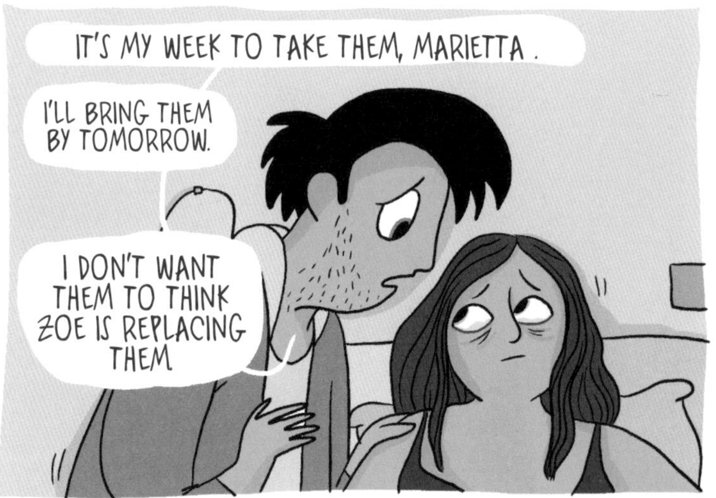
IT'S MY WEEK TO TAKE THEM, MARIETTA .
I'LL BRING THEM BY TOMORROW.
I DON'T WANT THEM TO THINK ZOE IS REPLACING THEM

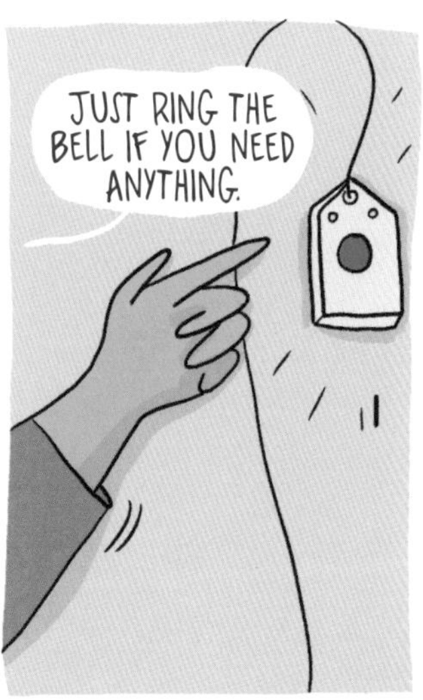
JUST RING THE BELL IF YOU NEED ANYTHING.

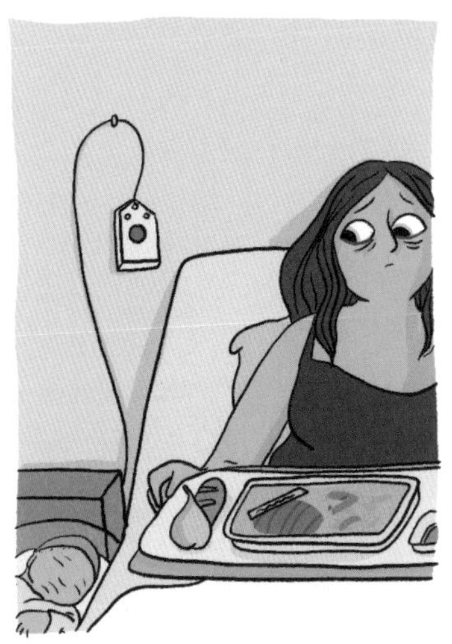

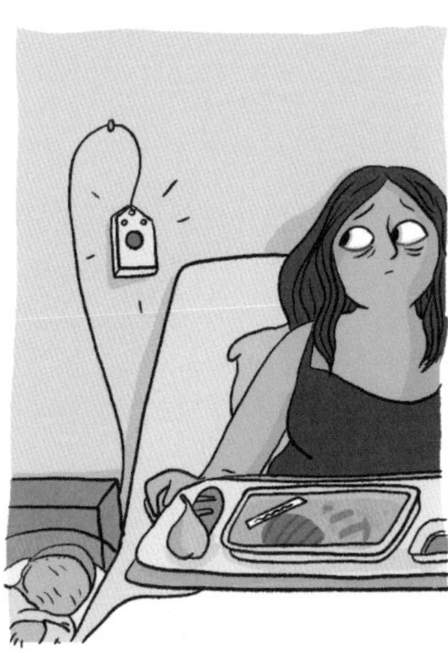

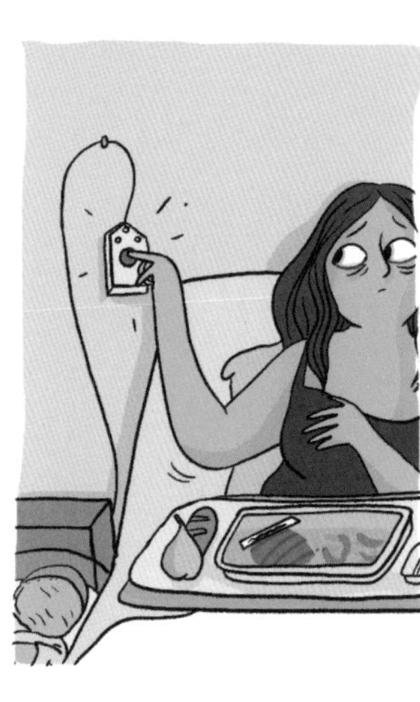

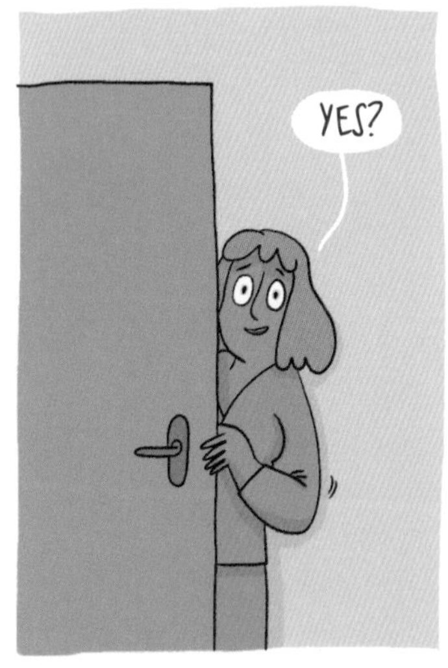
YES?

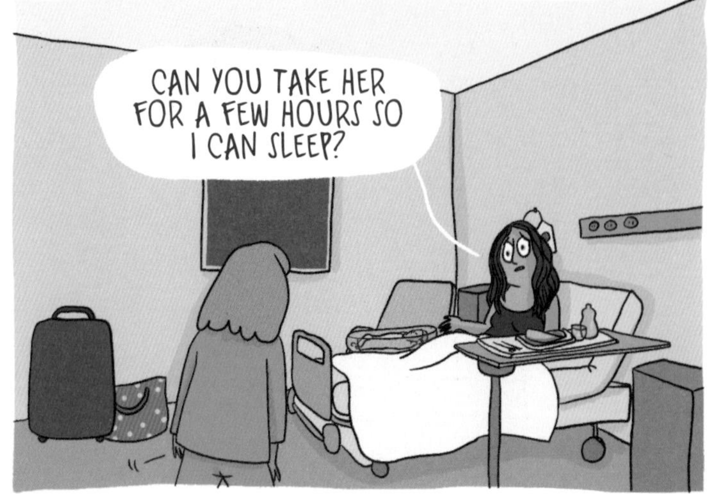
CAN YOU TAKE HER FOR A FEW HOURS SO I CAN SLEEP?

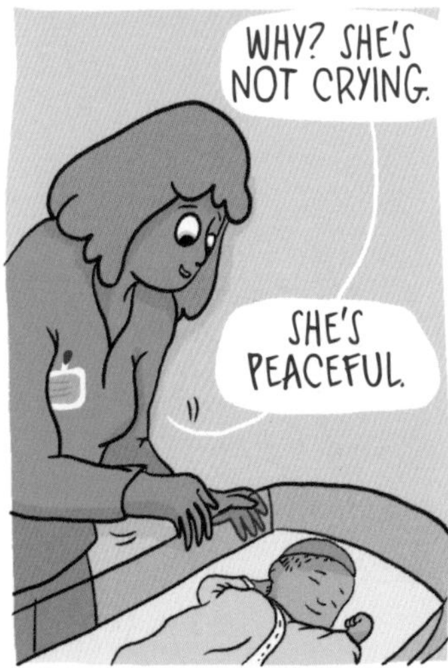
WHY? SHE'S NOT CRYING.
SHE'S PEACEFUL.

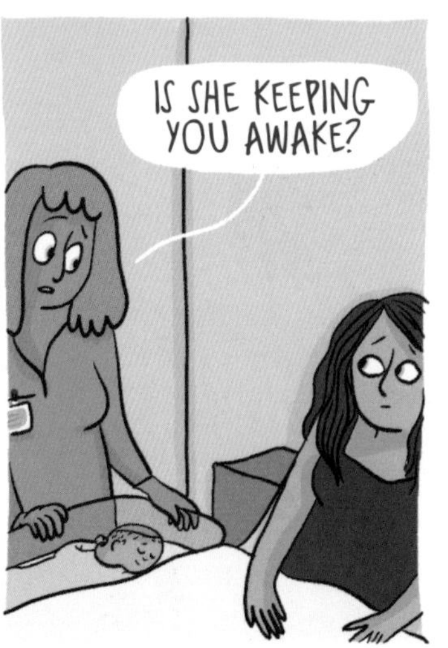
IS SHE KEEPING YOU AWAKE?

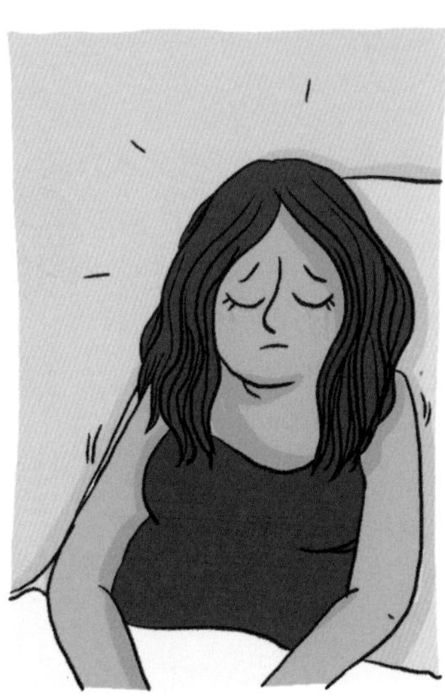

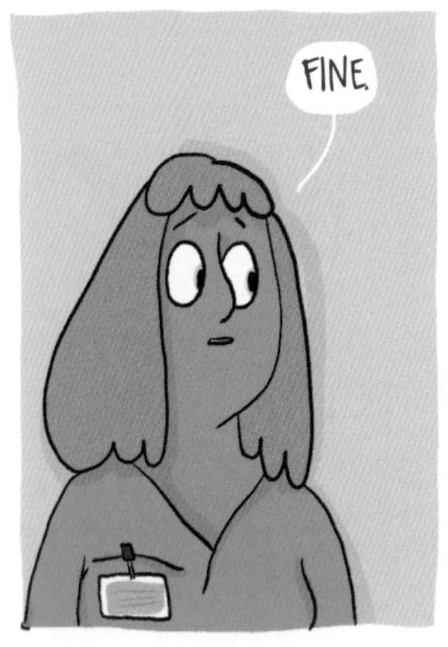
FINE.

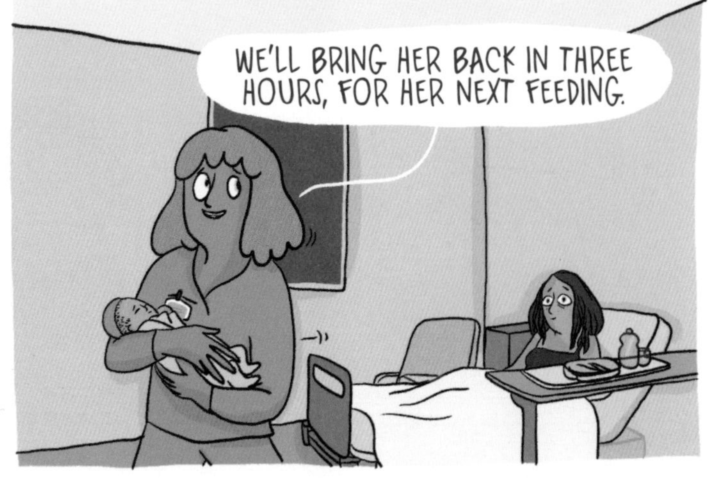
WE'LL BRING HER BACK IN THREE HOURS, FOR HER NEXT FEEDING.

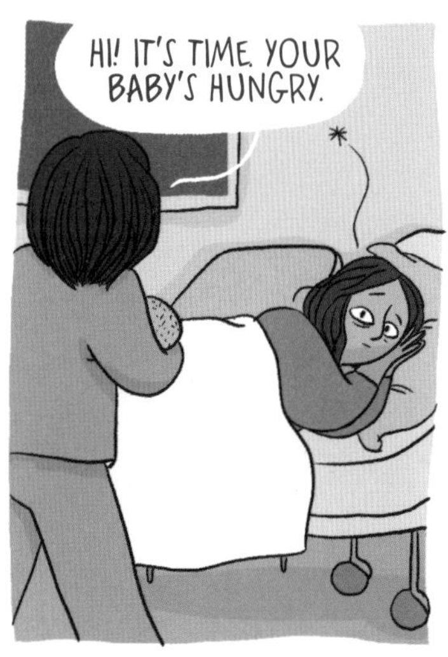
HI! IT'S TIME. YOUR BABY'S HUNGRY.

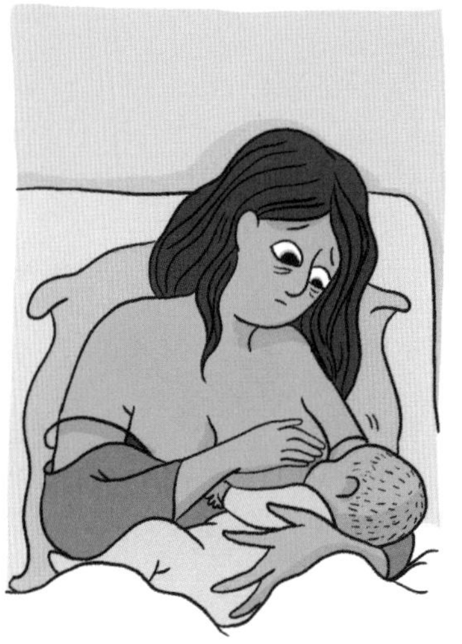

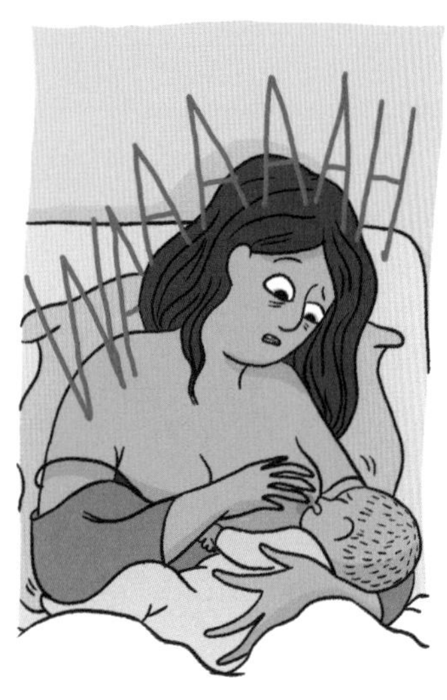
WAAAAAH

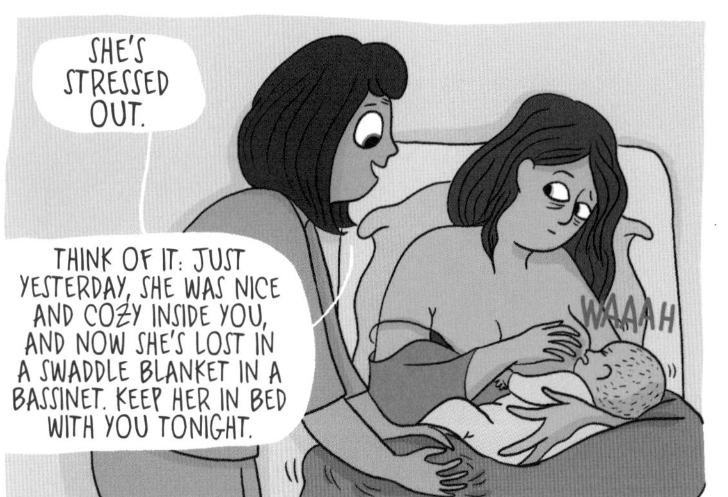
SHE'S STRESSED OUT.
THINK OF IT: JUST YESTERDAY, SHE WAS NICE AND COZY INSIDE YOU, AND NOW SHE'S LOST IN A SWADDLE BLANKET IN A BASSINET. KEEP HER IN BED WITH YOU TONIGHT.
WAAAH

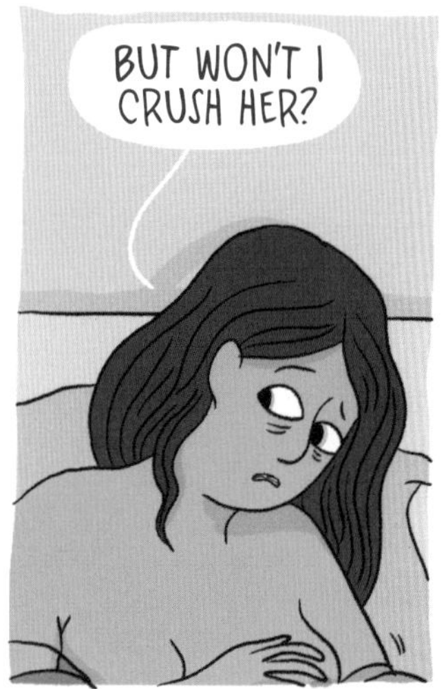
BUT WON'T I CRUSH HER?

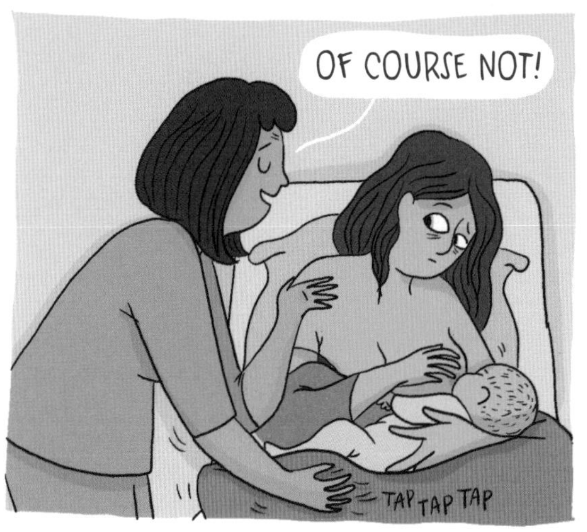
OF COURSE NOT!
TAP TAP TAP

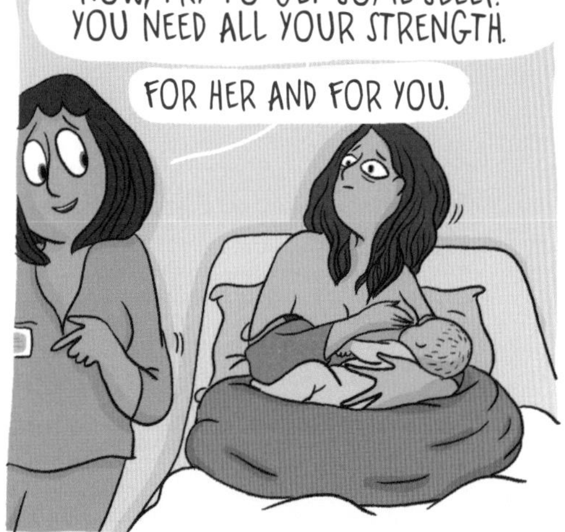
NOW, TRY TO GET SOME SLEEP. YOU NEED ALL YOUR STRENGTH.
FOR HER AND FOR YOU.

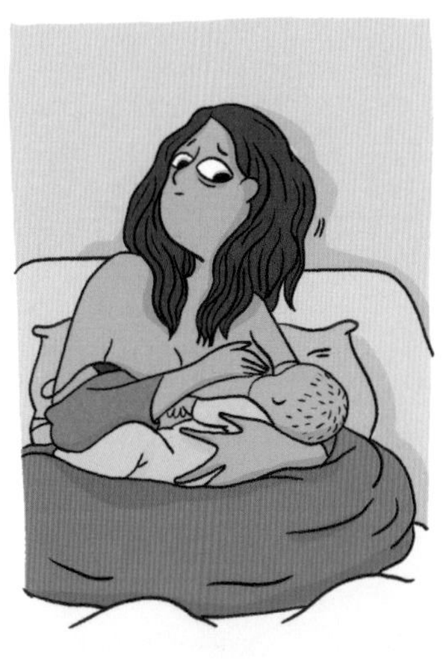

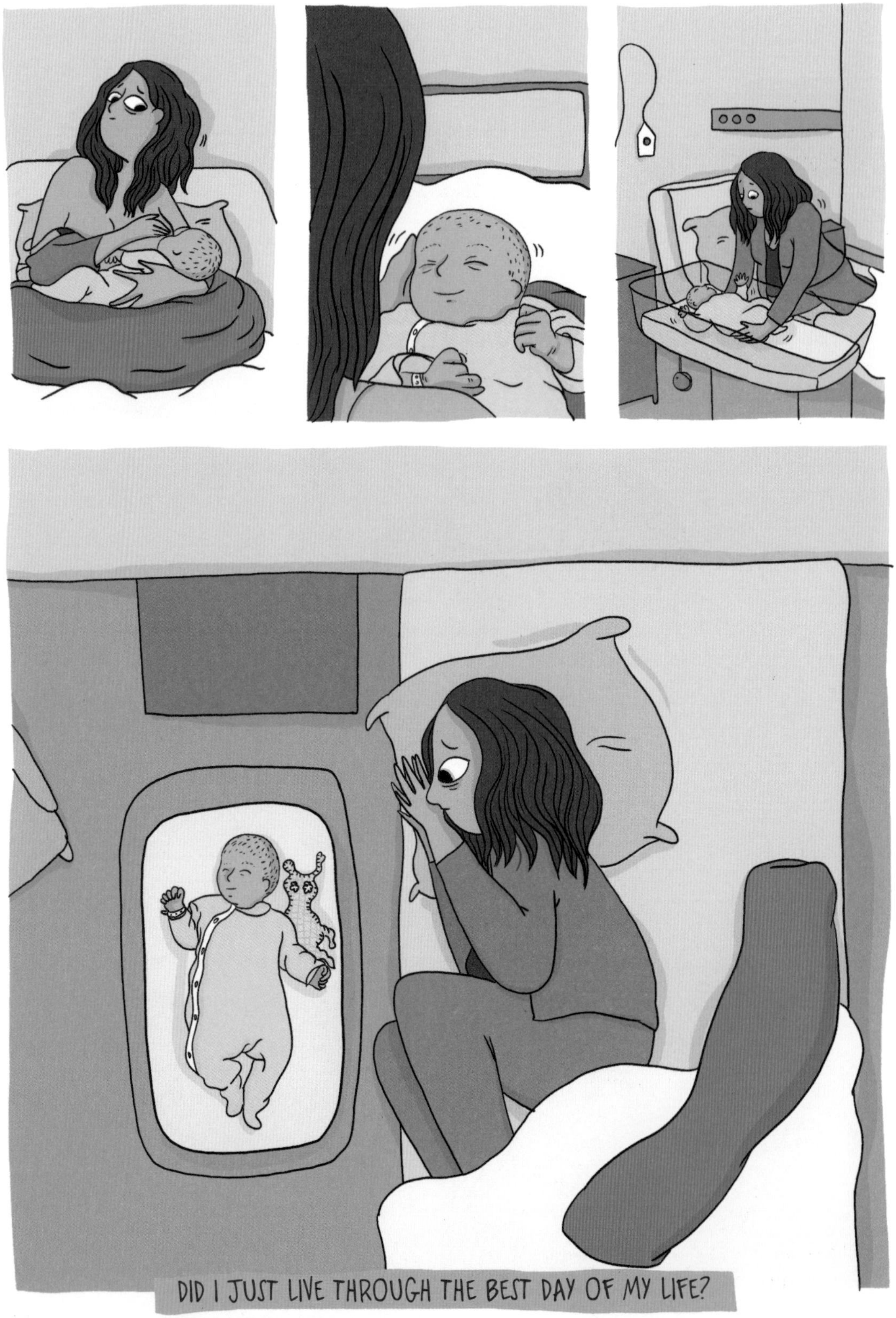

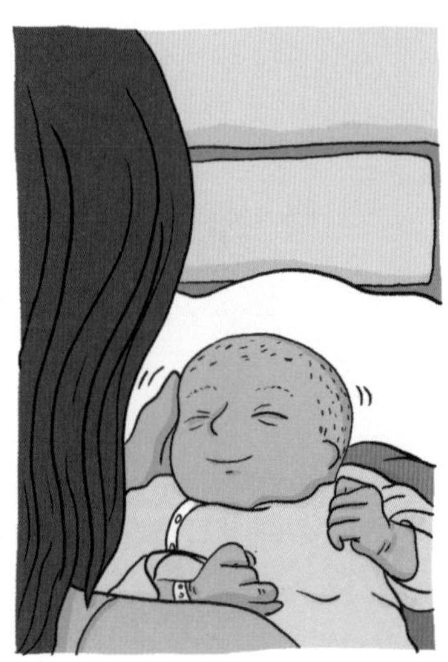

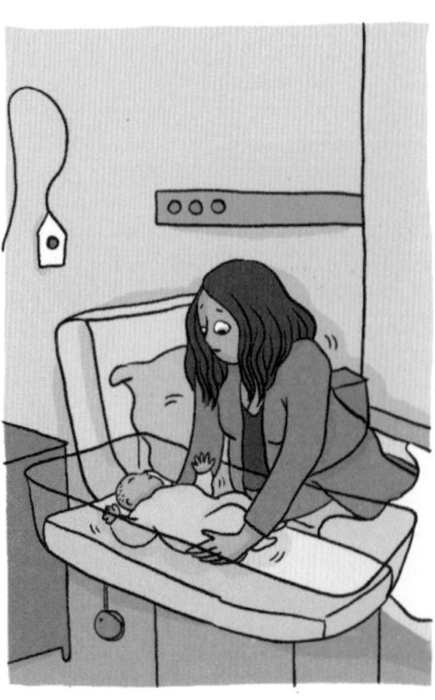

DID I JUST LIVE THROUGH THE BEST DAY OF MY LIFE?

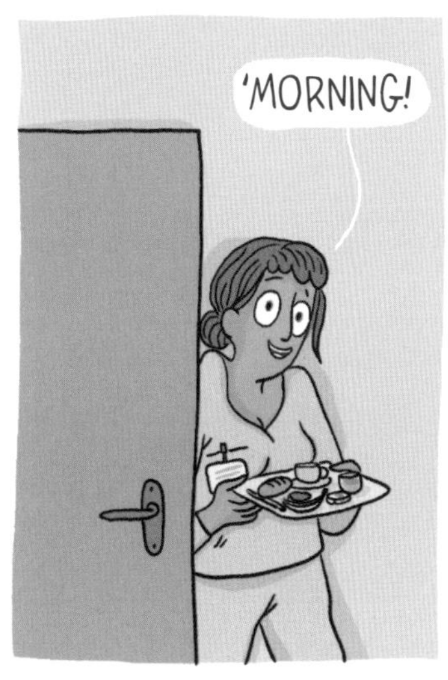
'MORNING!

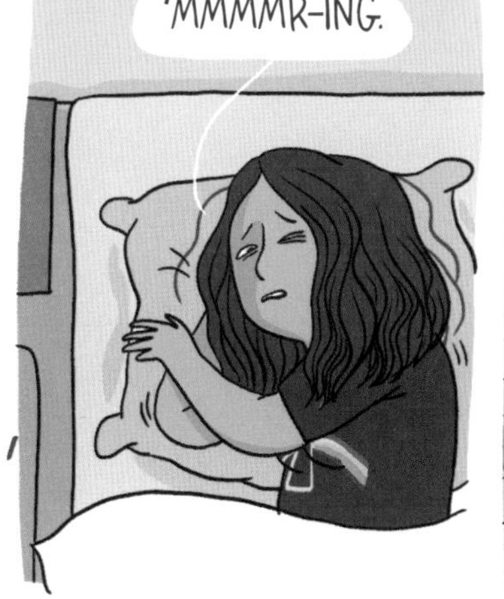
'MMMMR-ING.

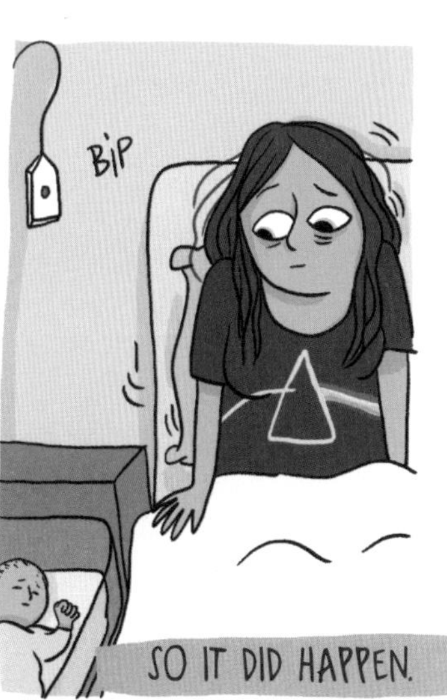
BIP
SO IT DID HAPPEN.

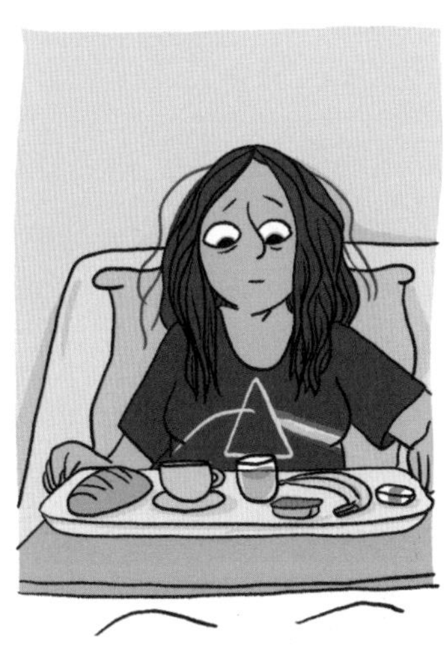

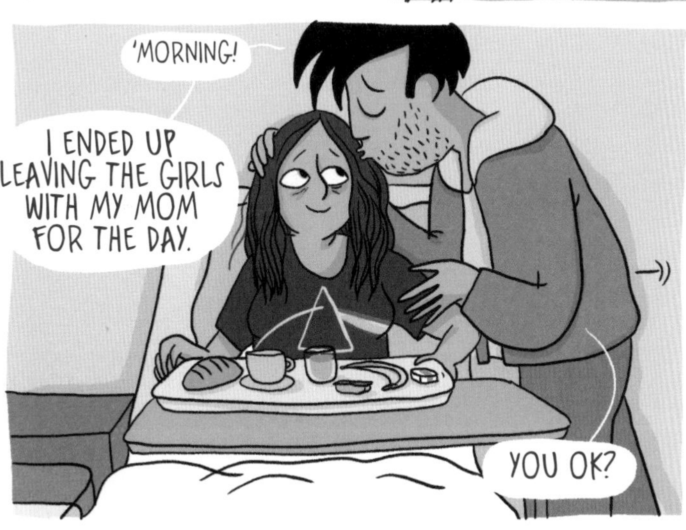
'MORNING!
I ENDED UP LEAVING THE GIRLS WITH MY MOM FOR THE DAY.
YOU OK?

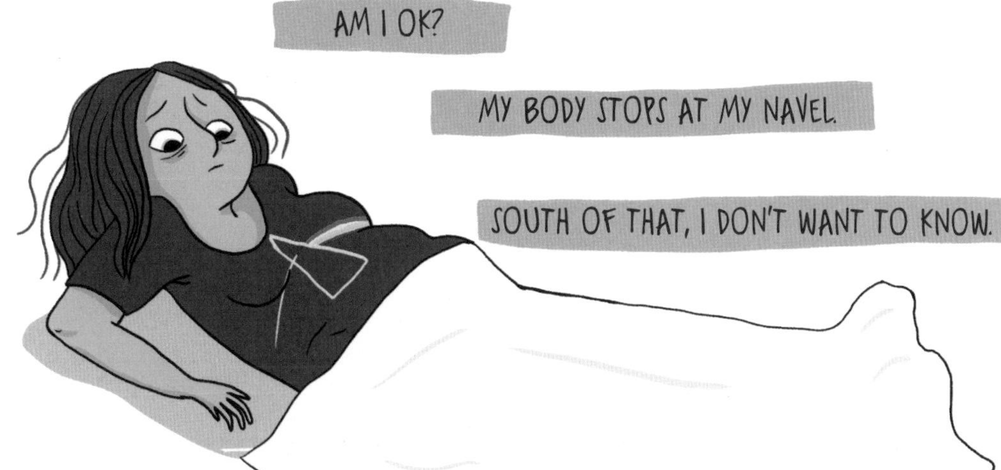
AM I OK?
MY BODY STOPS AT MY NAVEL.
SOUTH OF THAT, I DON'T WANT TO KNOW.

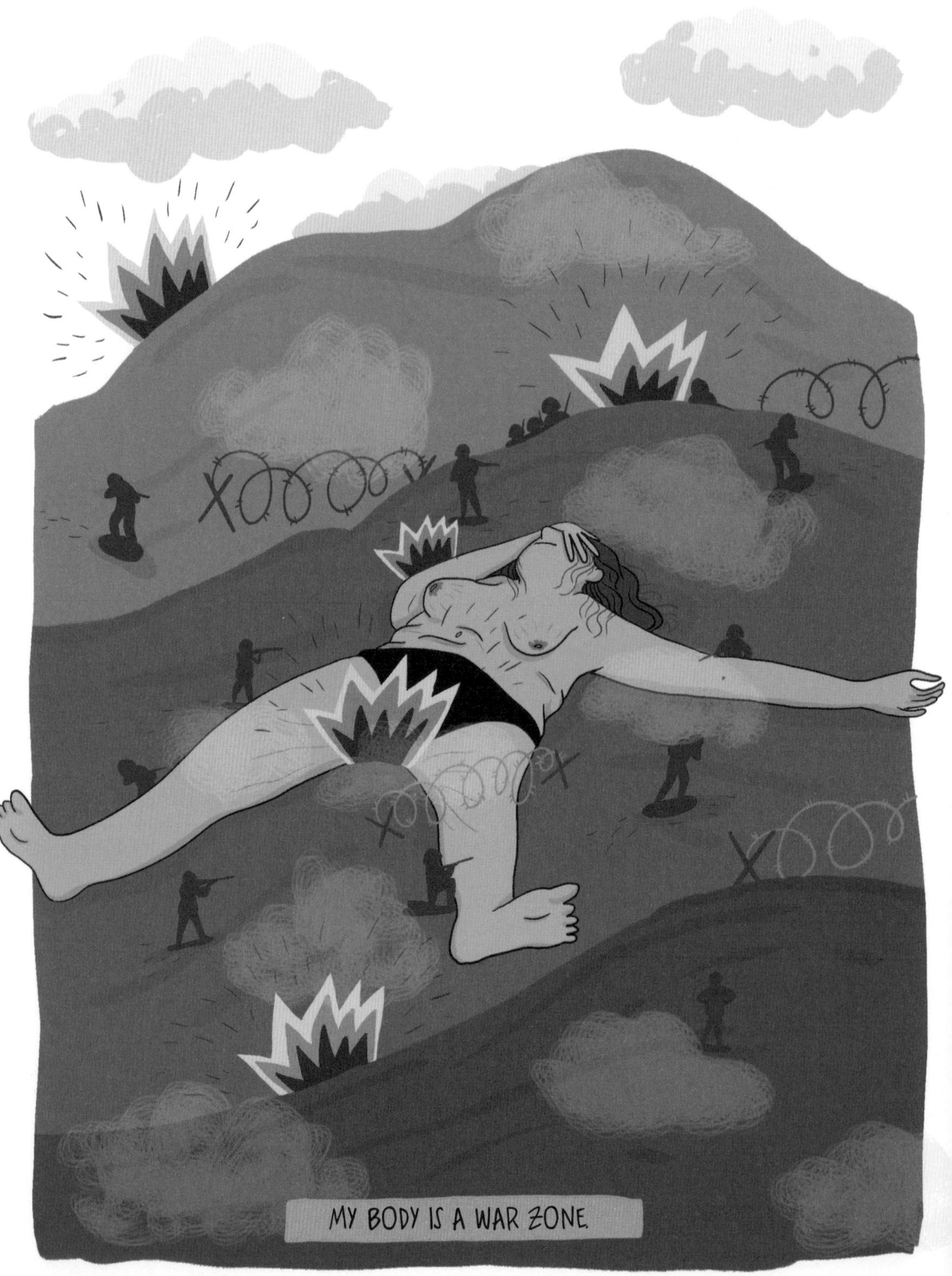
MY BODY IS A WAR ZONE.

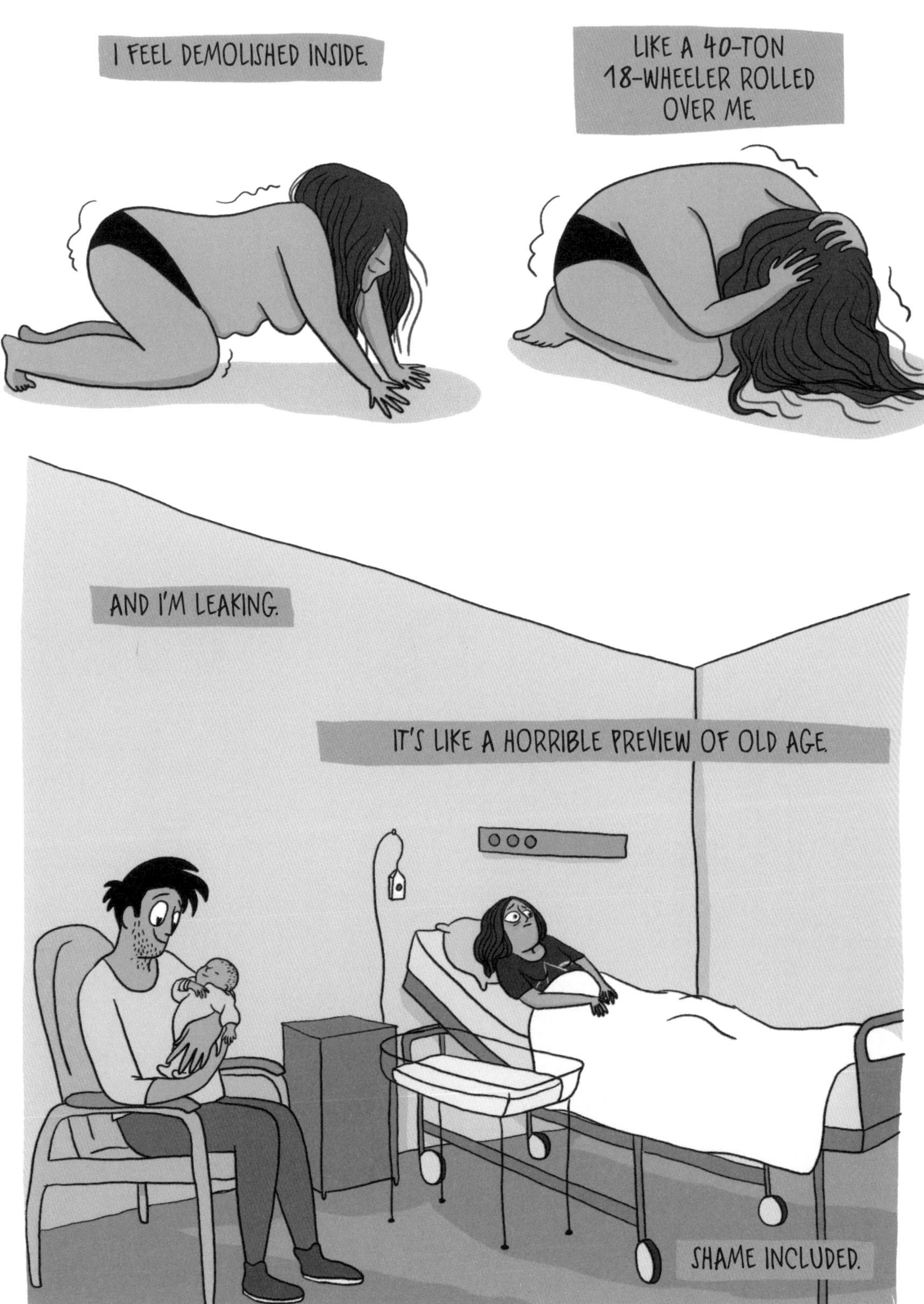
I FEEL DEMOLISHED INSIDE.
LIKE A 40-TON 18-WHEELER ROLLED OVER ME.
AND I'M LEAKING.
IT'S LIKE A HORRIBLE PREVIEW OF OLD AGE.
SHAME INCLUDED.

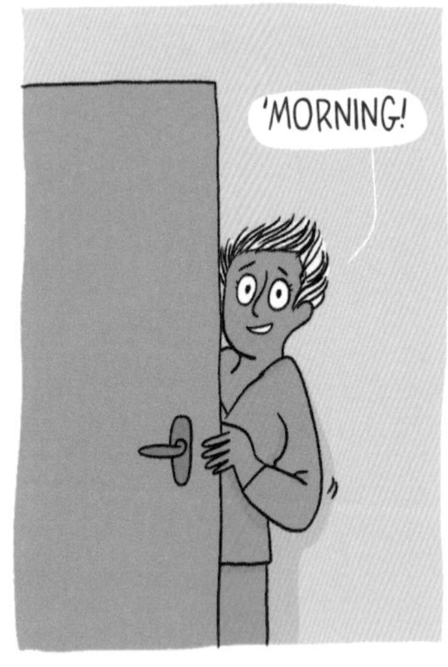
'MORNING!
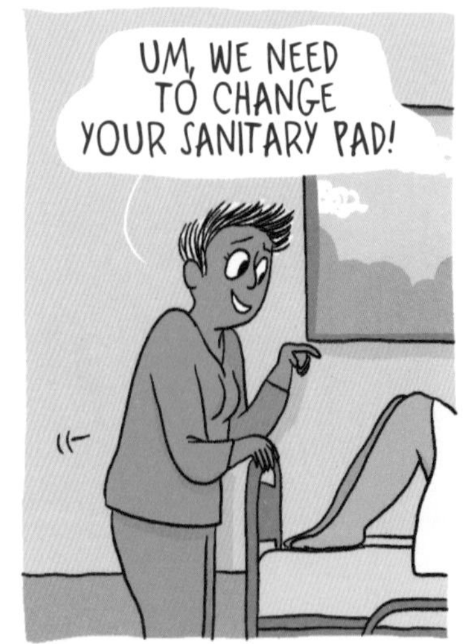
UM, WE NEED TO CHANGE YOUR SANITARY PAD!
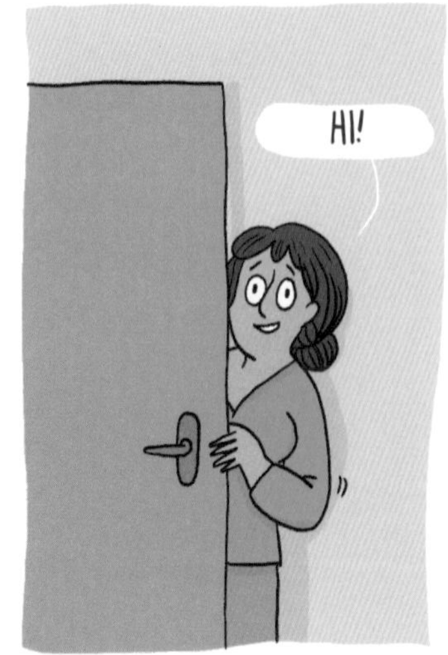
HI!
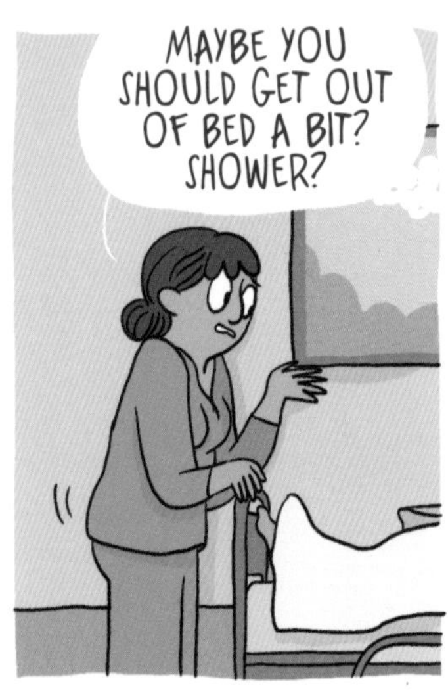
MAYBE YOU SHOULD GET OUT OF BED A BIT? SHOWER?
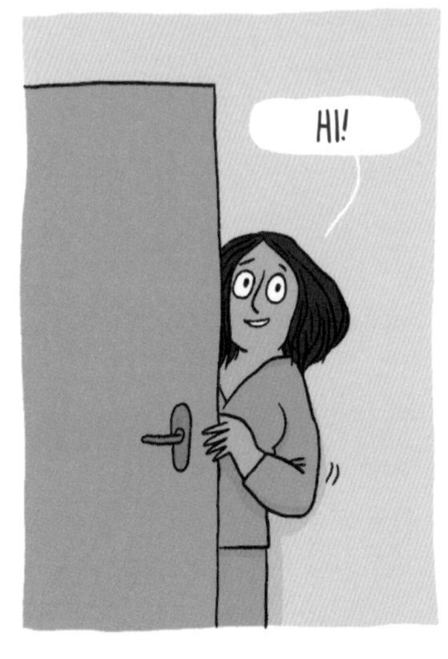
HI!
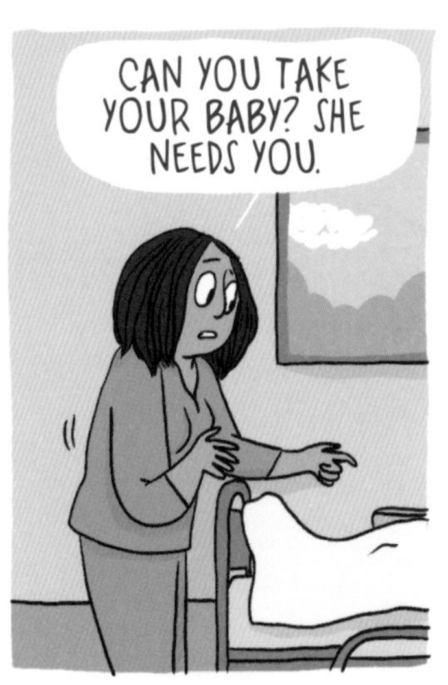
CAN YOU TAKE YOUR BABY? SHE NEEDS YOU.
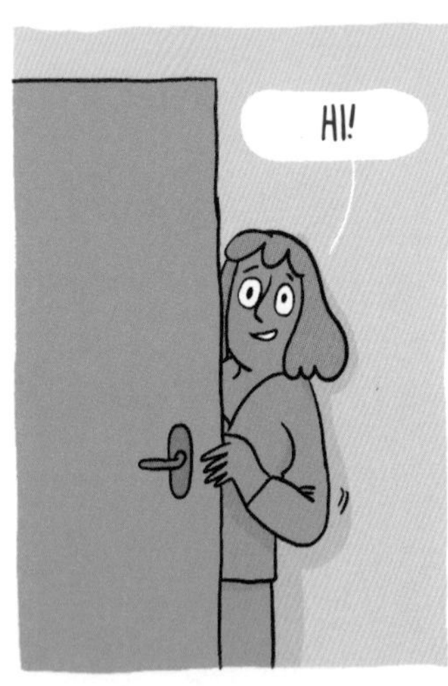
HI!
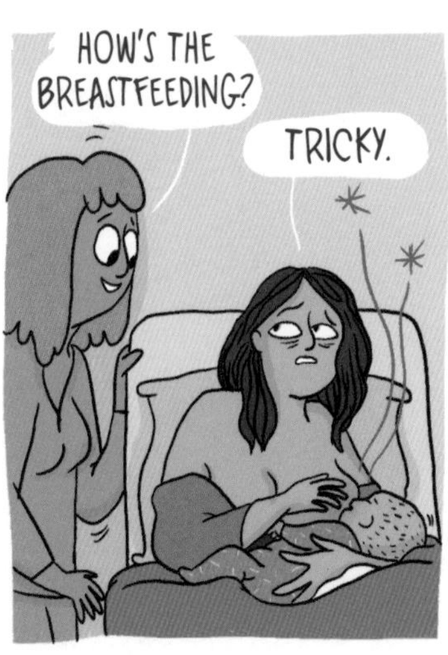
HOW'S THE BREASTFEEDING?
TRICKY.
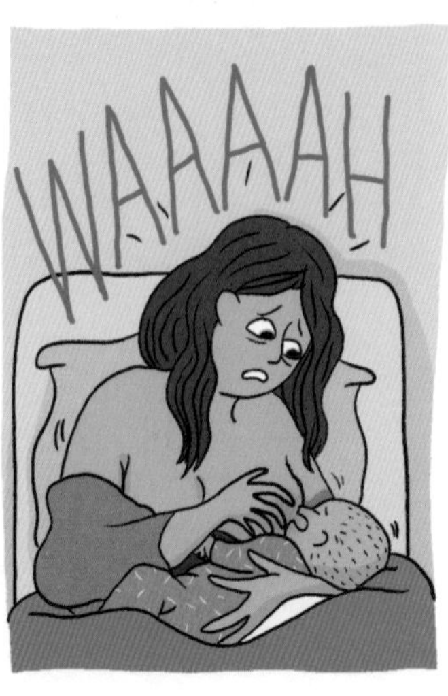
WAAAAH

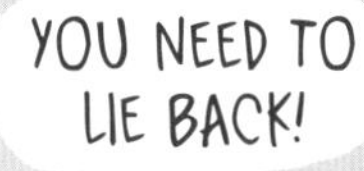
YOU NEED TO LIE BACK!

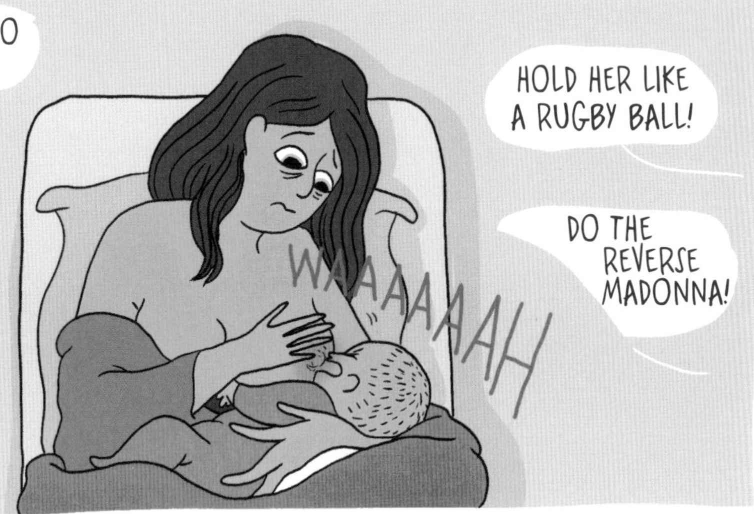
IT'LL BE EASIER IF YOU SIT UP!
TRY THE MADONNA POSITION.
HOLD HER LIKE A RUGBY BALL!
DO THE REVERSE MADONNA!
WAAAAAAAH

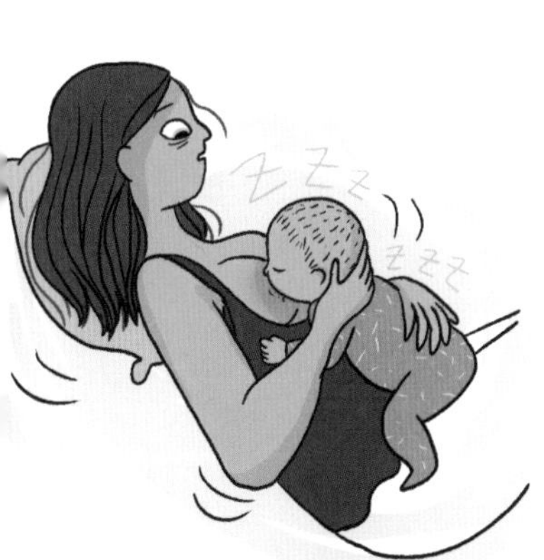

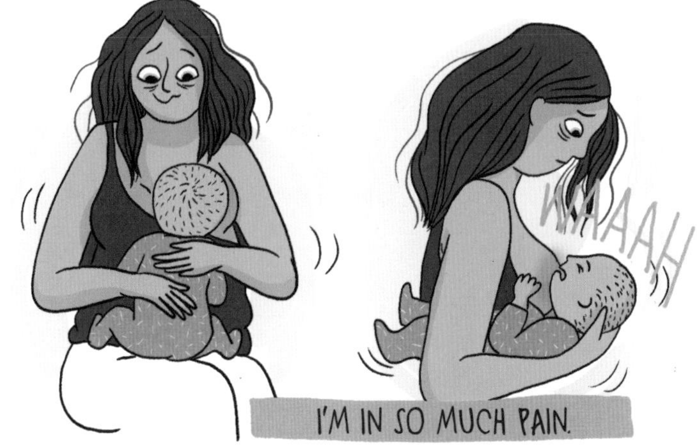
WAAAAH
I'M IN SO MUCH PAIN.

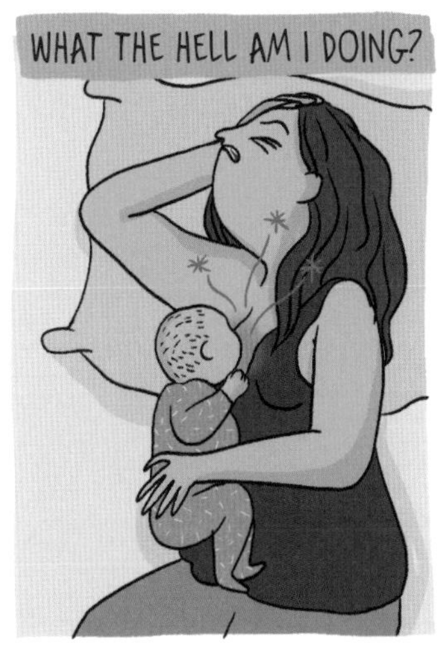
WHAT THE HELL AM I DOING?

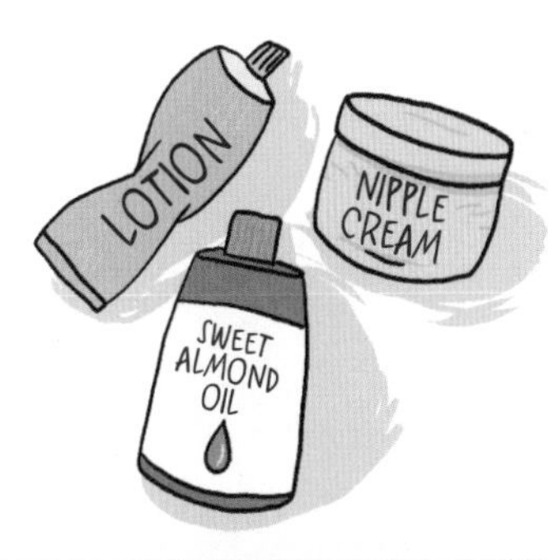
LOTION
NIPPLE CREAM
SWEET ALMOND OIL
MY NIPPLES ARE CRACKED AND THE LOTIONS DON'T WORK.

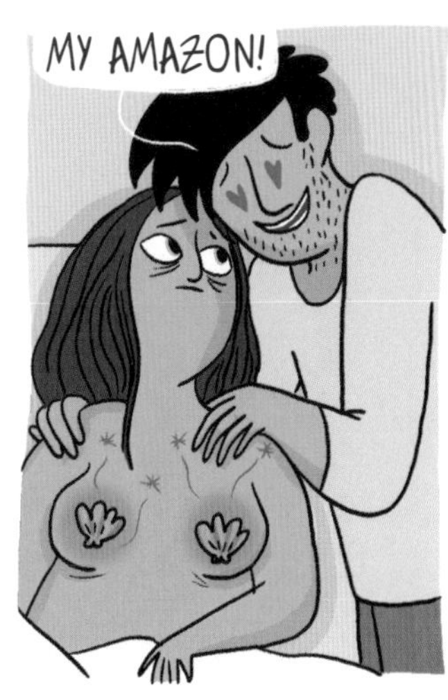
MY AMAZON!

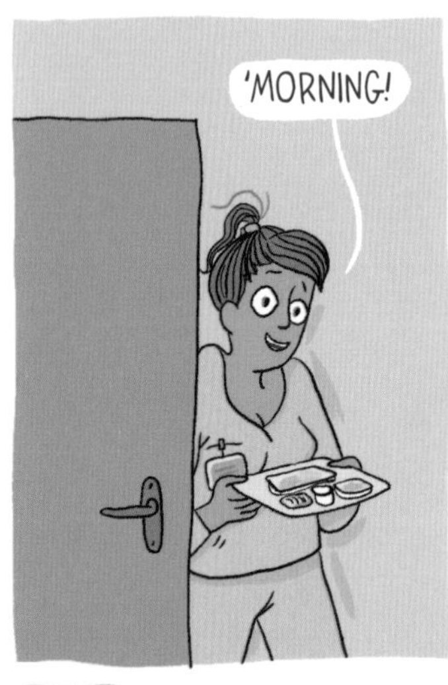

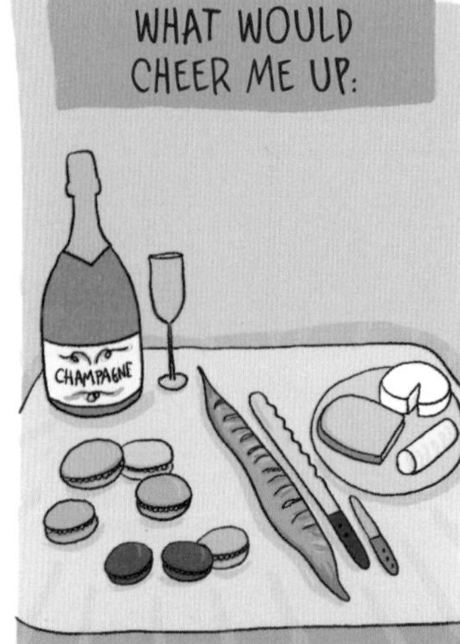

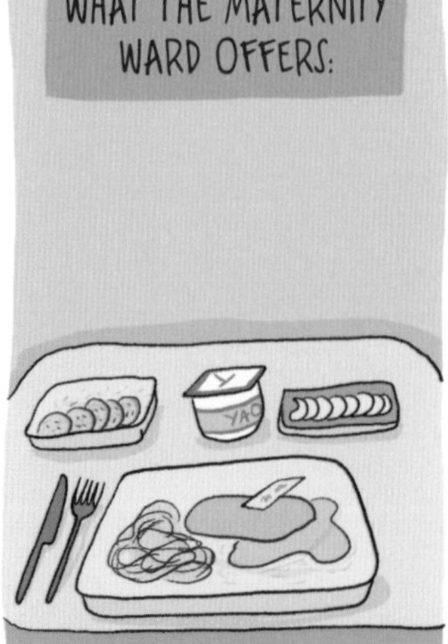

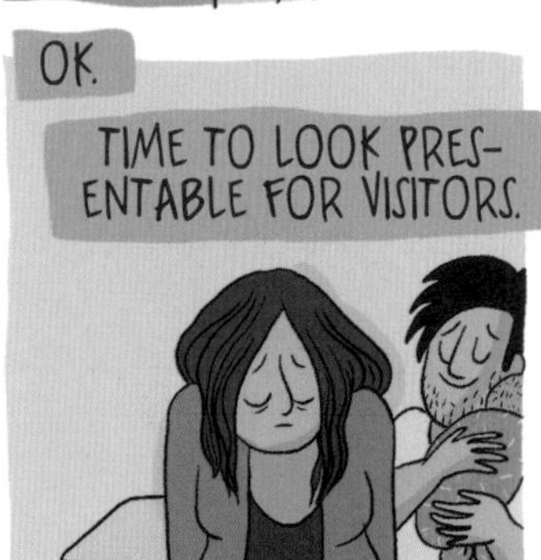

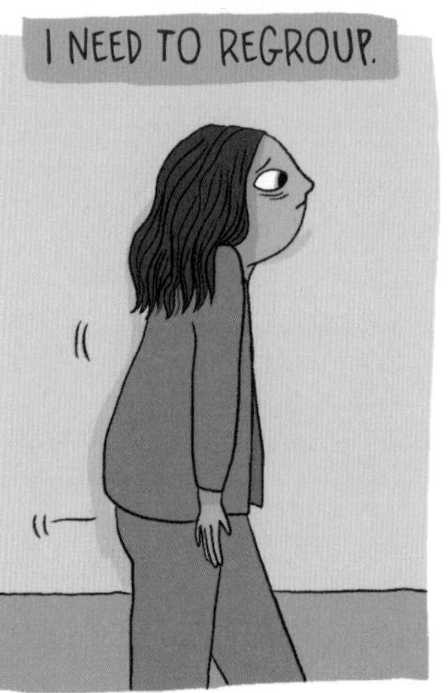

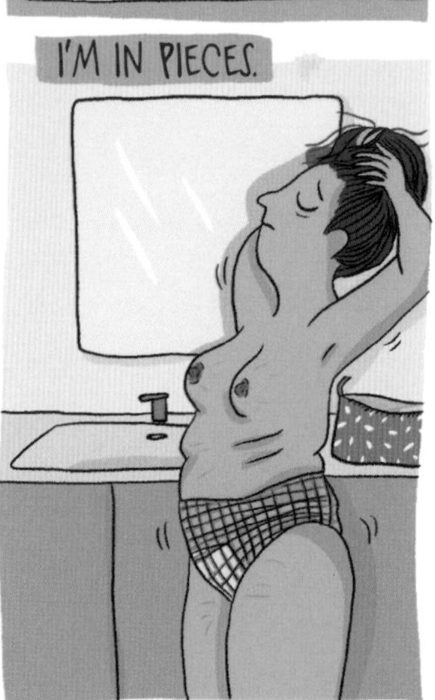

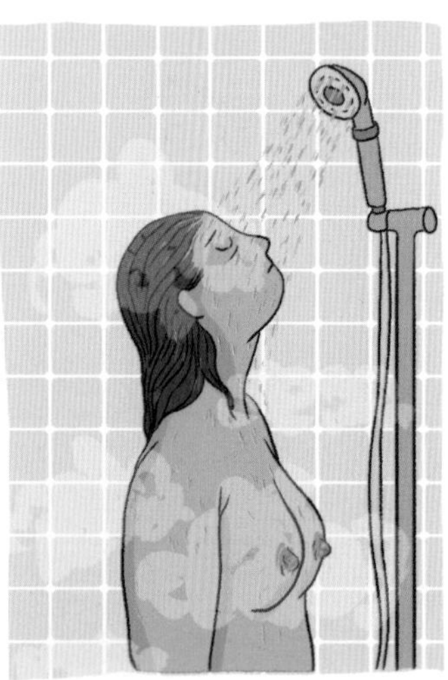

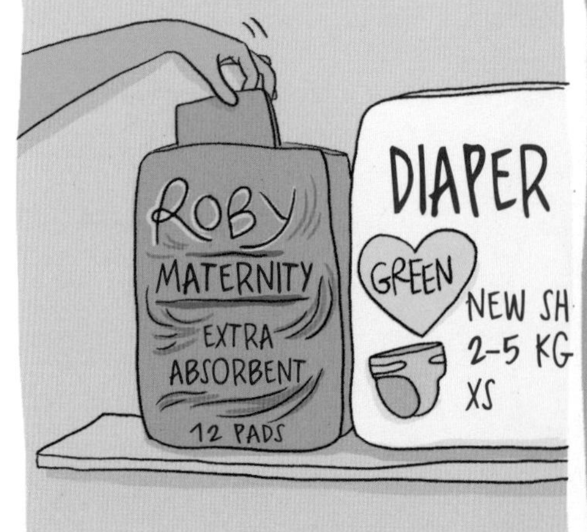

THERE ARE DIAPERS FOR ME AND DIAPERS FOR ZOE IN HERE.

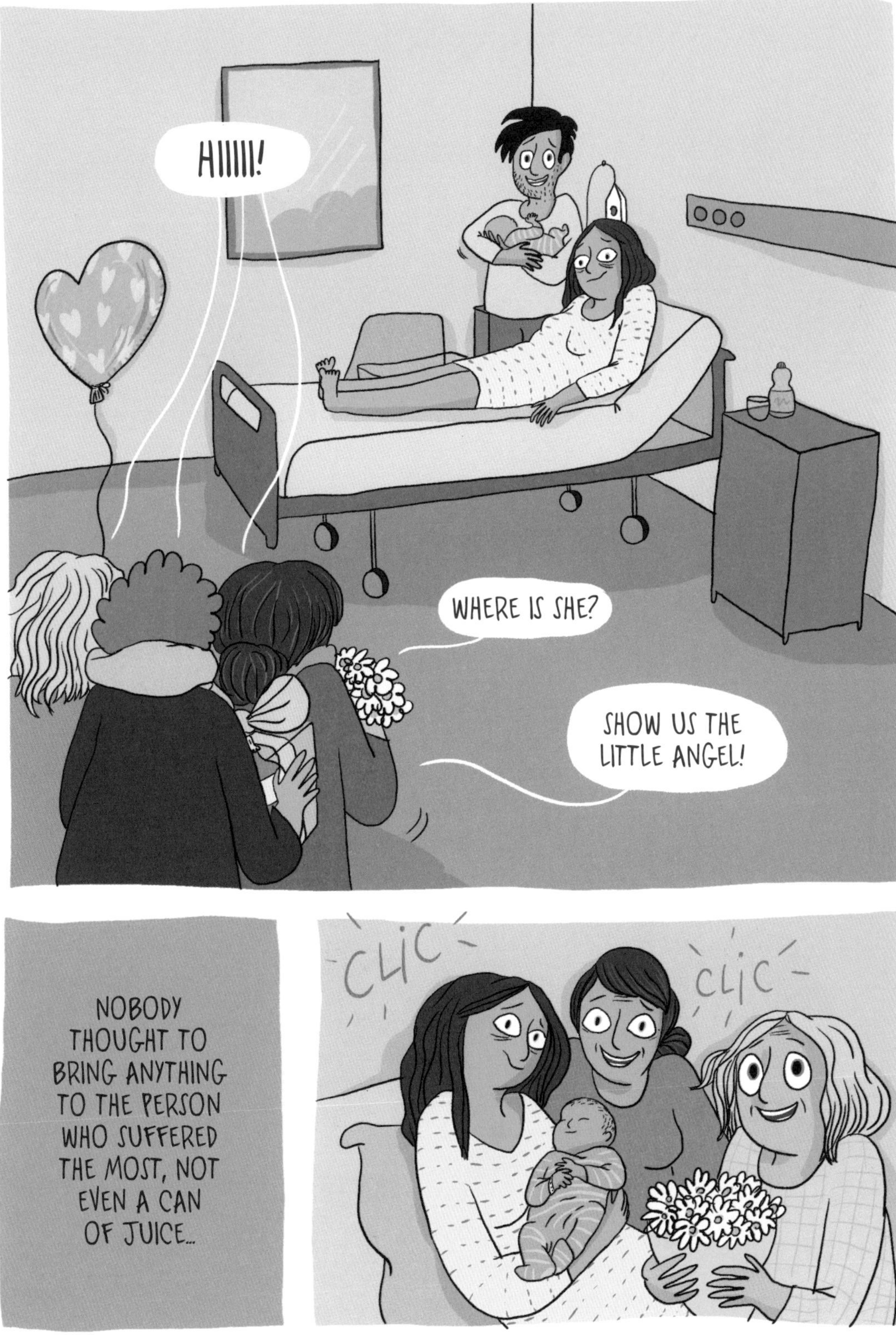

HIIIII!

WHERE IS SHE?

SHOW US THE LITTLE ANGEL!

NOBODY THOUGHT TO BRING ANYTHING TO THE PERSON WHO SUFFERED THE MOST, NOT EVEN A CAN OF JUICE...

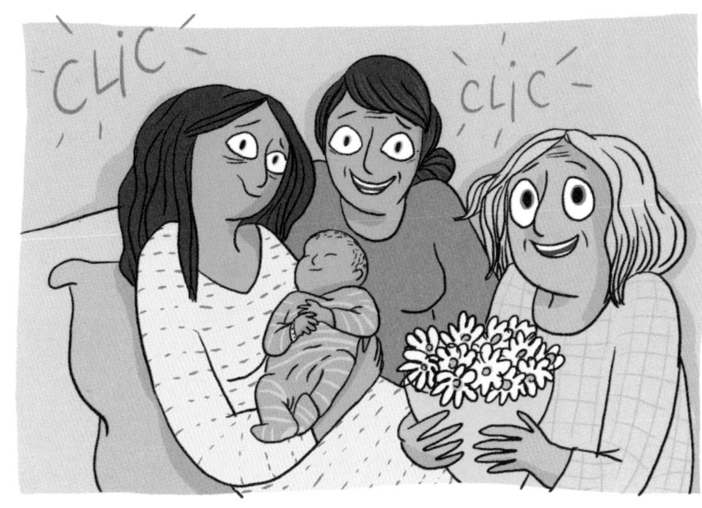

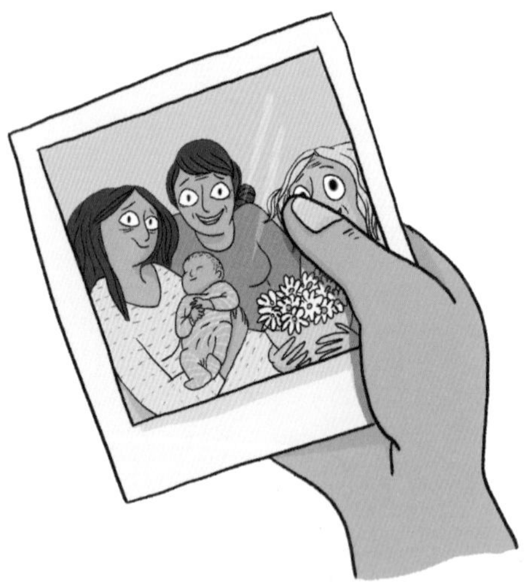

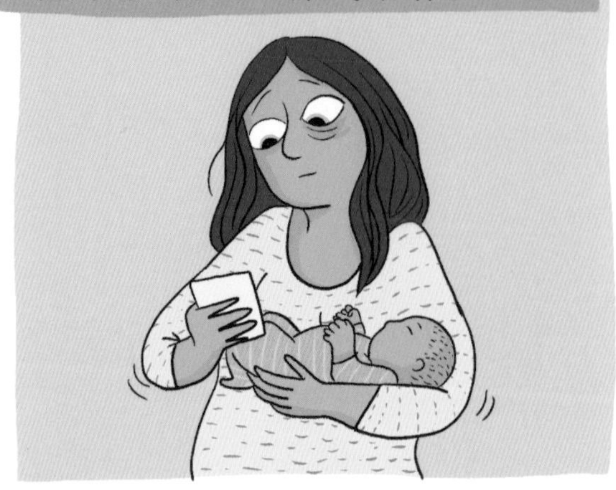

I FANTASIZE ABOUT HIRING A PROXY MOM

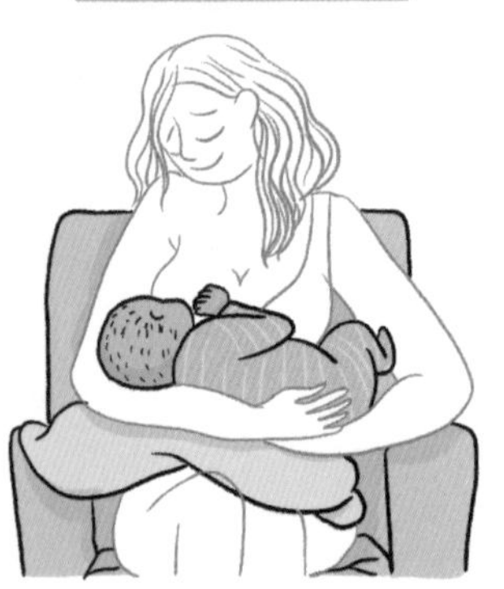

WHO WOULD BREASTFEED EFFORTLESSLY.

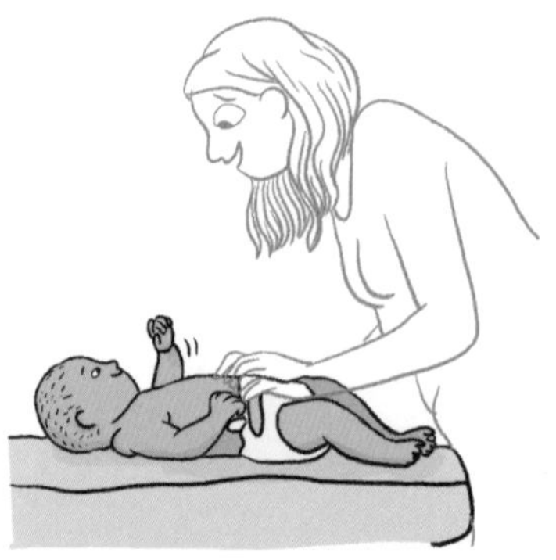

AND GET ZOE TO BE QUIET.

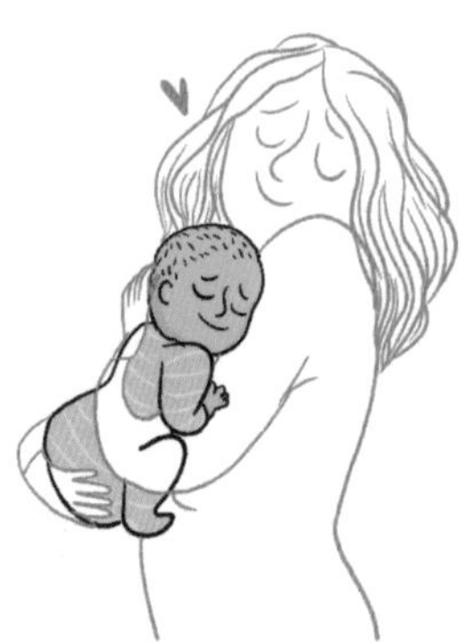

A WONDER-MOM VERSION OF MARIETTA

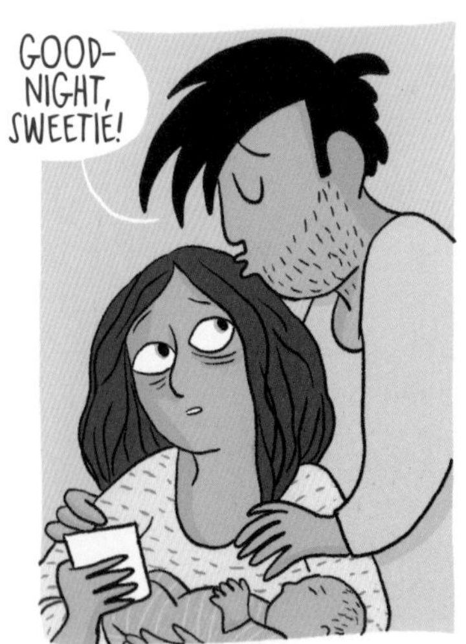

GOOD-NIGHT, SWEETIE!

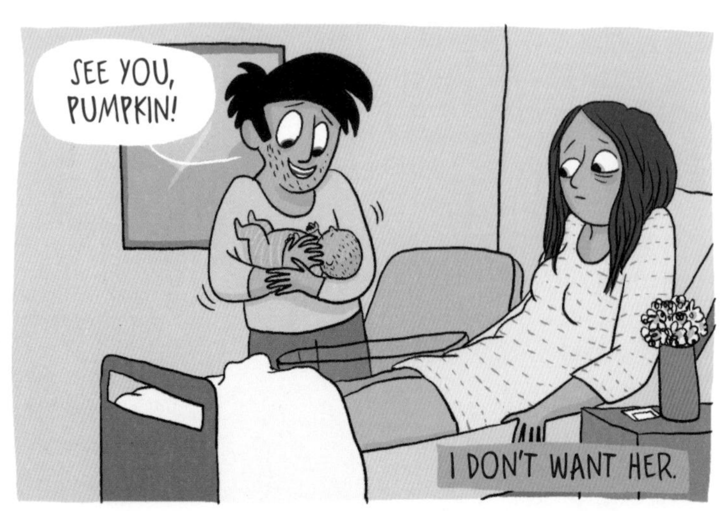

SEE YOU, PUMPKIN!
I DON'T WANT HER.

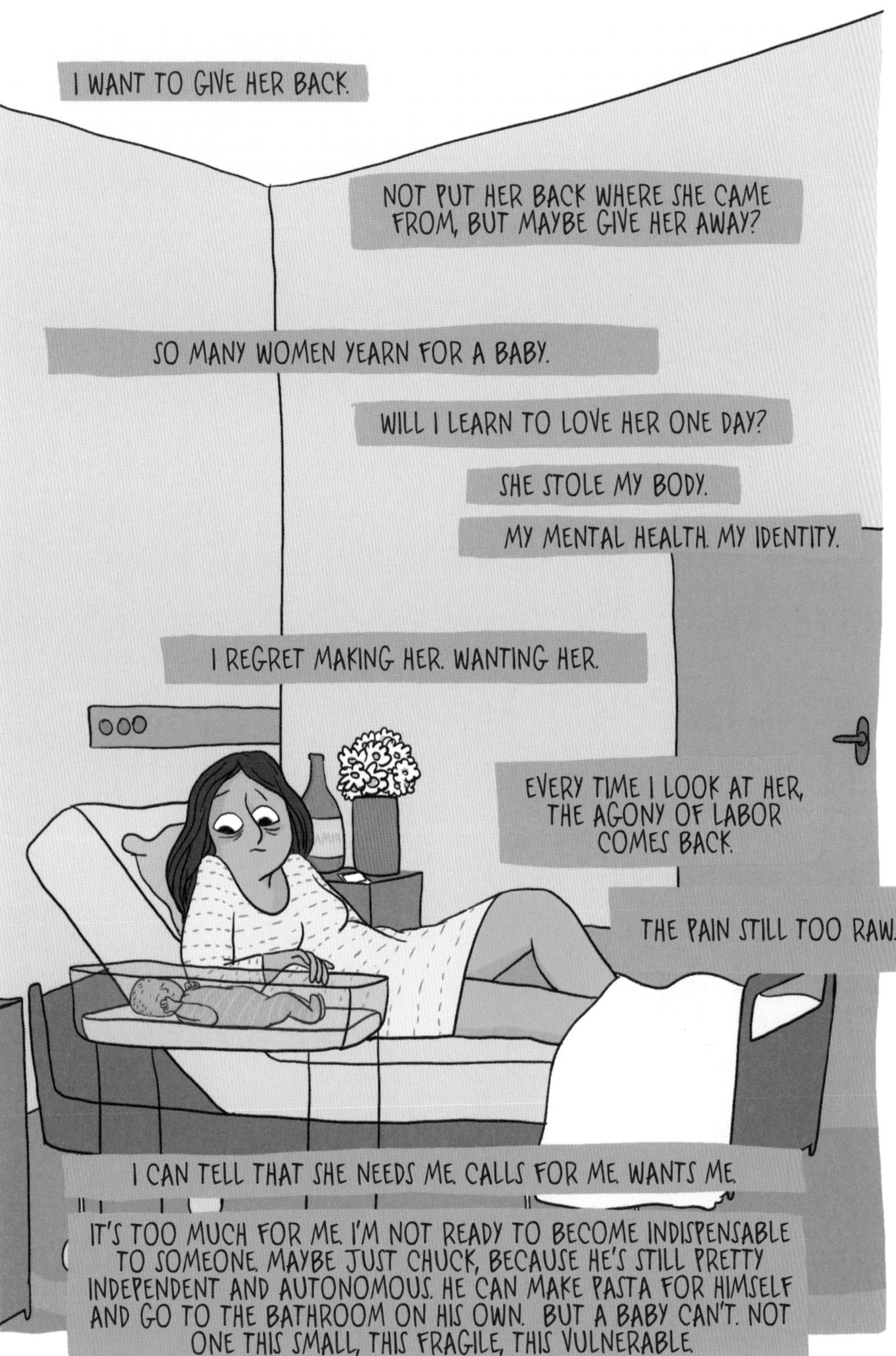
I WANT TO GIVE HER BACK.
NOT PUT HER BACK WHERE SHE CAME FROM, BUT MAYBE GIVE HER AWAY?
SO MANY WOMEN YEARN FOR A BABY.
WILL I LEARN TO LOVE HER ONE DAY?
SHE STOLE MY BODY.
MY MENTAL HEALTH. MY IDENTITY.
I REGRET MAKING HER. WANTING HER.
EVERY TIME I LOOK AT HER, THE AGONY OF LABOR COMES BACK.
THE PAIN STILL TOO RAW...
I CAN TELL THAT SHE NEEDS ME. CALLS FOR ME. WANTS ME.
IT'S TOO MUCH FOR ME. I'M NOT READY TO BECOME INDISPENSABLE TO SOMEONE. MAYBE JUST CHUCK, BECAUSE HE'S STILL PRETTY INDEPENDENT AND AUTONOMOUS. HE CAN MAKE PASTA FOR HIMSELF AND GO TO THE BATHROOM ON HIS OWN. BUT A BABY CAN'T. NOT ONE THIS SMALL, THIS FRAGILE, THIS VULNERABLE.

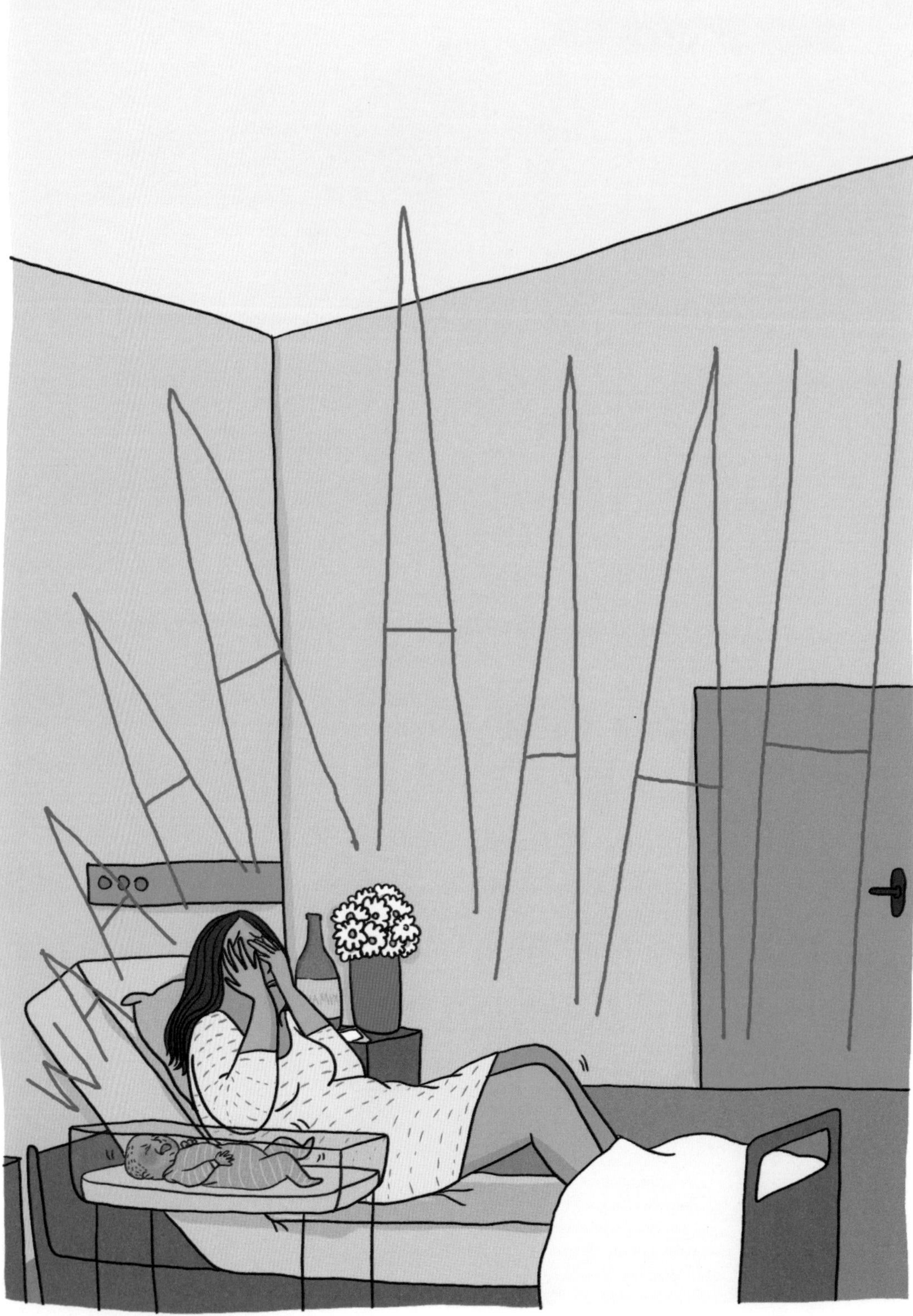
WAAAAAAAH

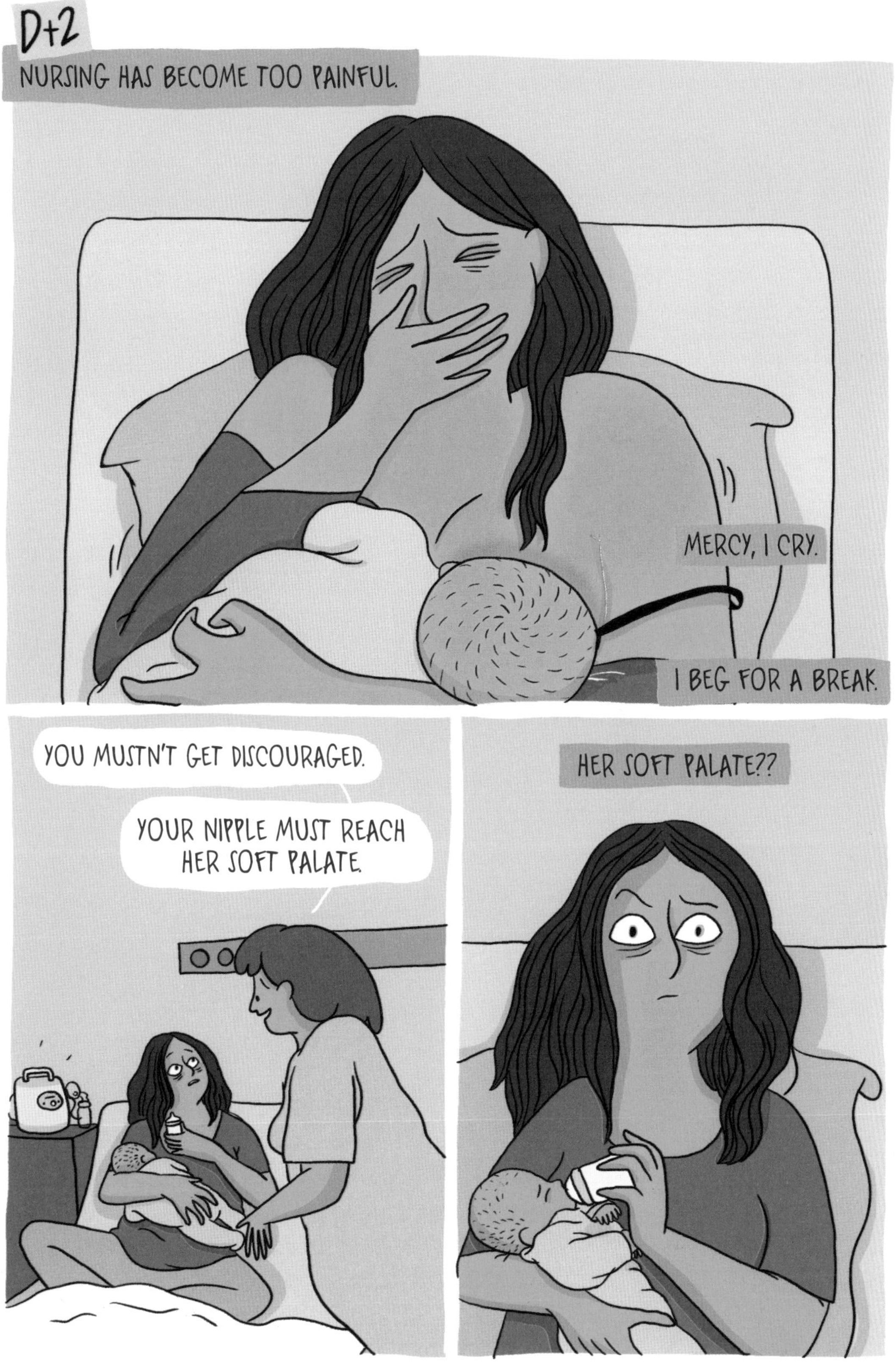

D+2

NURSING HAS BECOME TOO PAINFUL.

MERCY, I CRY.

I BEG FOR A BREAK.

YOU MUSTN'T GET DISCOURAGED.
YOUR NIPPLE MUST REACH HER SOFT PALATE.

HER SOFT PALATE??

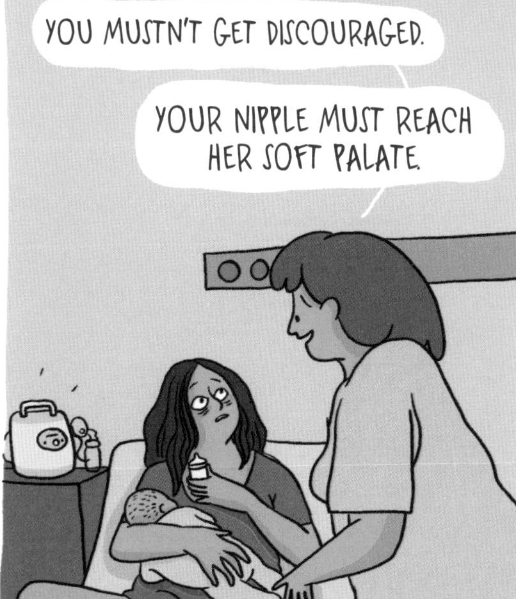

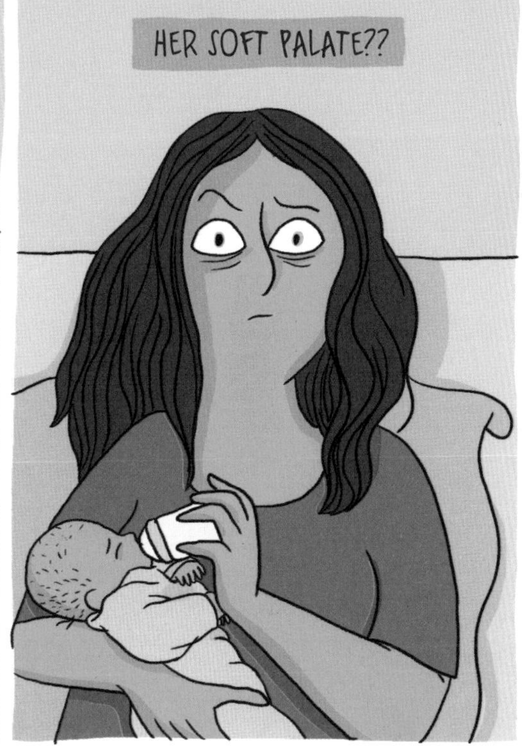

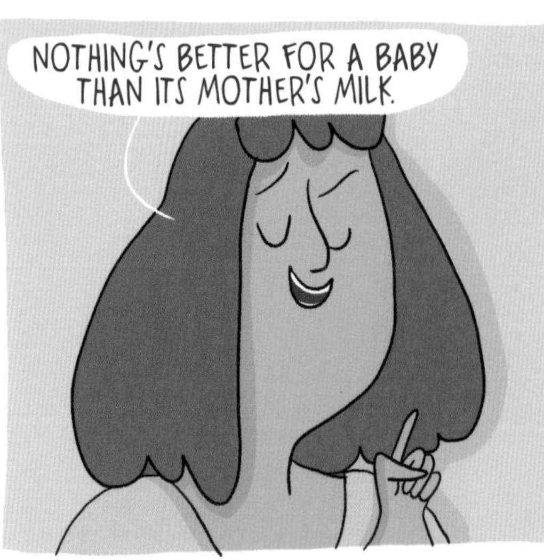
NOTHING'S BETTER FOR A BABY THAN ITS MOTHER'S MILK.
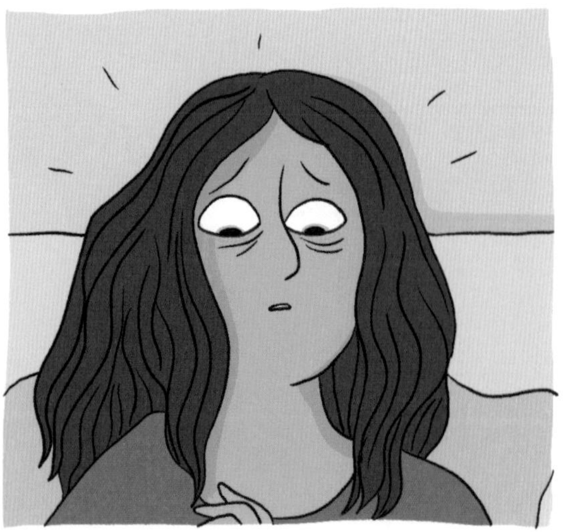
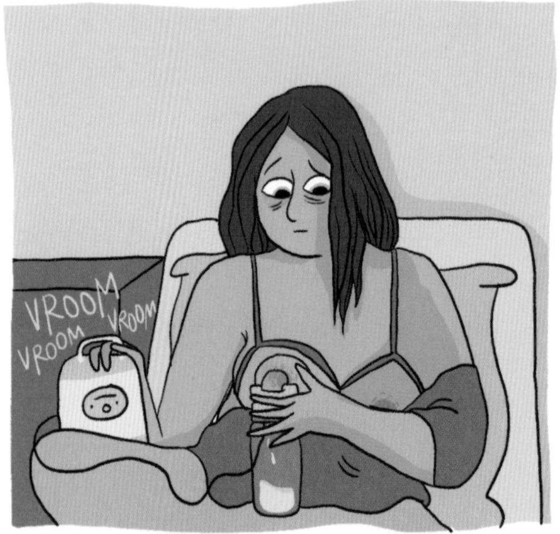
VROOM
VROOM
VROOM
VROOM
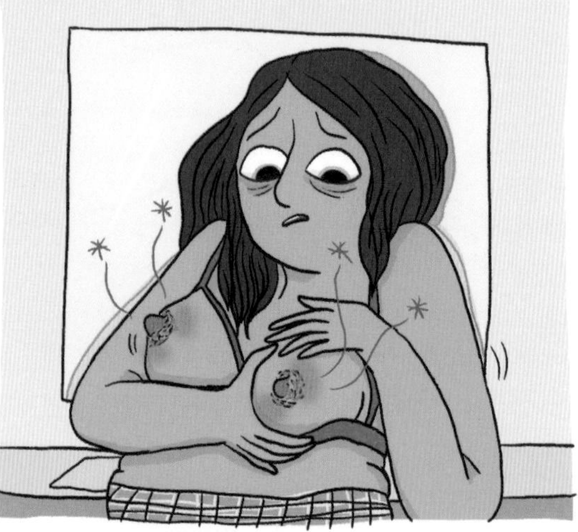
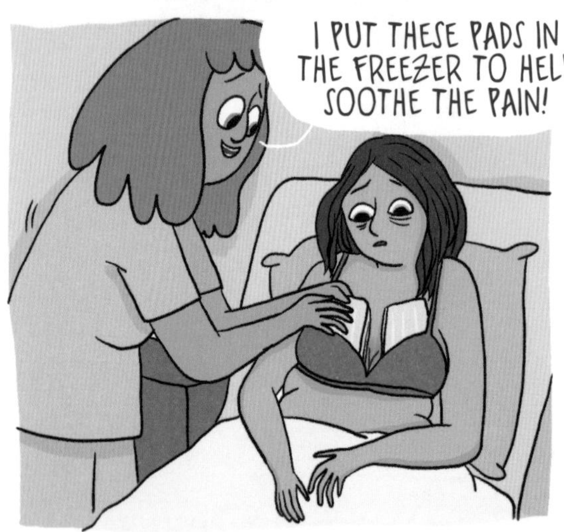
I PUT THESE PADS IN THE FREEZER TO HELP SOOTHE THE PAIN!
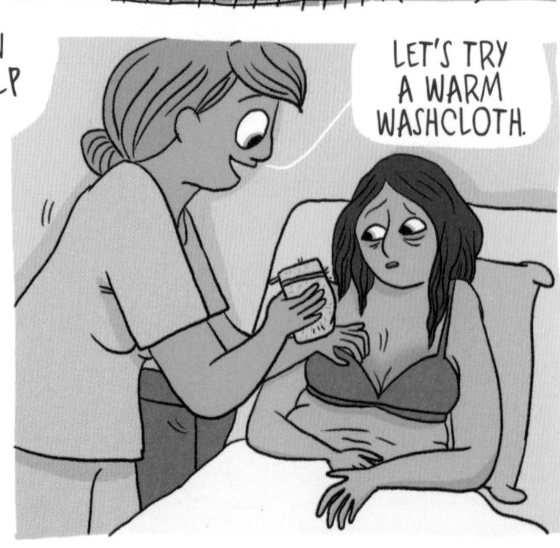
LET'S TRY A WARM WASHCLOTH.

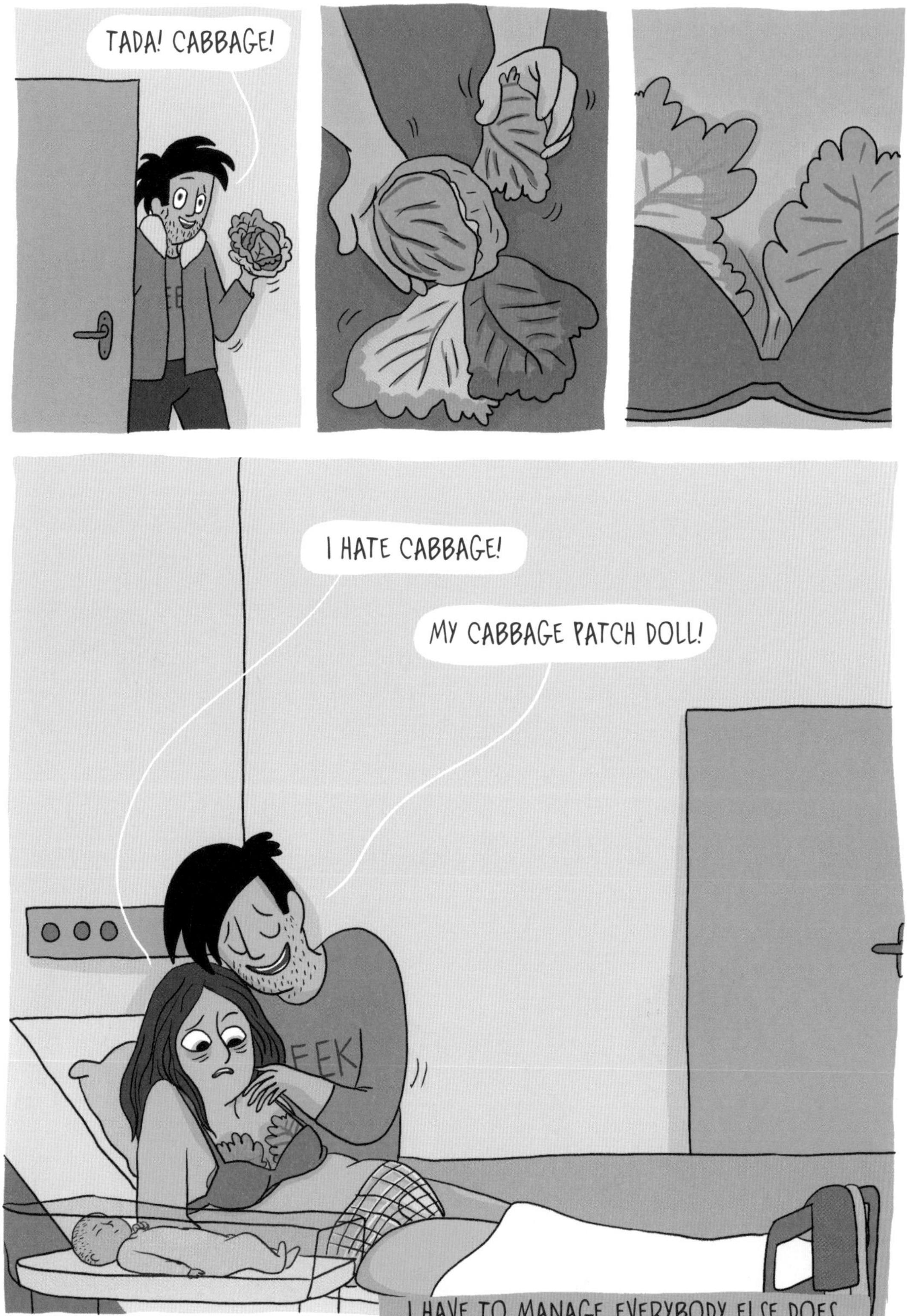

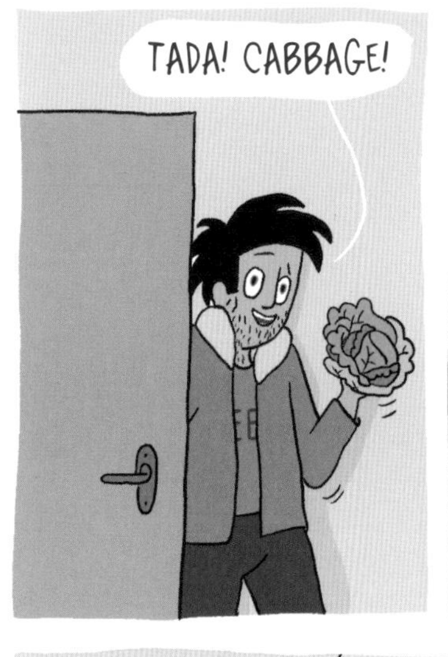

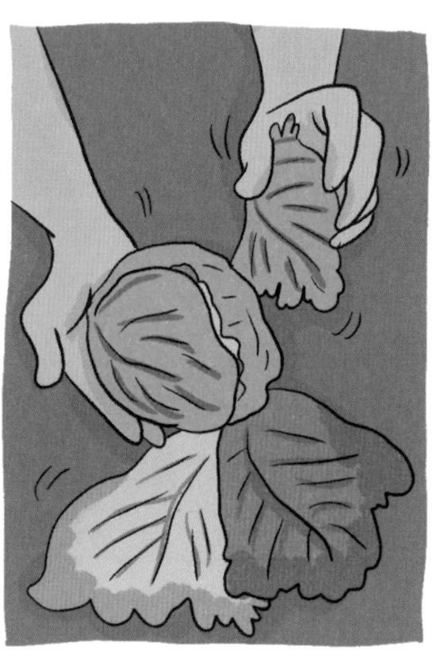

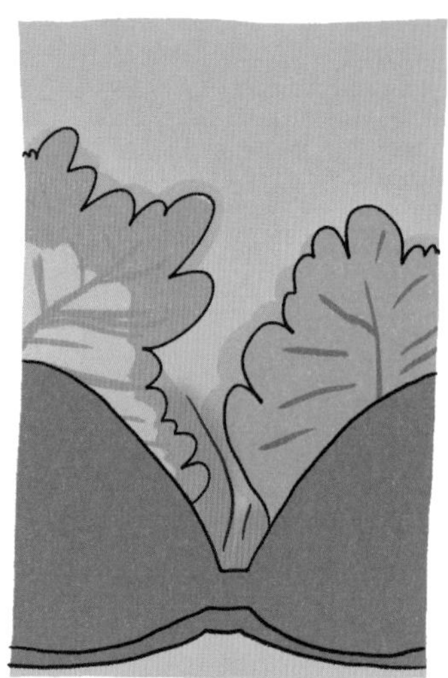

I HATE CABBAGE!

MY CABBAGE PATCH DOLL!

I HAVE TO MANAGE. EVERYBODY ELSE DOES.

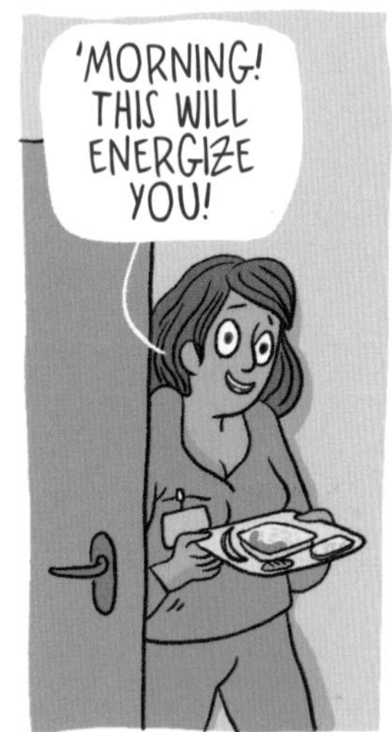
'MORNING! THIS WILL ENERGIZE YOU!

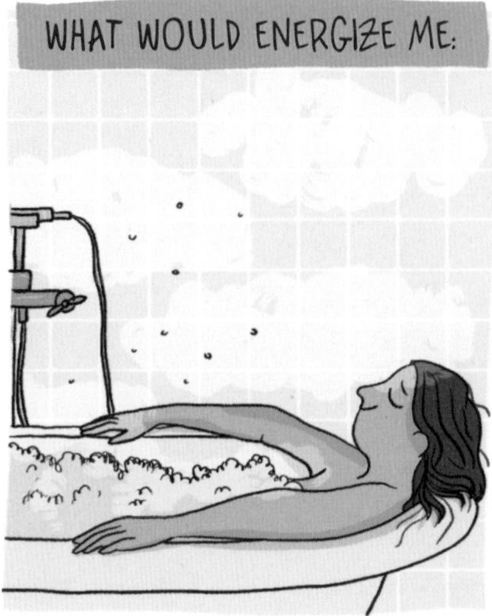
WHAT WOULD ENERGIZE ME:

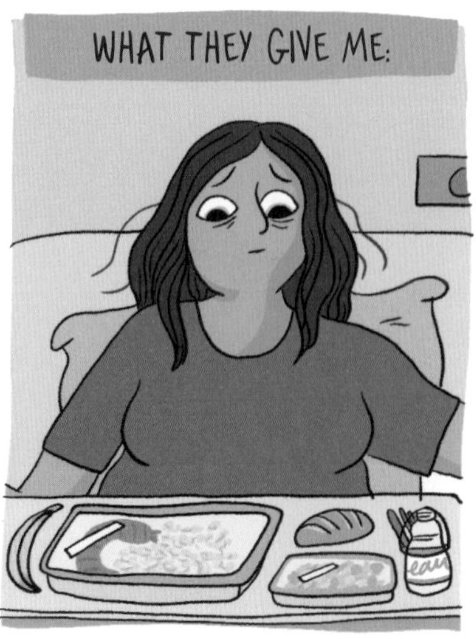
WHAT THEY GIVE ME:

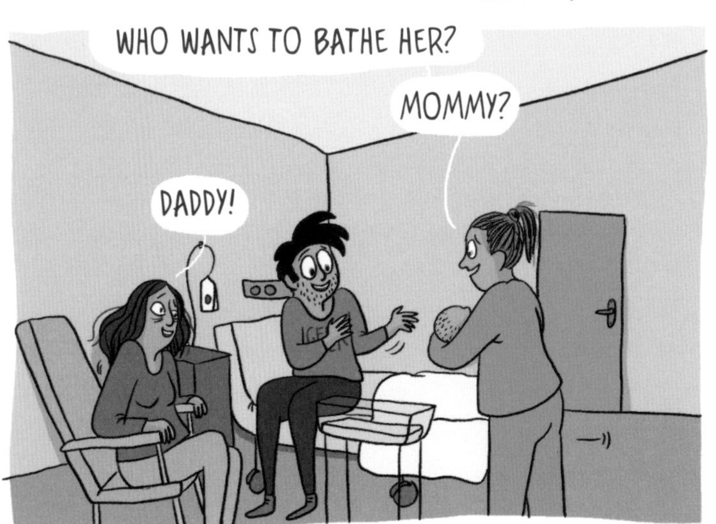
WHO WANTS TO BATHE HER?
MOMMY?
DADDY!

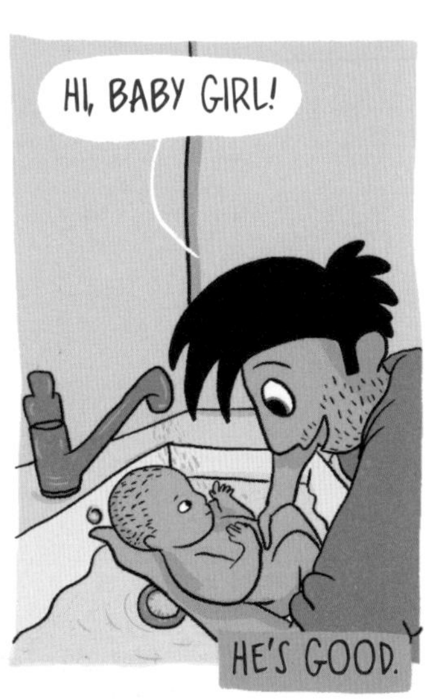
HI, BABY GIRL!
HE'S GOOD.

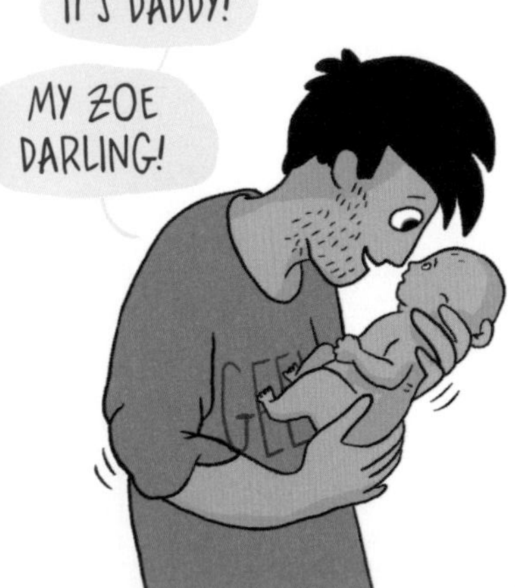
IT'S DADDY!
MY ZOE DARLING!

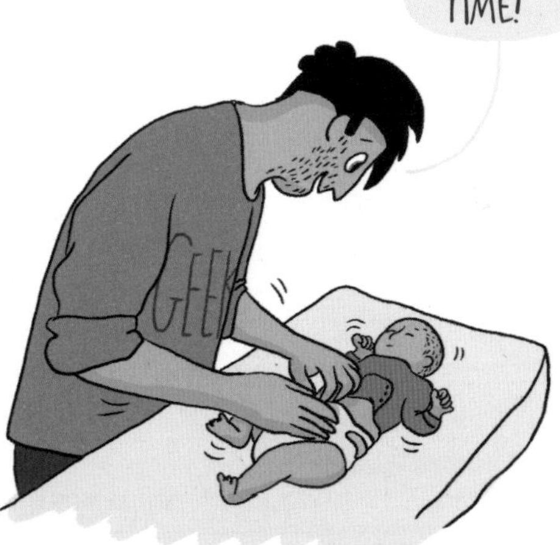
DIAPER TIME!

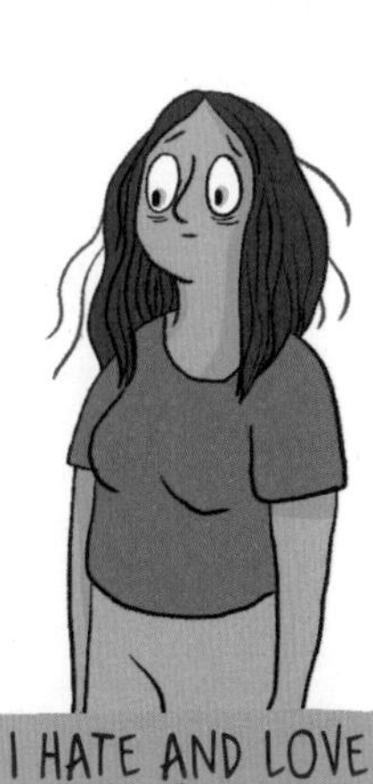
I HATE AND LOVE HIM EQUALLY.

NO, I THINK I HATE HIM A BIT MORE THAN I LOVE HIM AND WITH ZOE, I'M BOUND TO HIM FOREVER

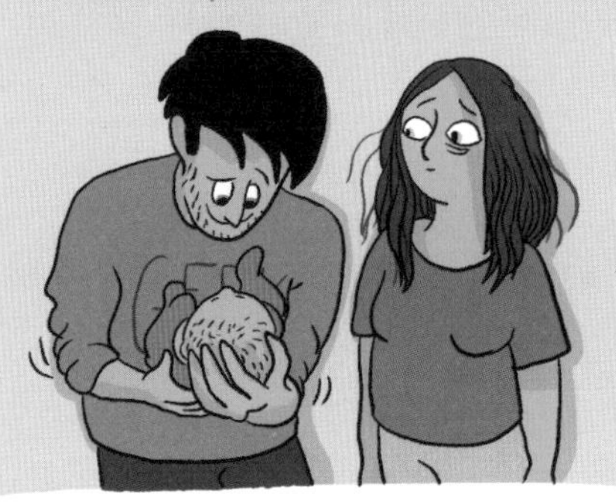

YOU'VE DONE THIS BEFORE, WITH YOUR DAUGHTERS. NO WONDER YOU MANAGE SO WELL!

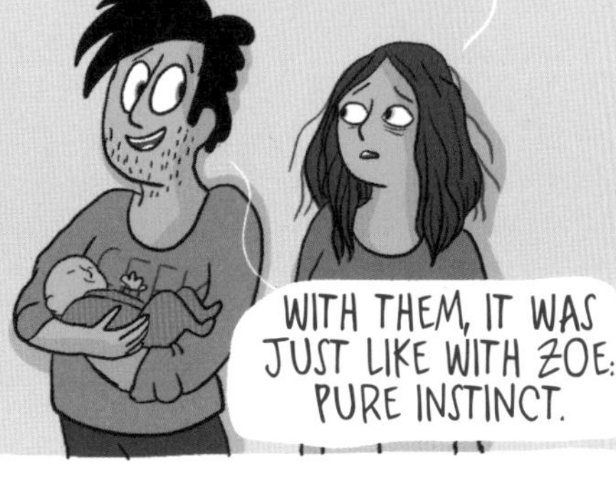

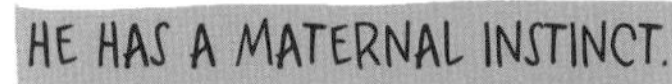

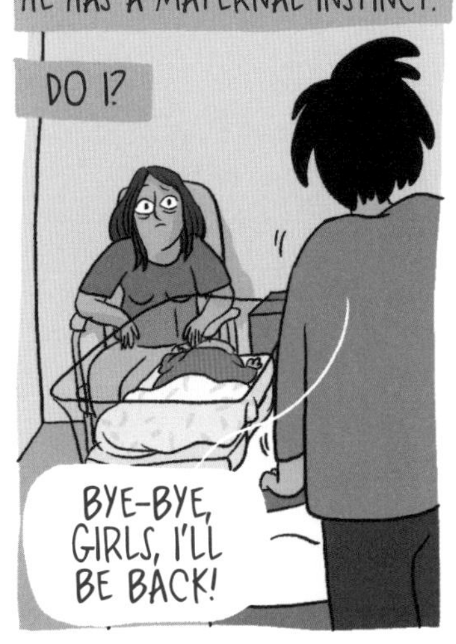

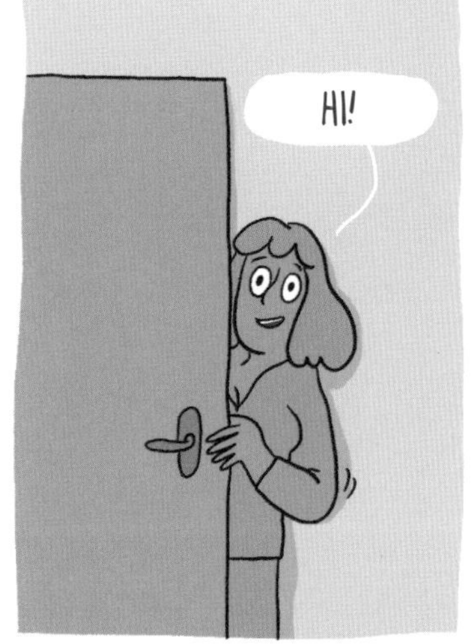

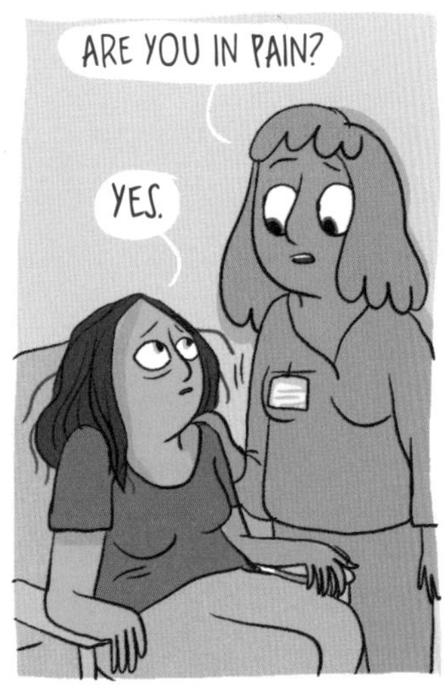

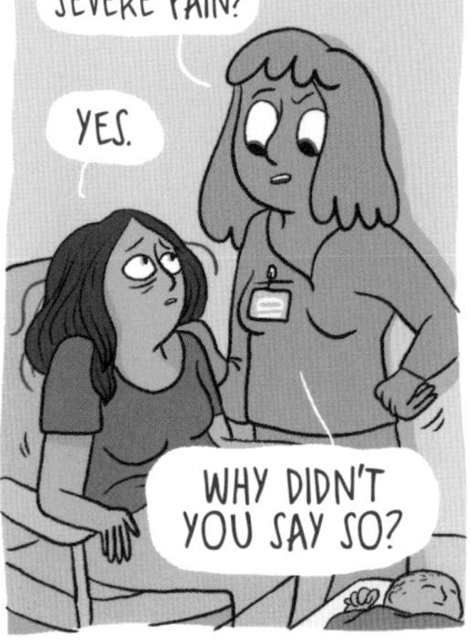

WHY?!

BECAUSE I WAS TAUGHT NOT TO COMPLAIN. BECAUSE NOBODY BELIEVED ME WHEN I USED TO SAY I HAD PAINFUL MENSTRUAL CRAMPS. BECAUSE I DON'T FULLY EXIST. BECAUSE WHAT MATTERS IS MY BABY. BECAUSE SUFFERING IS PART OF GIVING BIRTH. BECAUSE BEING A WOMAN MEANS PRETENDING IT'S NO BIG DEAL.

BECAUSE NOBODY ASKED ME.

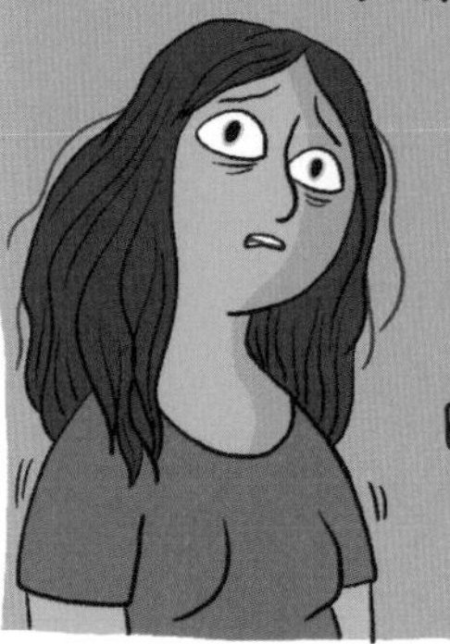

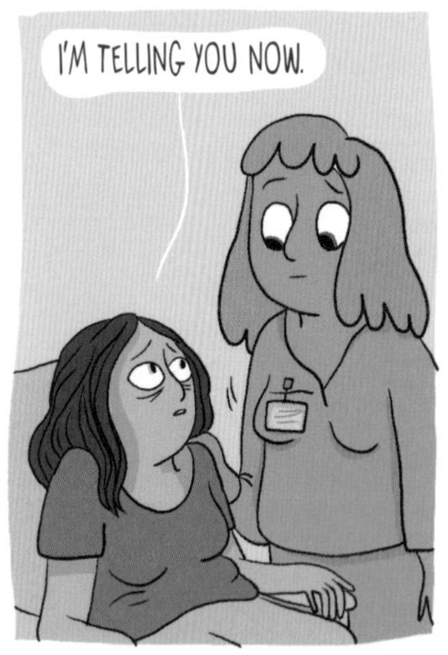
I'M TELLING YOU NOW.

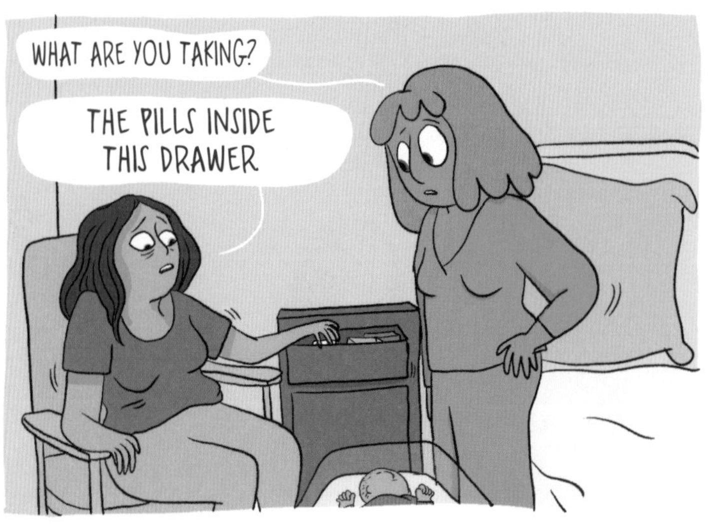
WHAT ARE YOU TAKING?
THE PILLS INSIDE THIS DRAWER

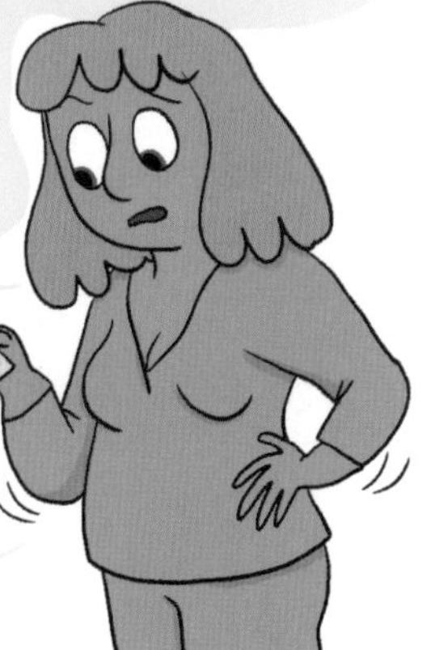
THIS IS WHAT WE GIVE EVERYONE. THEN WE ADJUST, BASED ON THE PAIN. IT CAN EVEN REQUIRE MORPHINE! I'LL GIVE YOU SOMETHING THAT'LL MAKE YOU FEEL BETTER VERY QUICKLY.
YOU'LL BE MUCH MORE FUNC-TIONAL.

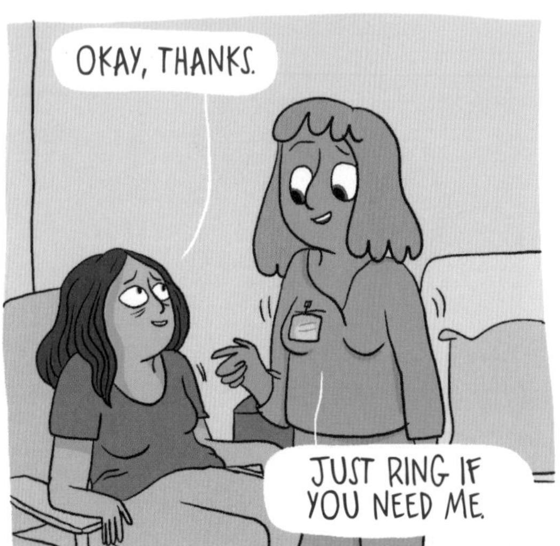
OKAY, THANKS.
JUST RING IF YOU NEED ME.

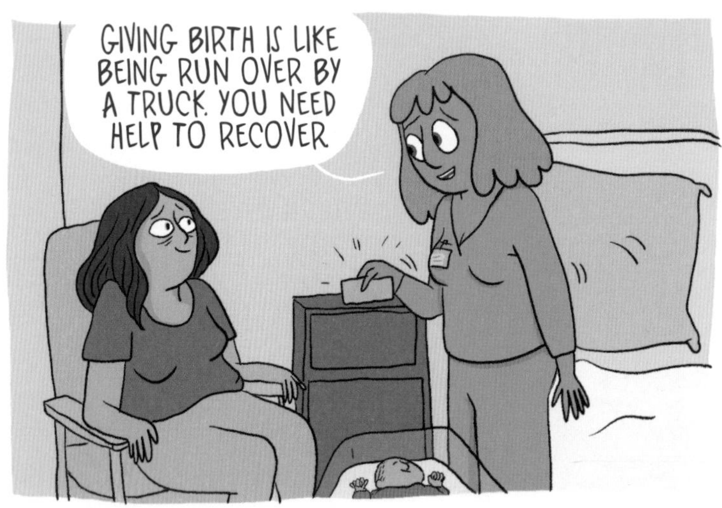
GIVING BIRTH IS LIKE BEING RUN OVER BY A TRUCK. YOU NEED HELP TO RECOVER

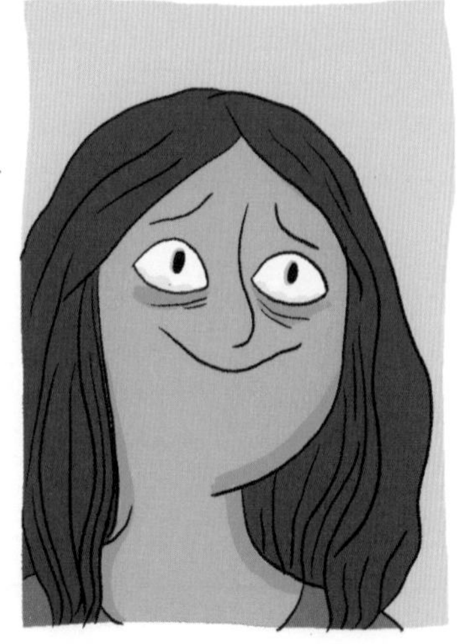

HERE SHE IS! YOUR LITTLE SISTER!
IT HADN'T DAWNED ON ME: ZOE HAS TWO SISTERS.

SHE'S CROSS-EYED!

ZOE HASN'T RECOVERED HER BIRTH WEIGHT.

DRINK, LITTLE BABY.

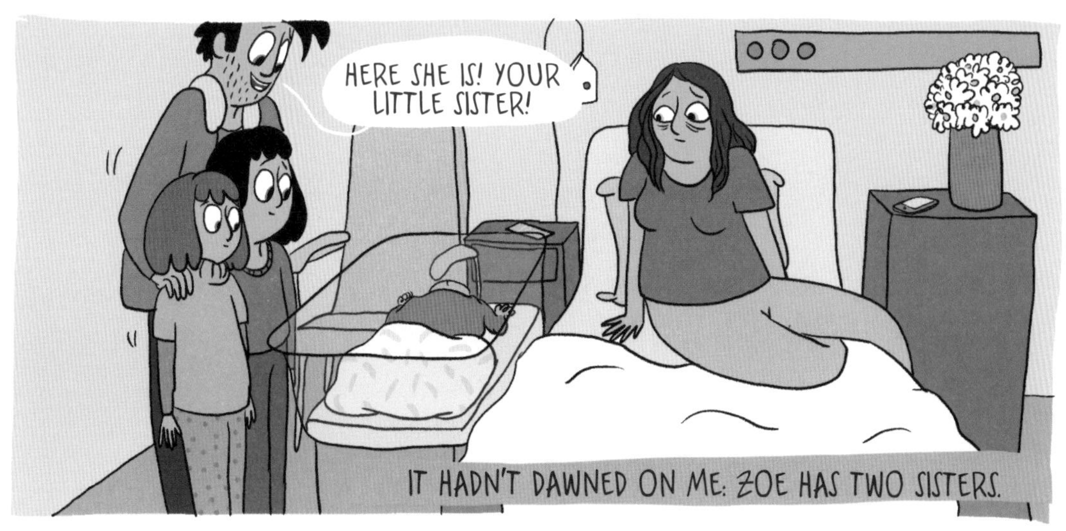

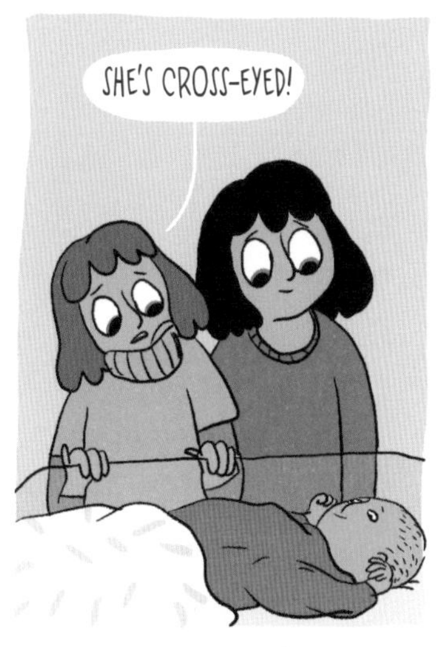

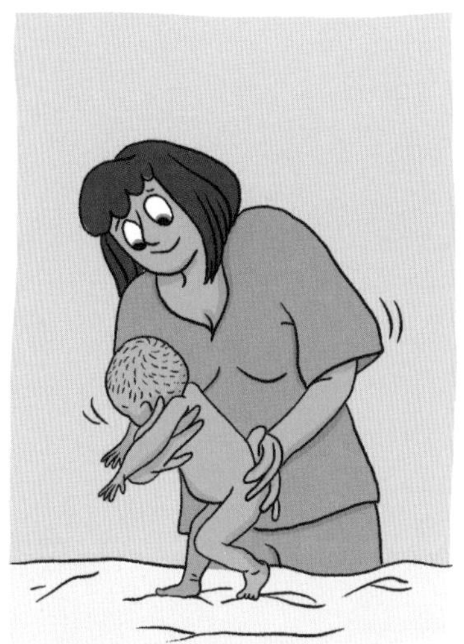

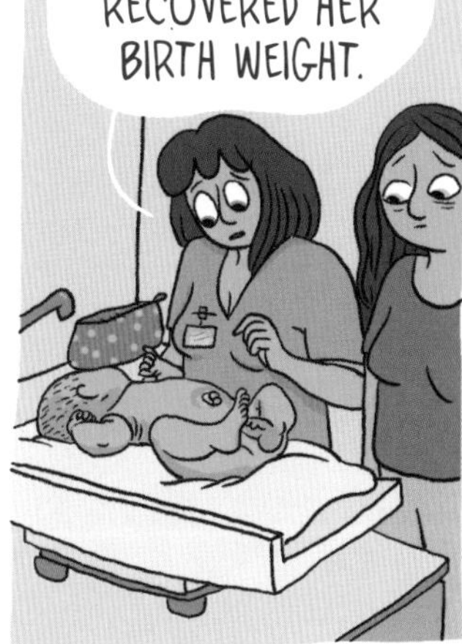

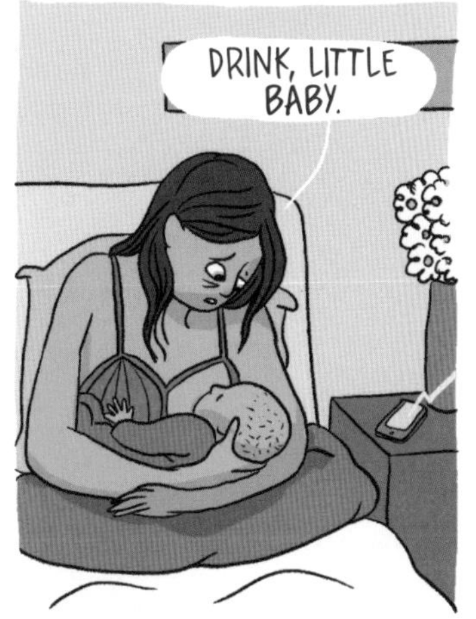

A MIGRANT FROM NIGERIA CALLED HER BABY GIRL GIFT AFTER GIVING BIRTH ON A SHIP THAT RESCUED HER IN THE MEDITERRANEAN SEA. OTHER MIGRANT WOMEN GAVE THEIR BABIES NAMES LIKE LUCKY, HOPE, ANGELA MERKEL AND DIGNITY, IN HONOR OF THE SHIP THAT SAVED ONE OF THEIR OWN.

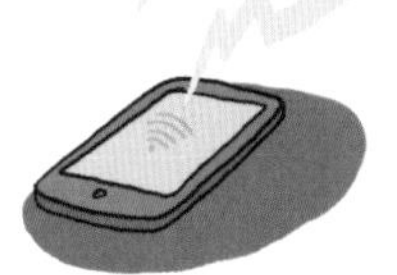

WAAAAAAH

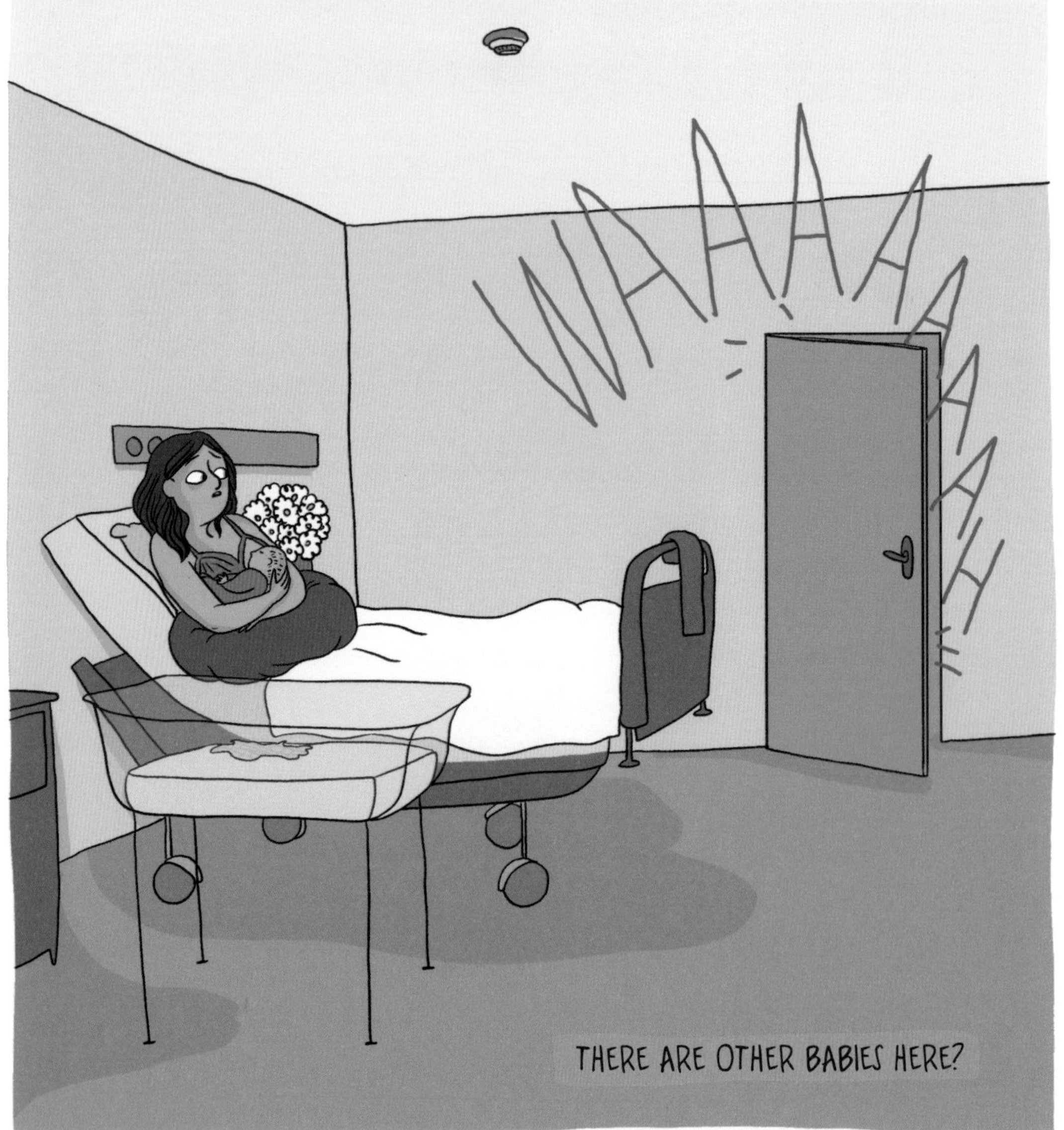
WAAAAAAAAAAH
THERE ARE OTHER BABIES HERE?

D+3

EVERYBODY WILL GIVE YOU ADVICE.

I ASSUME THEY ALREADY DO.

SO I'LL PITCH IN TOO. HERE'S MY ADVICE: JUST SAY YES.

WHEN SOMEONE RELATES AN ANECDOTE, OR RECOMMENDS THIS OR THAT, OR SWEARS TO HAVE A MIRACLE SOLUTION FOR A PROBLEM, JUST GO ALONG.

THEN THEY'LL LEAVE YOU ALONE. "YES" IS OFTEN A BETTER SHIELD THAN "NO."

SO I SHOULD SAY YES TO THIS TIP?

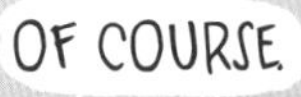

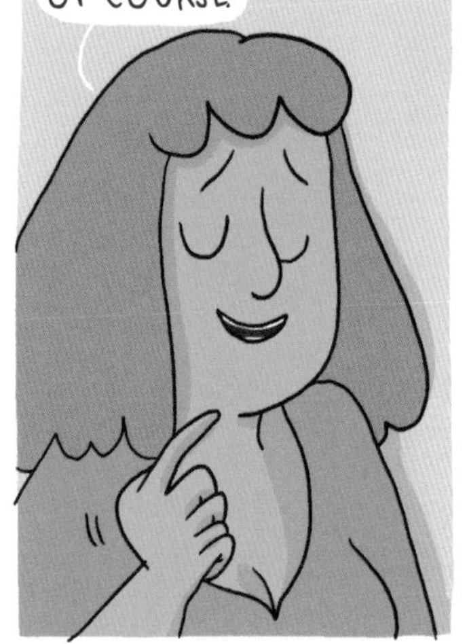

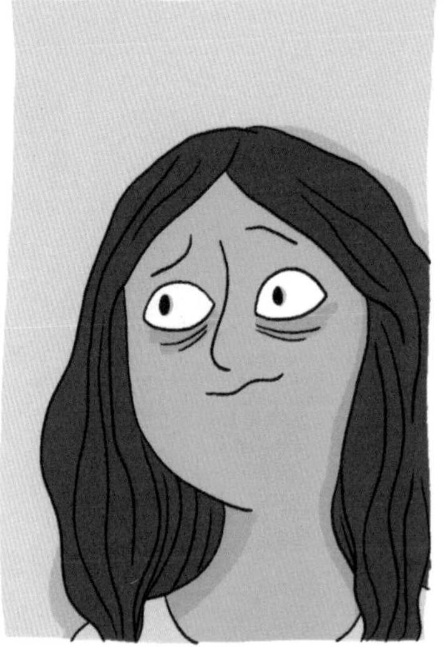

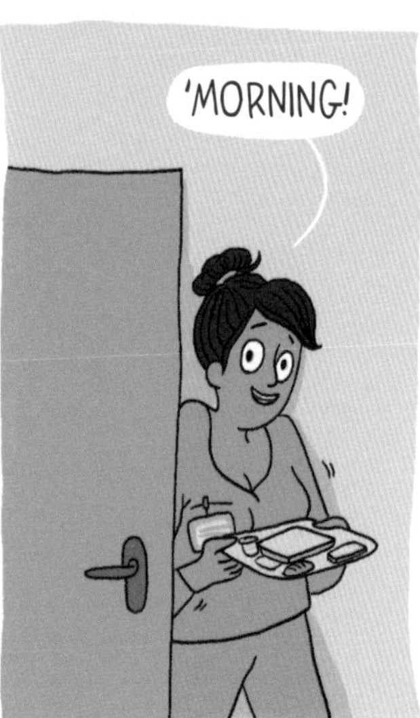

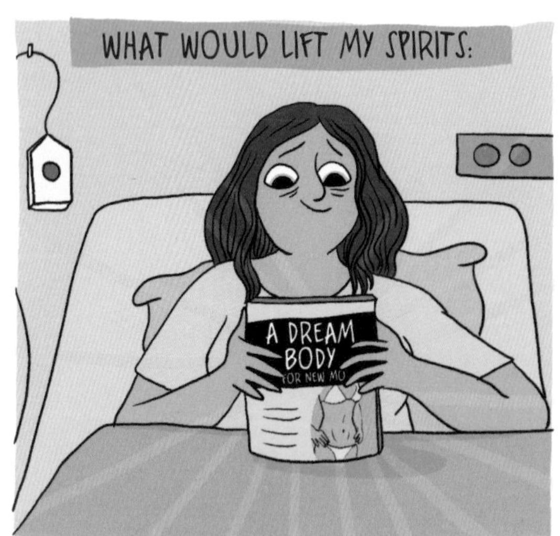
WHAT WOULD LIFT MY SPIRITS:
A DREAM BODY

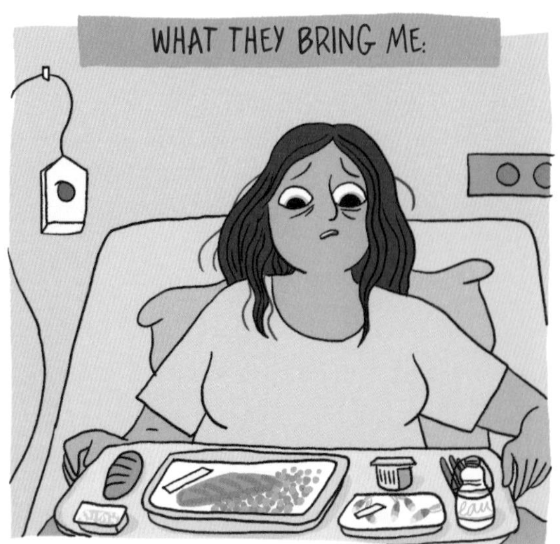
WHAT THEY BRING ME:

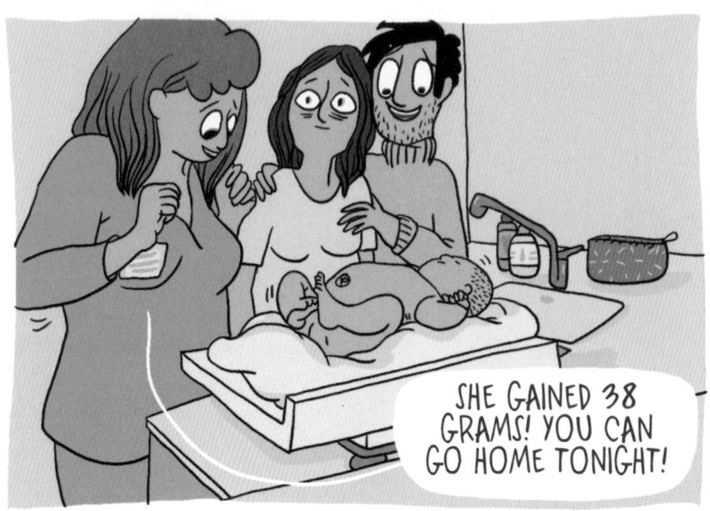
SHE GAINED 38 GRAMS! YOU CAN GO HOME TONIGHT!

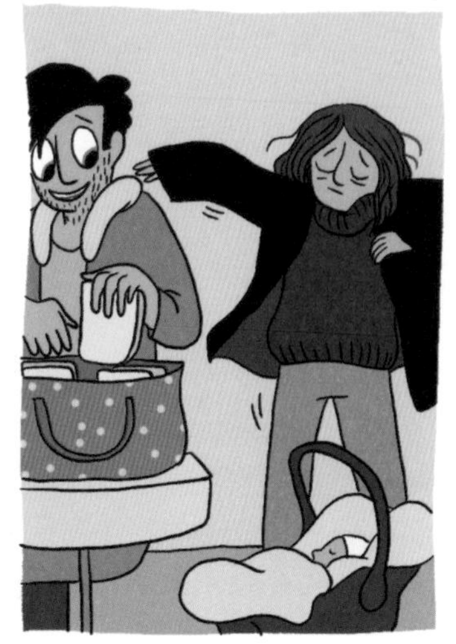

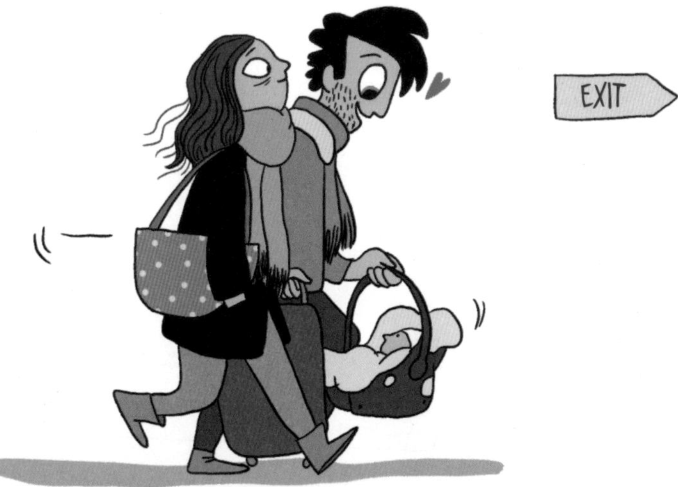
EXIT

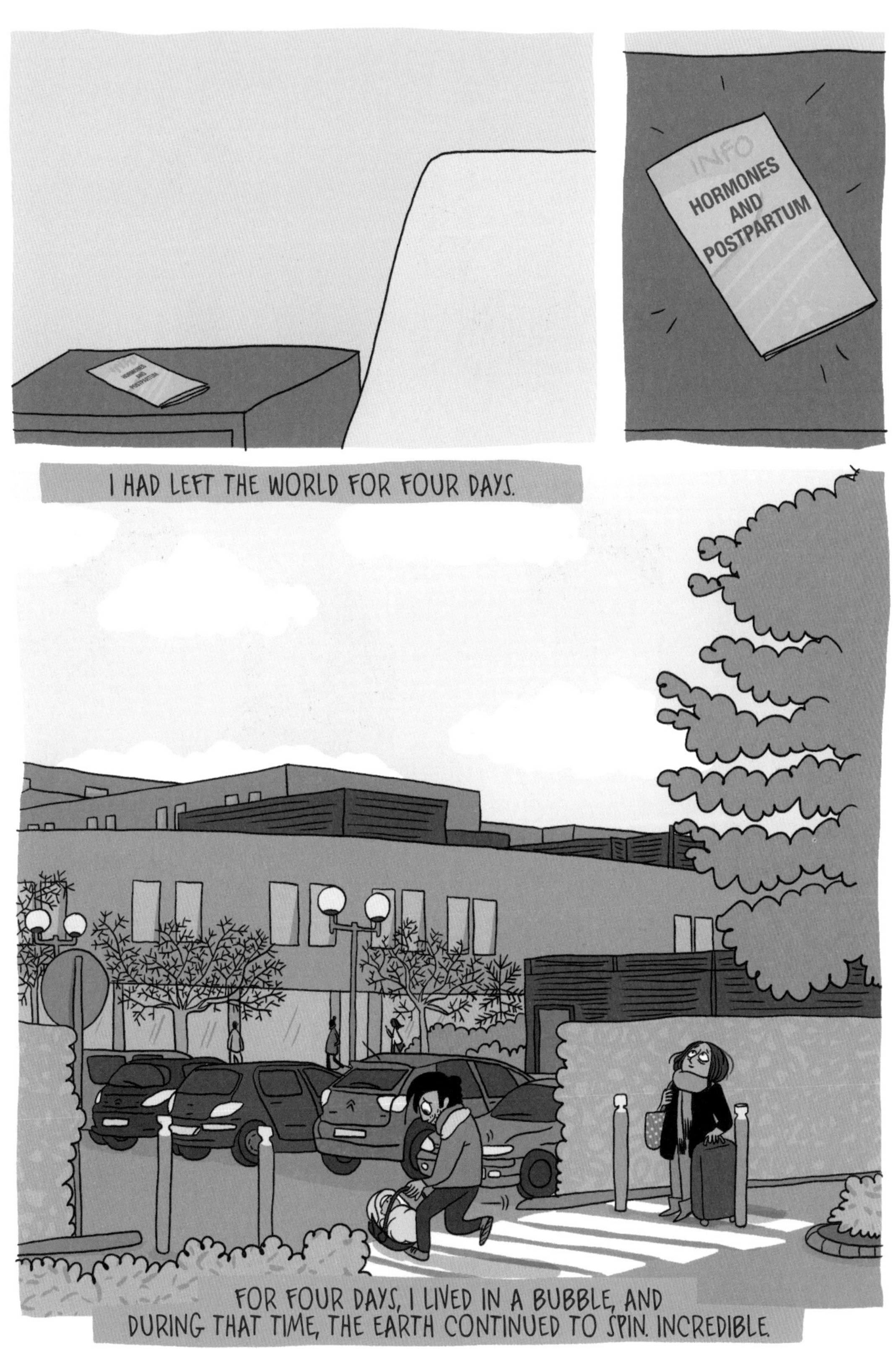
INFO
HORMONES
AND
POSTPARTUM
I HAD LEFT THE WORLD FOR FOUR DAYS.
FOR FOUR DAYS, I LIVED IN A BUBBLE, AND
DURING THAT TIME, THE EARTH CONTINUED TO SPIN. INCREDIBLE.

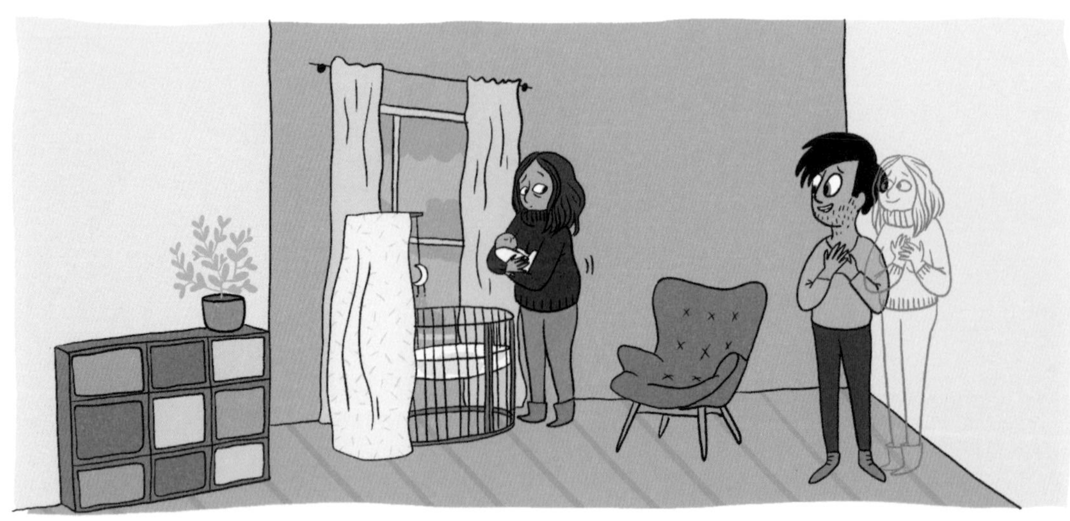

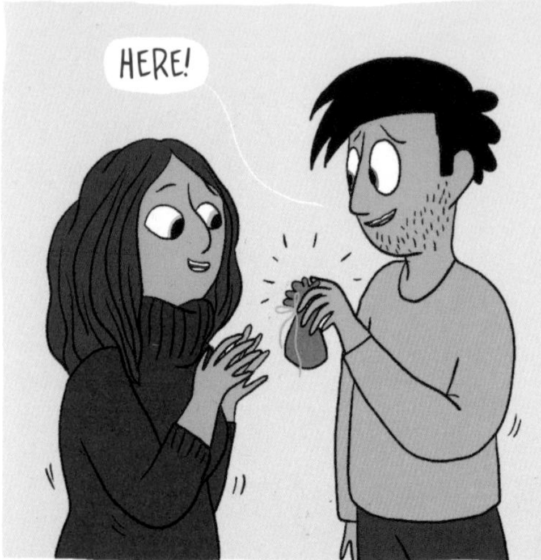

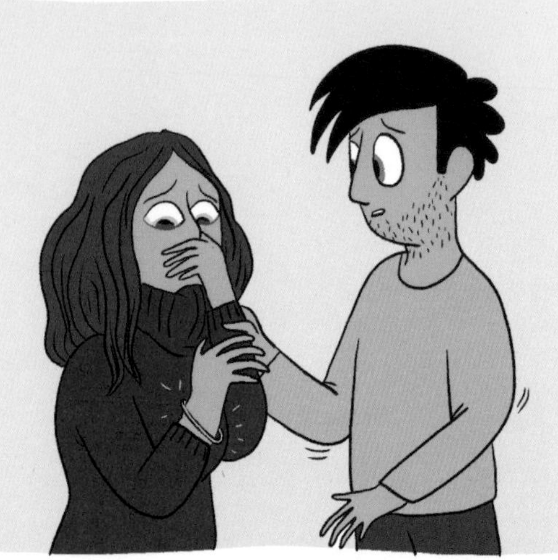

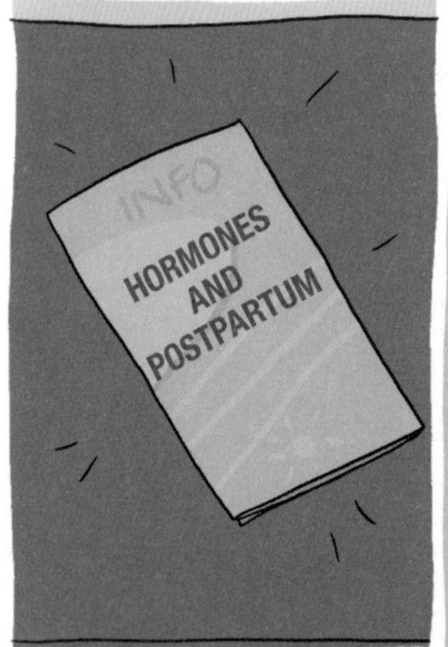

HORMONES AND POSTPARTUM

AFTER GIVING BIRTH, YOUR BODY PRODUCES DIFFERENT HORMONES. PROLACTIN IS RESPONSIBLE FOR LACTATION. OTHER HORMONES ENABLE YOUR UTERUS TO RETURN TO ITS ORIGINAL SIZE AND ITS LINING TO REGENERATE. THEY ALSO AFFECT YOUR SWEAT GLANDS, YOUR SLEEP (MAKING YOU A LIGHT SLEEPER), AND CAUSE A DROP IN ESTROGEN AND PROGESTERONE, THUS TAKING YOU ON AN EMOTIONAL ROLLERCOASTER.

ANYTHING AND EVERYTHING CAN TRIGGER TEARS IN ME:

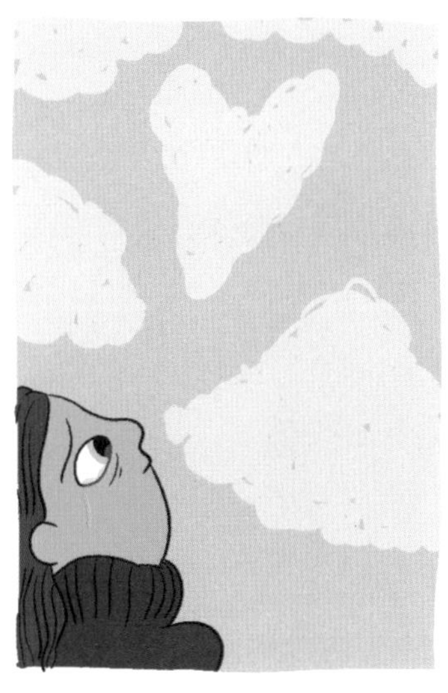

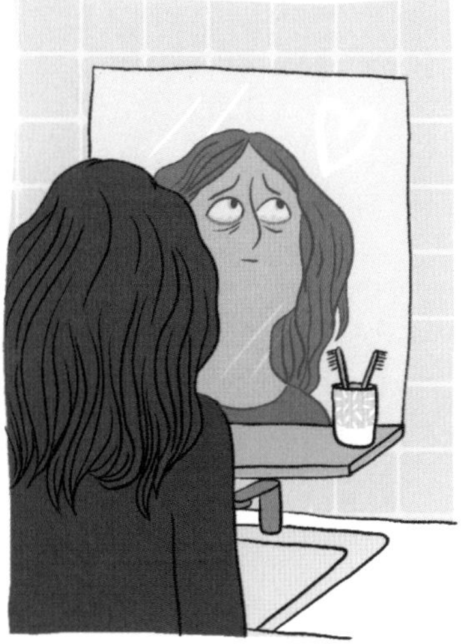

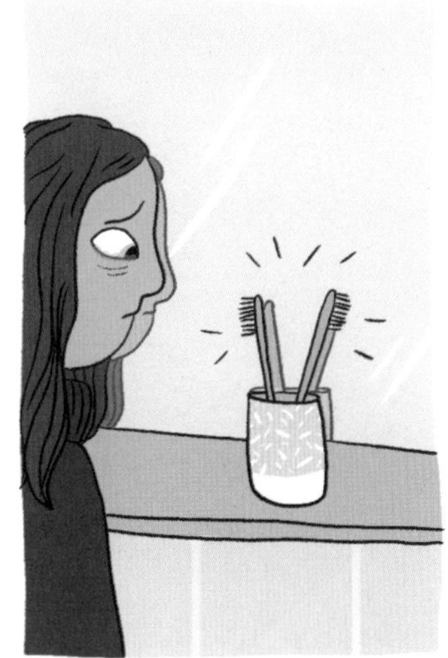

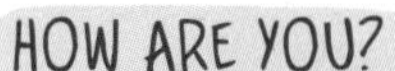

HOW ARE YOU?

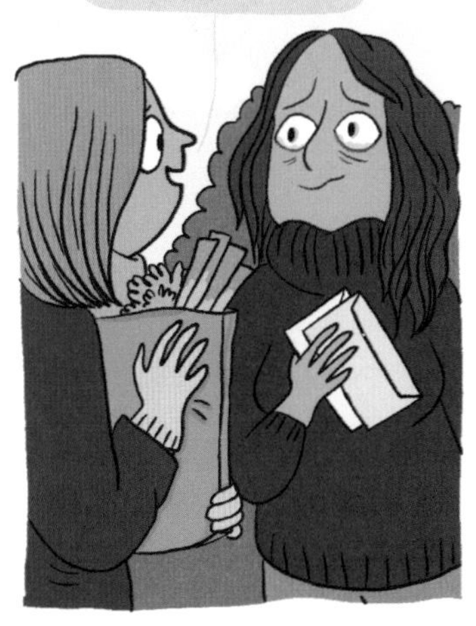

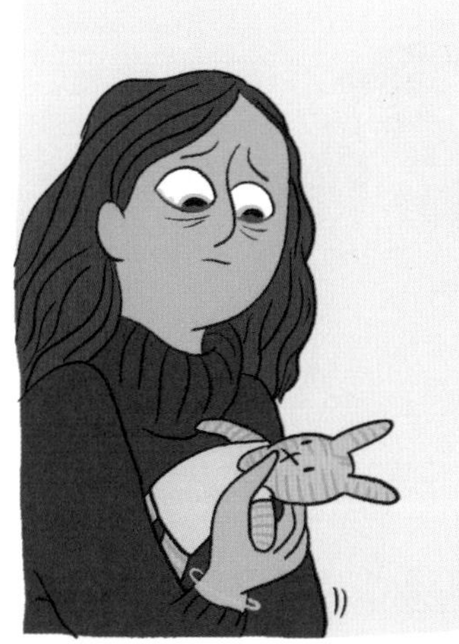

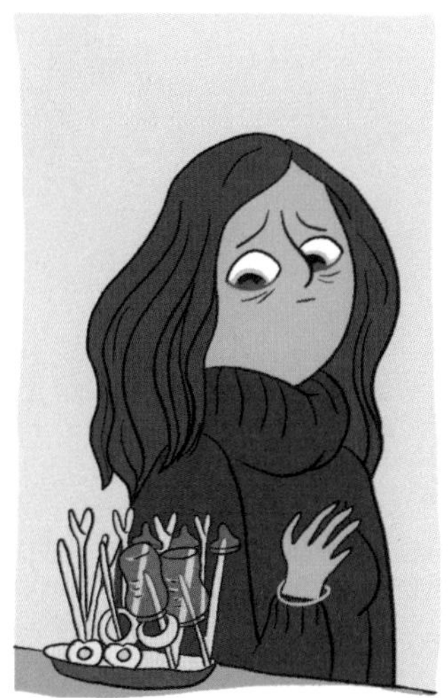

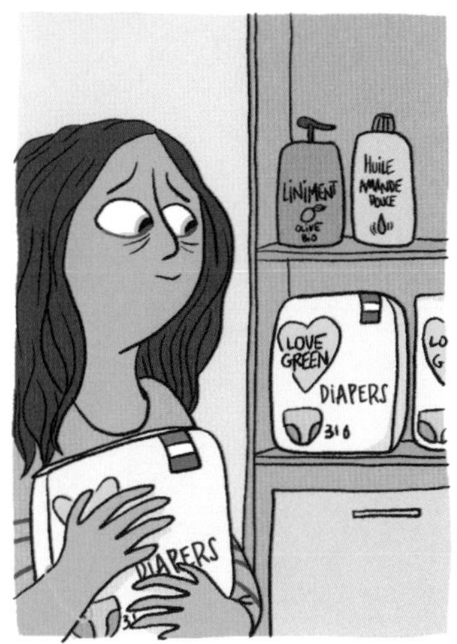

LINIMENT
HUILE AMANDE DOUCE
LOVE GREEN
DIAPERS
DIAPERS

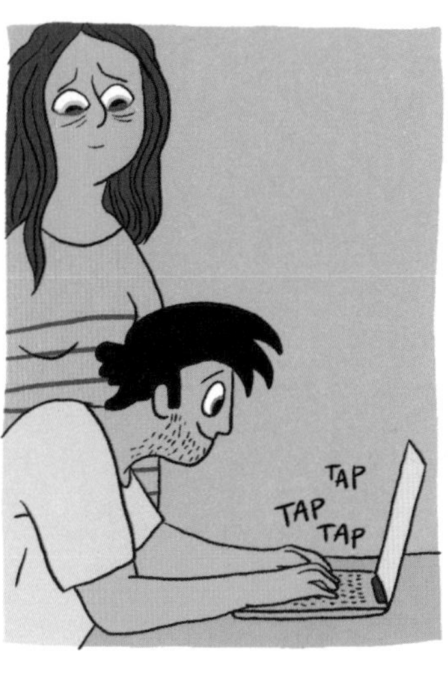

TAP
TAP
TAP

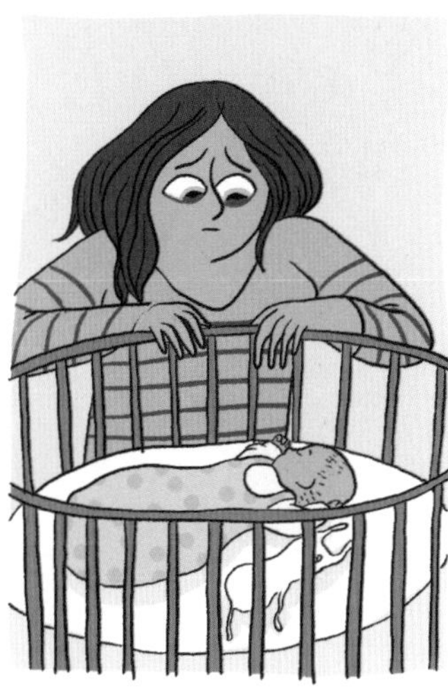

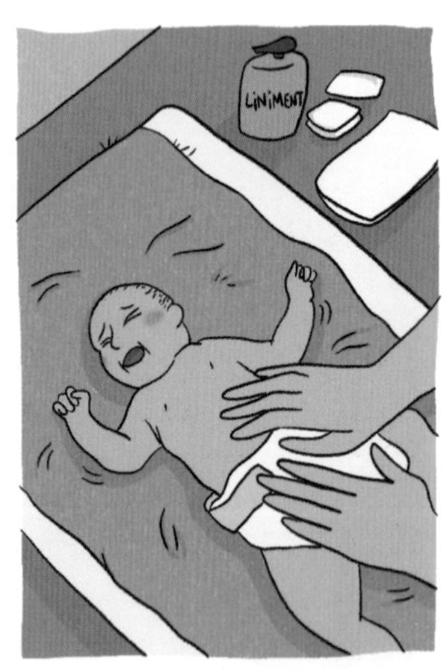
LINIMENT

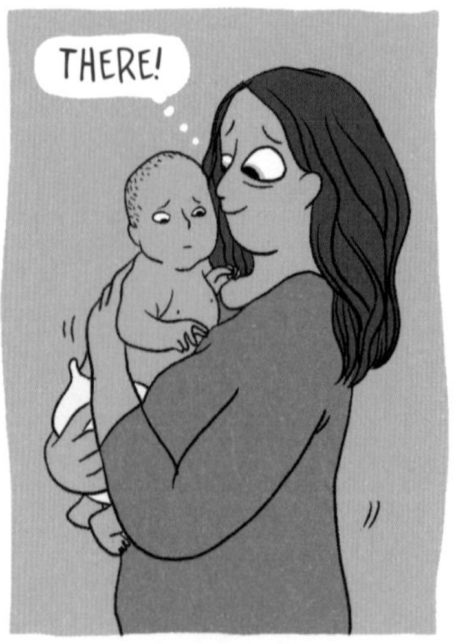
THERE!

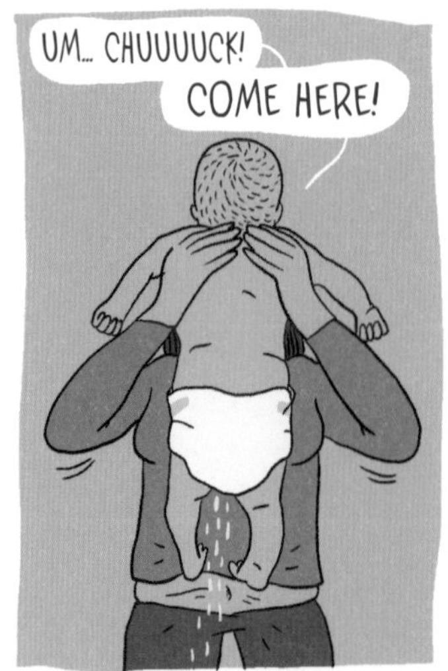
UM... CHUUUUCK!
COME HERE!

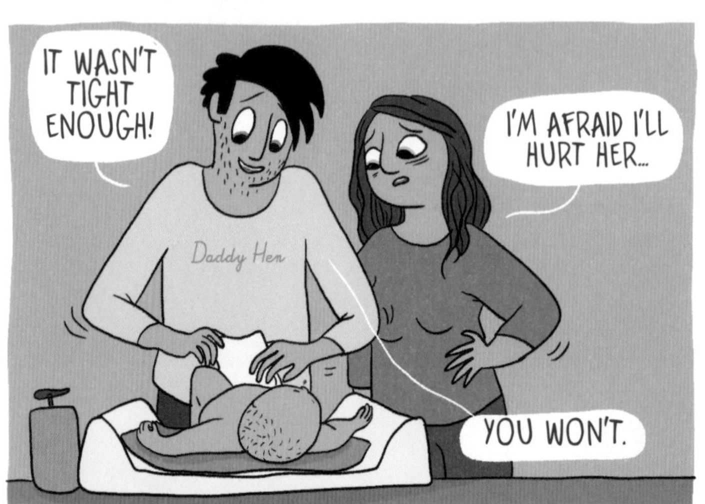
IT WASN'T TIGHT ENOUGH!
Daddy Hen
I'M AFRAID I'LL HURT HER...
YOU WON'T.

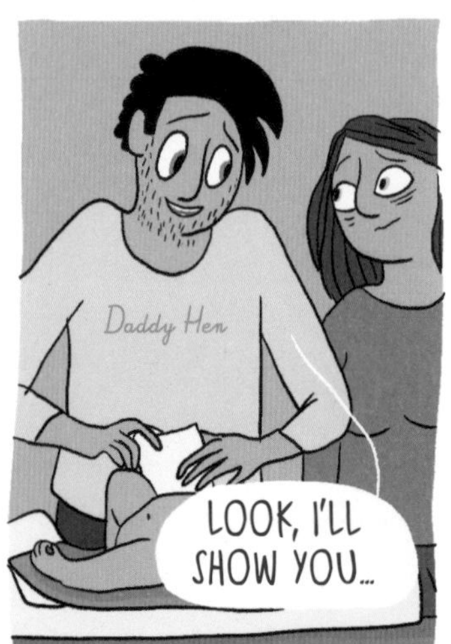
Daddy Hen
LOOK, I'LL SHOW YOU...

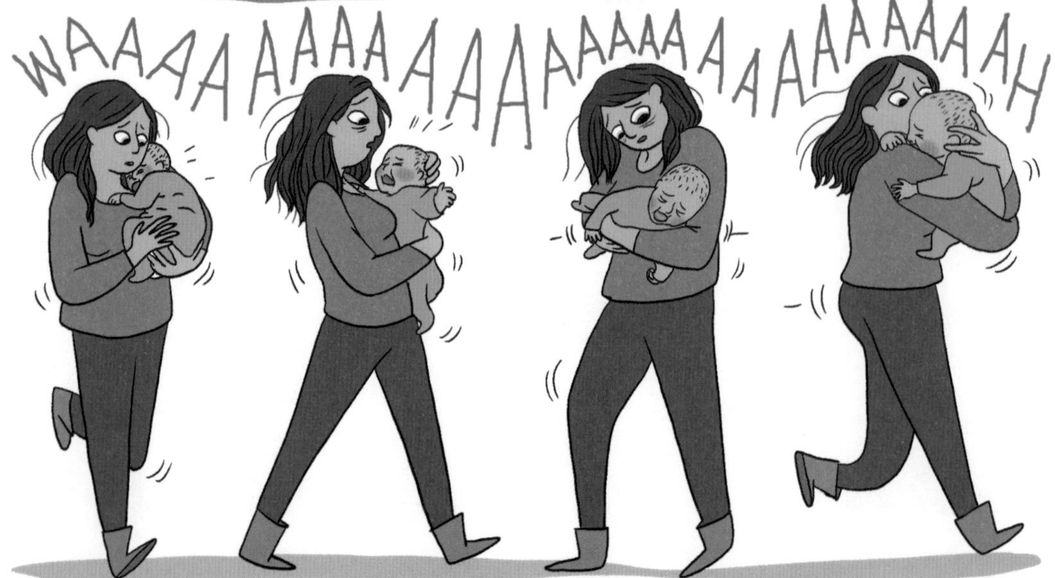
WAAAAAAAAAAAAAAAAAAAAAAAAAH

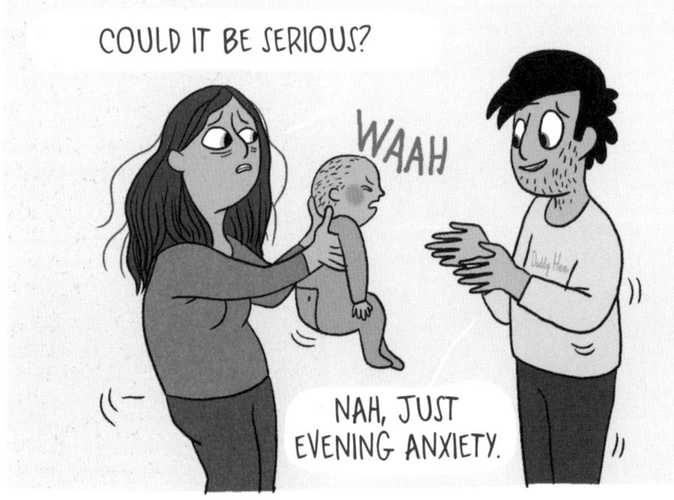
COULD IT BE SERIOUS?
WAAH
NAH, JUST EVENING ANXIETY.

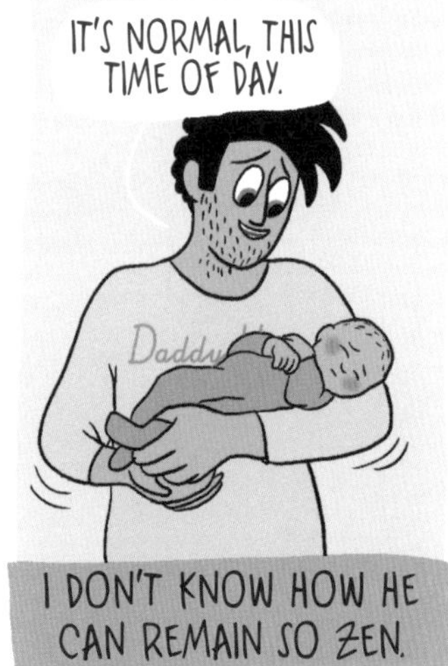
IT'S NORMAL, THIS TIME OF DAY.
I DON'T KNOW HOW HE CAN REMAIN SO ZEN.

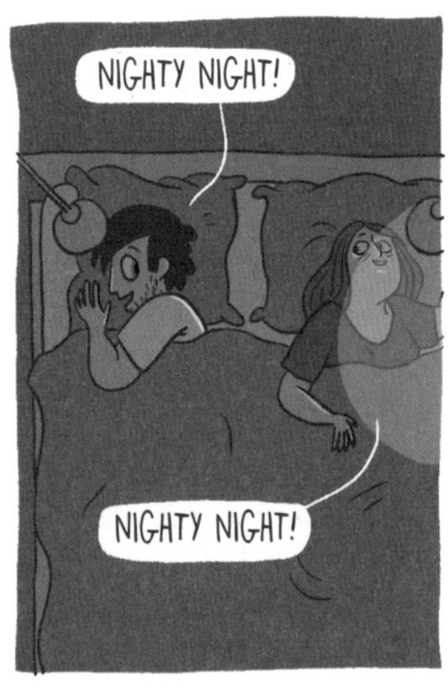
NIGHTY NIGHT!
NIGHTY NIGHT!

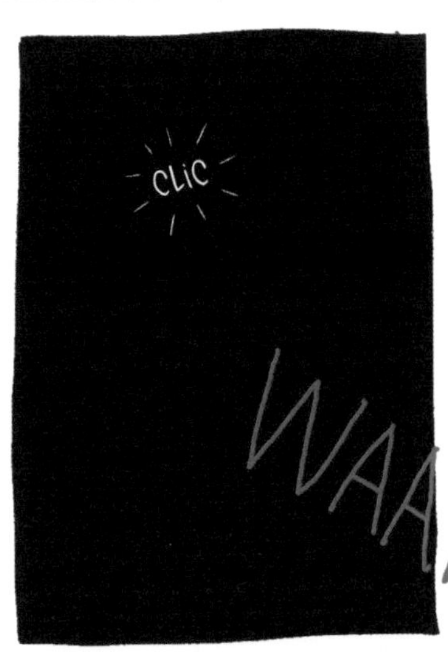
CLIC

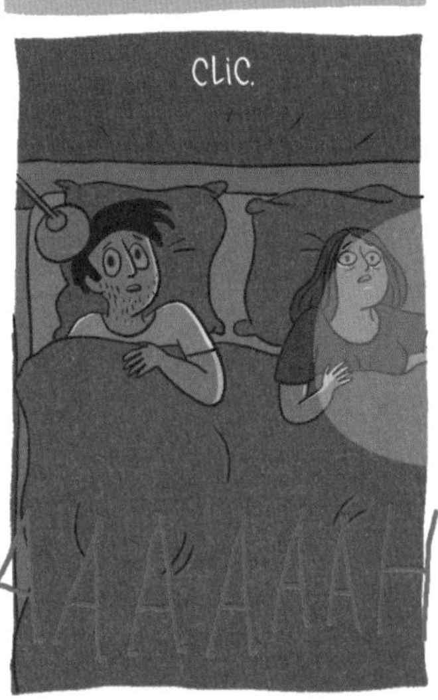
CLIC.
WAAAAAAAAH

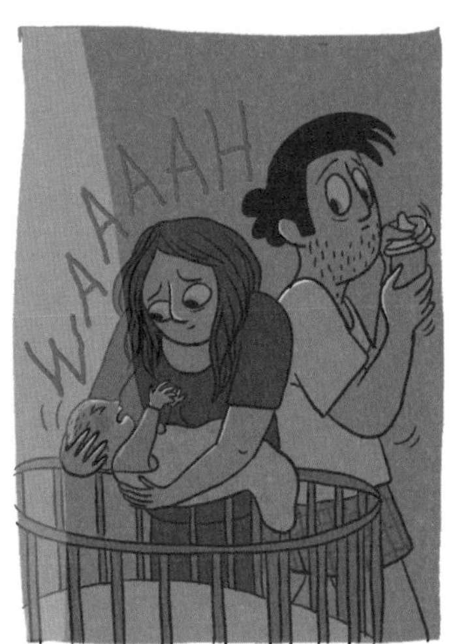
WAAAAH

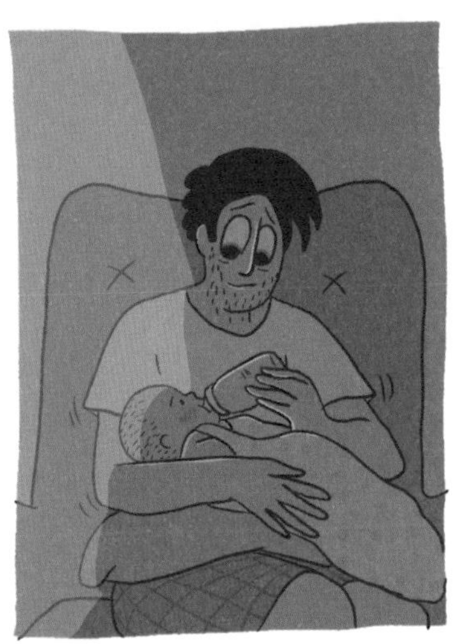

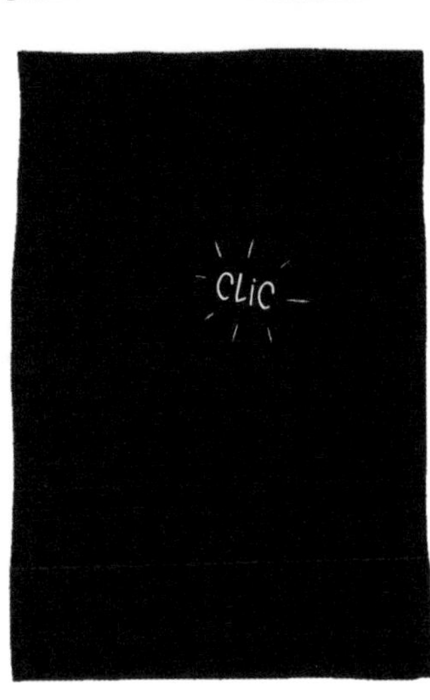
CLIC

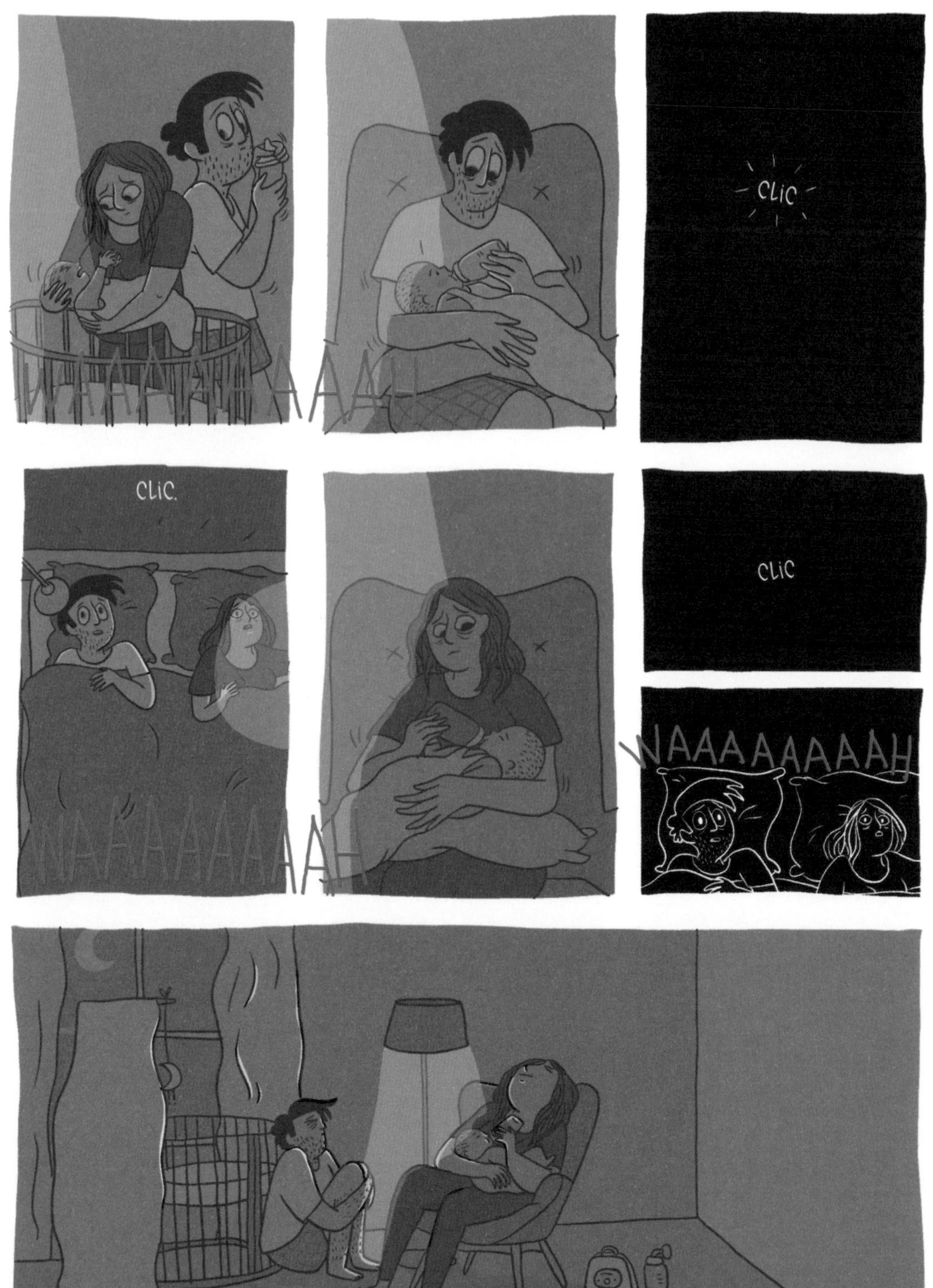

WAAAAAAAAAH
CLIC
CLIC.
WAAAAAAAAAH
CLIC
WAAAAAAAAH
THIS MUST BE WHAT HELL IS LIKE.

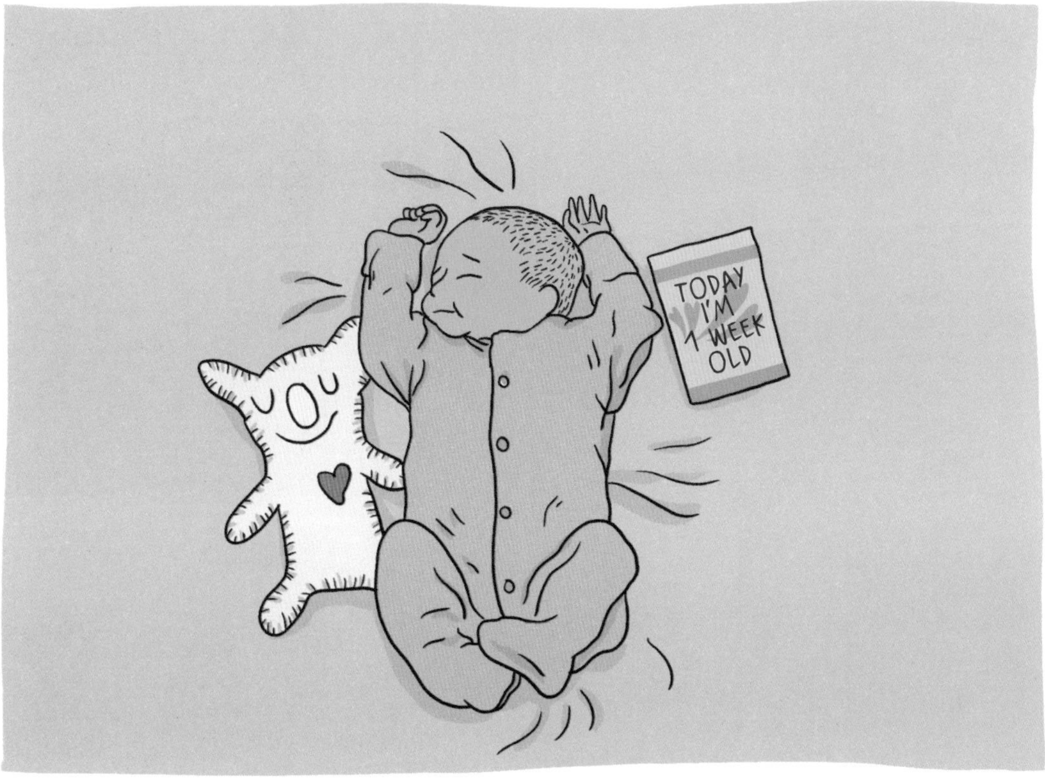

I MISS BEING PREGNANT.

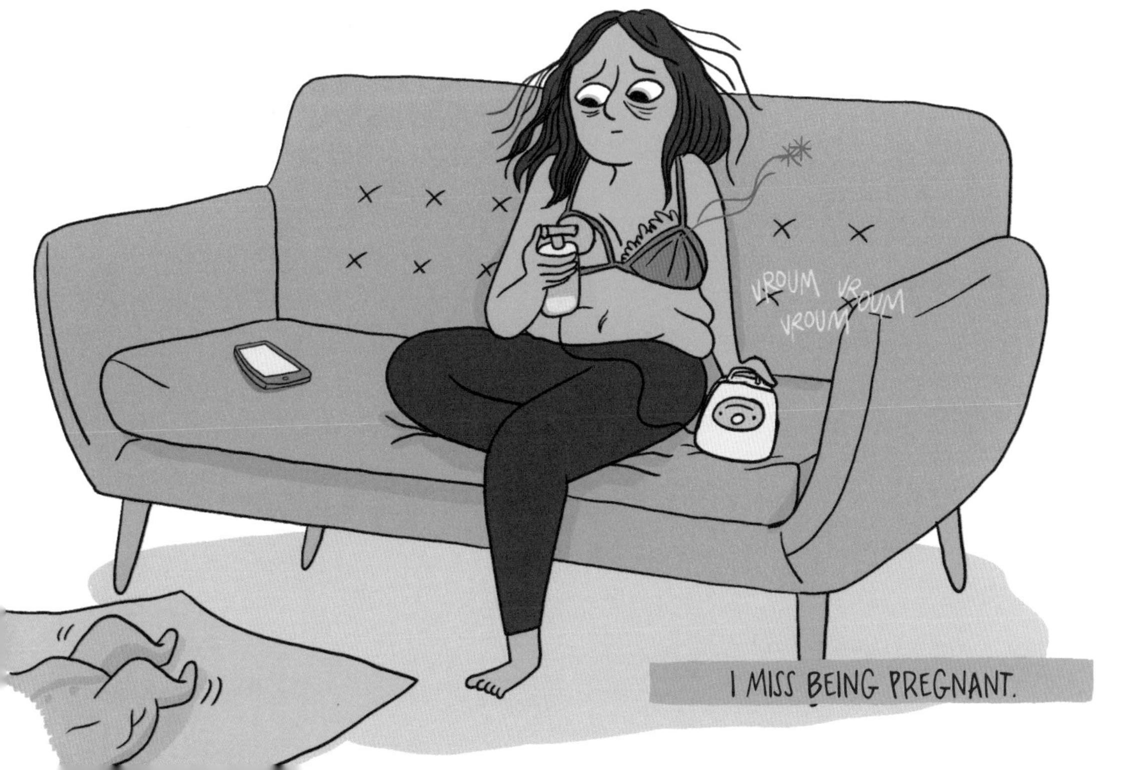

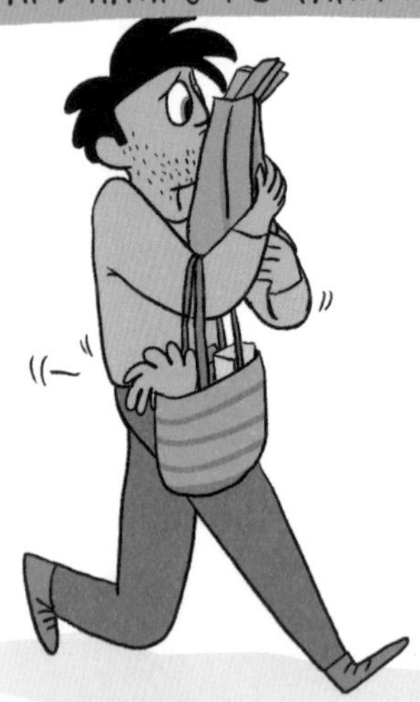
AND HAVING NO PARENTAL RESPONSIBILITIES.

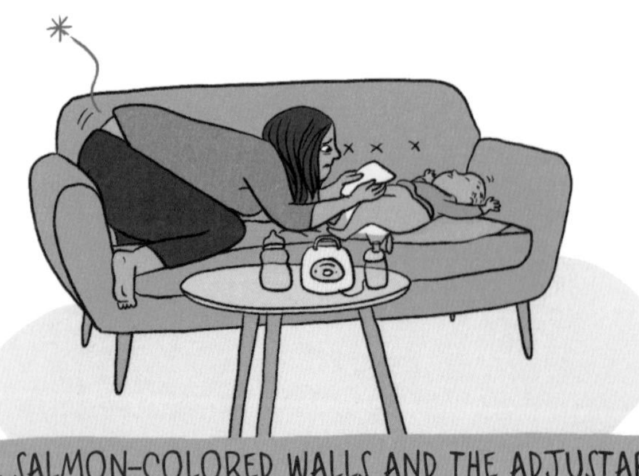
I MISS THE SALMON-COLORED WALLS AND THE ADJUSTABLE BED, THE YELLOW SHEETS AND THE SEE-THROUGH BASSINET.

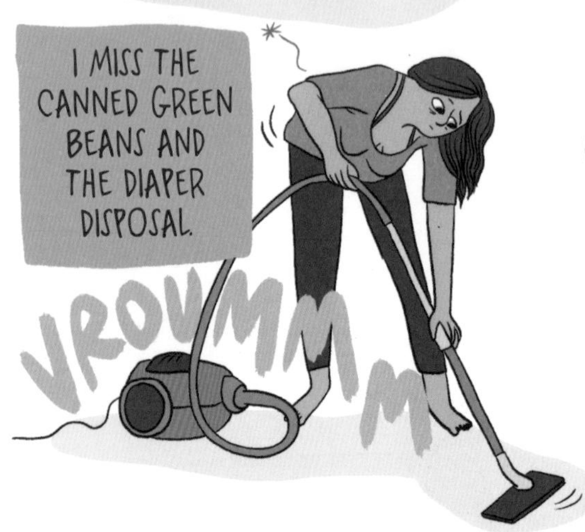
I MISS THE CANNED GREEN BEANS AND THE DIAPER DISPOSAL.
VROUMMMM

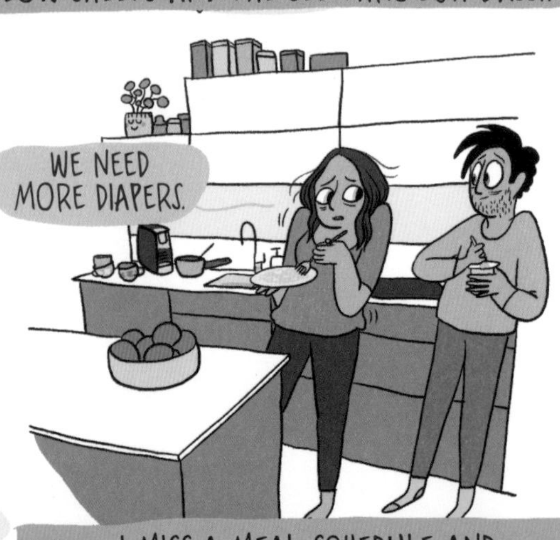
WE NEED MORE DIAPERS.
I MISS A MEAL SCHEDULE AND A HOUSECLEANING STAFF.

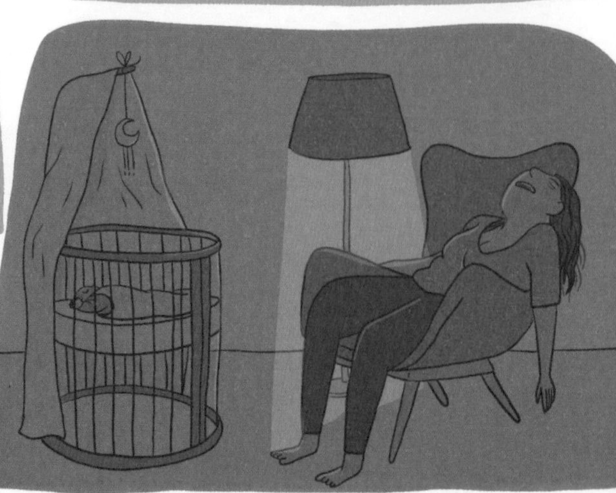
I MISS USING A REMOTE TO TURN OFF THE LIGHTS. I MISS THE BELL I CAN RING AT ALL HOURS.

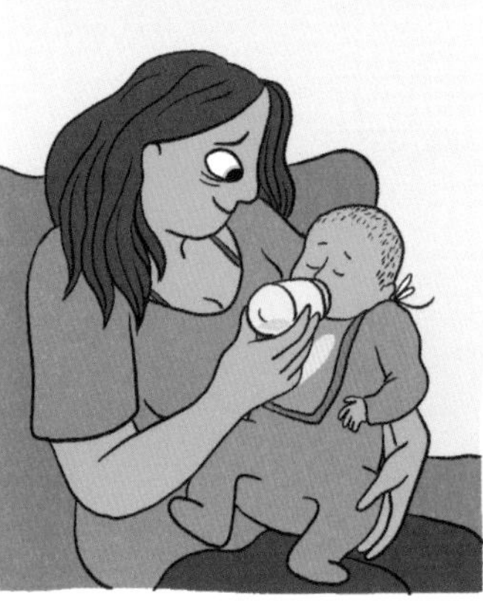
SOMETIMES, IT'S NEAT.

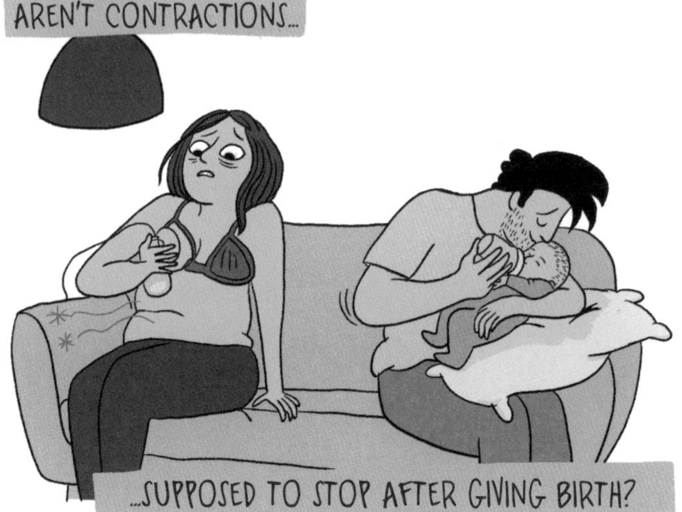
AREN'T CONTRACTIONS...
...SUPPOSED TO STOP AFTER GIVING BIRTH?

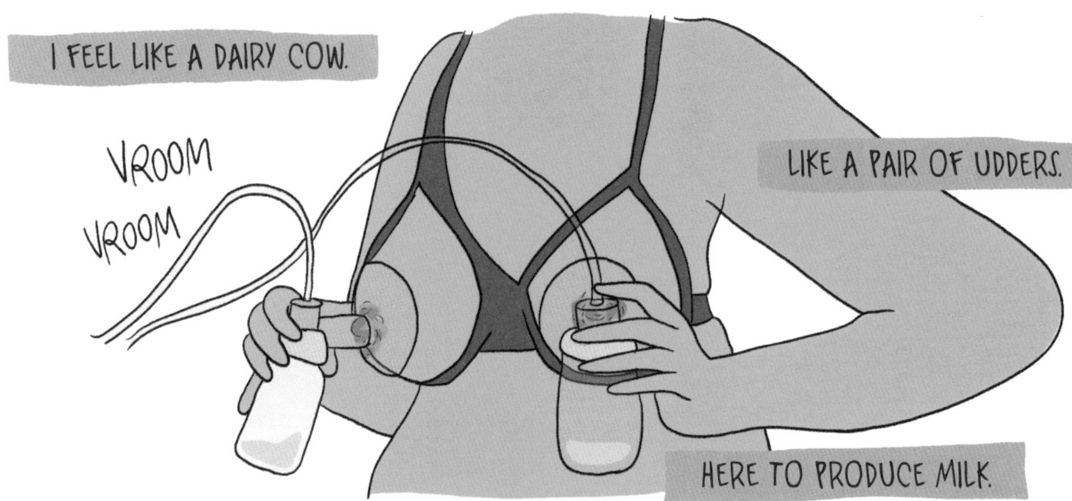
I FEEL LIKE A DAIRY COW.
VROOM
VROOM
LIKE A PAIR OF UDDERS.
HERE TO PRODUCE MILK.

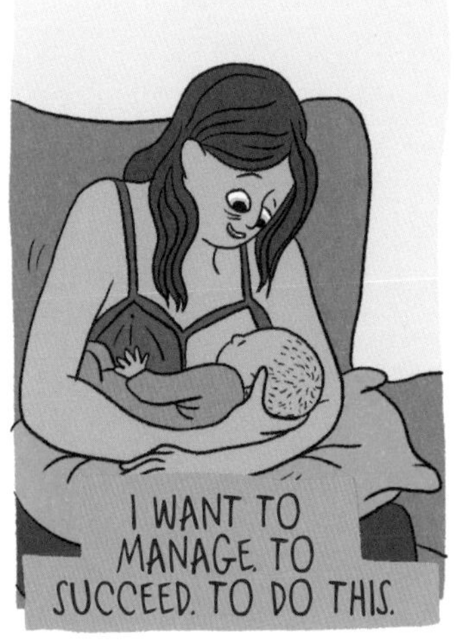
I WANT TO MANAGE. TO SUCCEED. TO DO THIS.

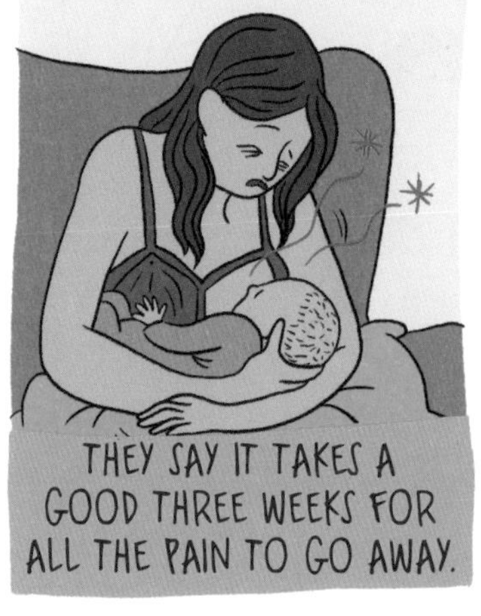
THEY SAY IT TAKES A GOOD THREE WEEKS FOR ALL THE PAIN TO GO AWAY.

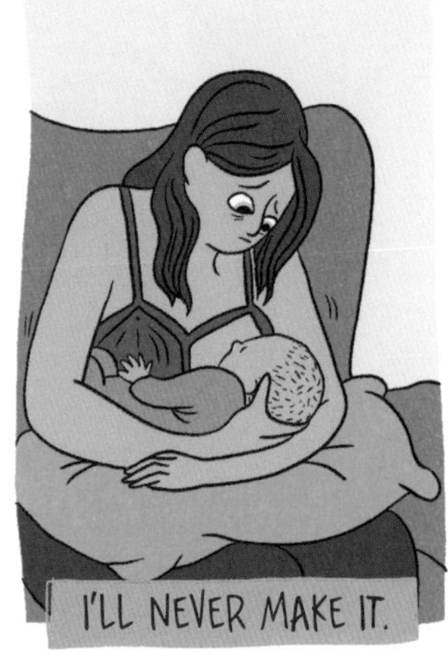
I'LL NEVER MAKE IT.

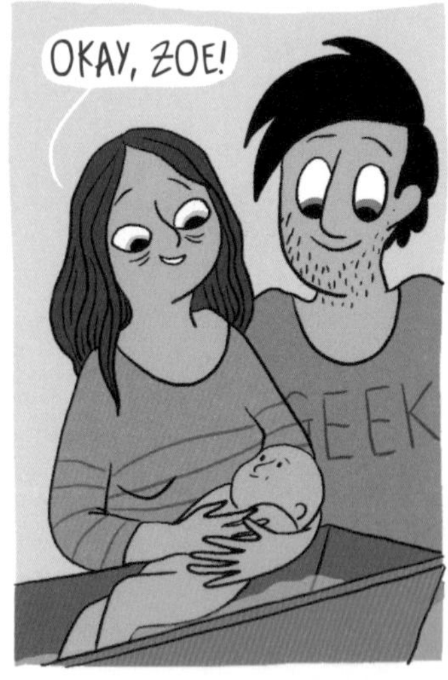

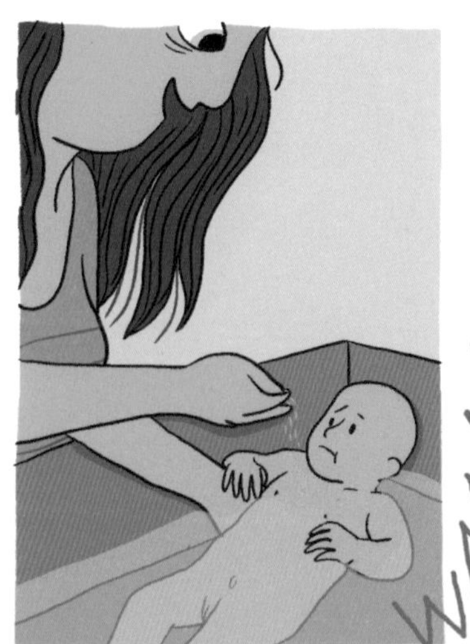

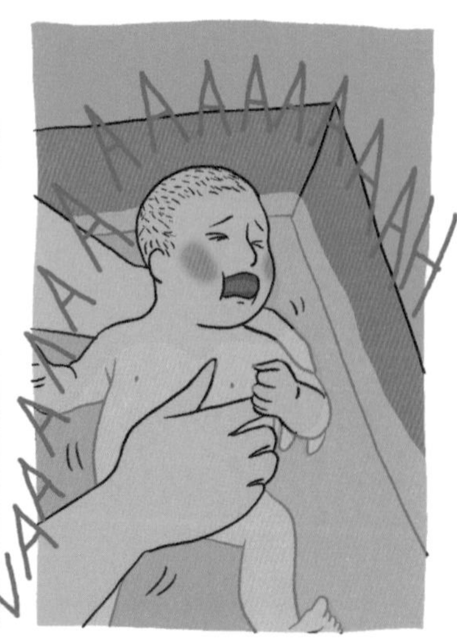

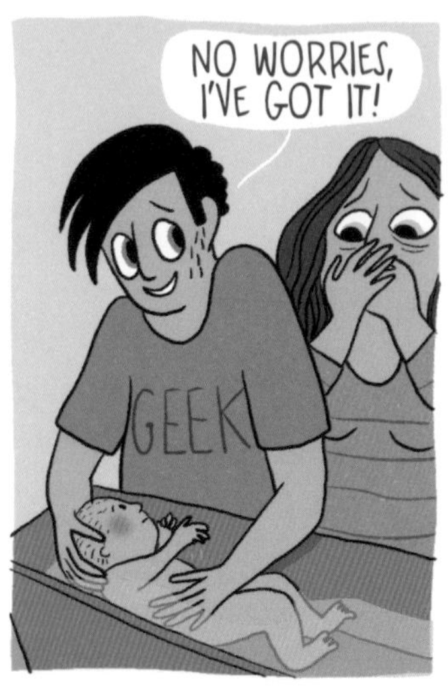

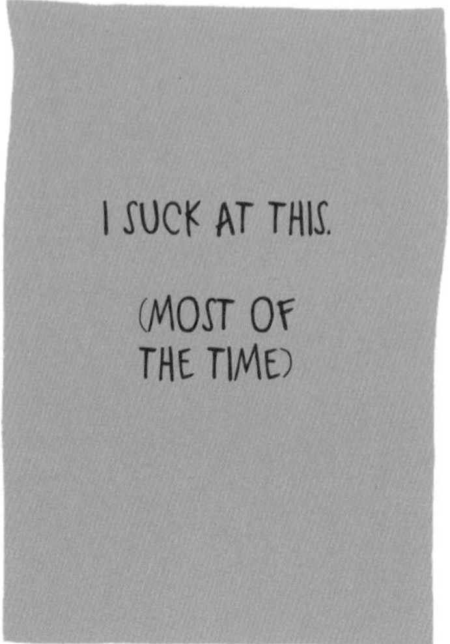

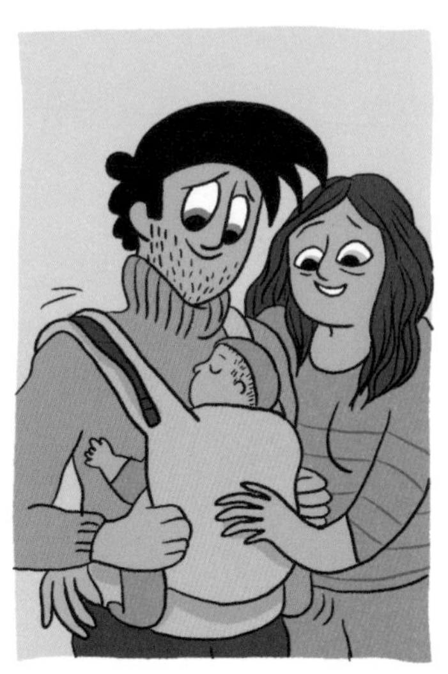

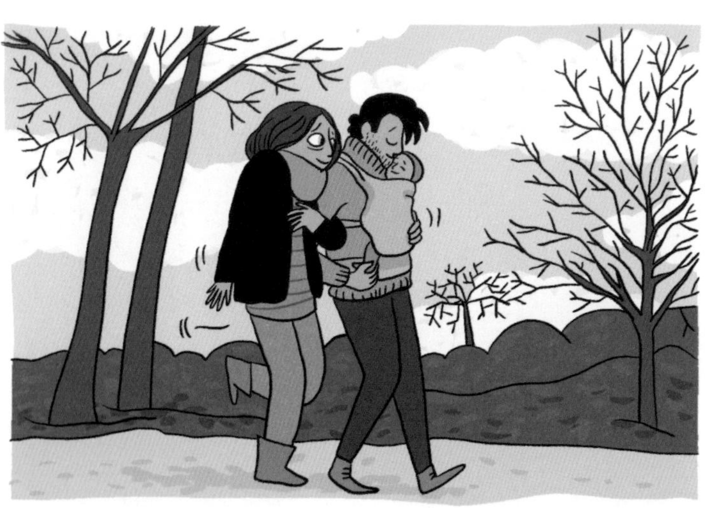

I FEEL GOOD.

(FOR TWO MINUTES)

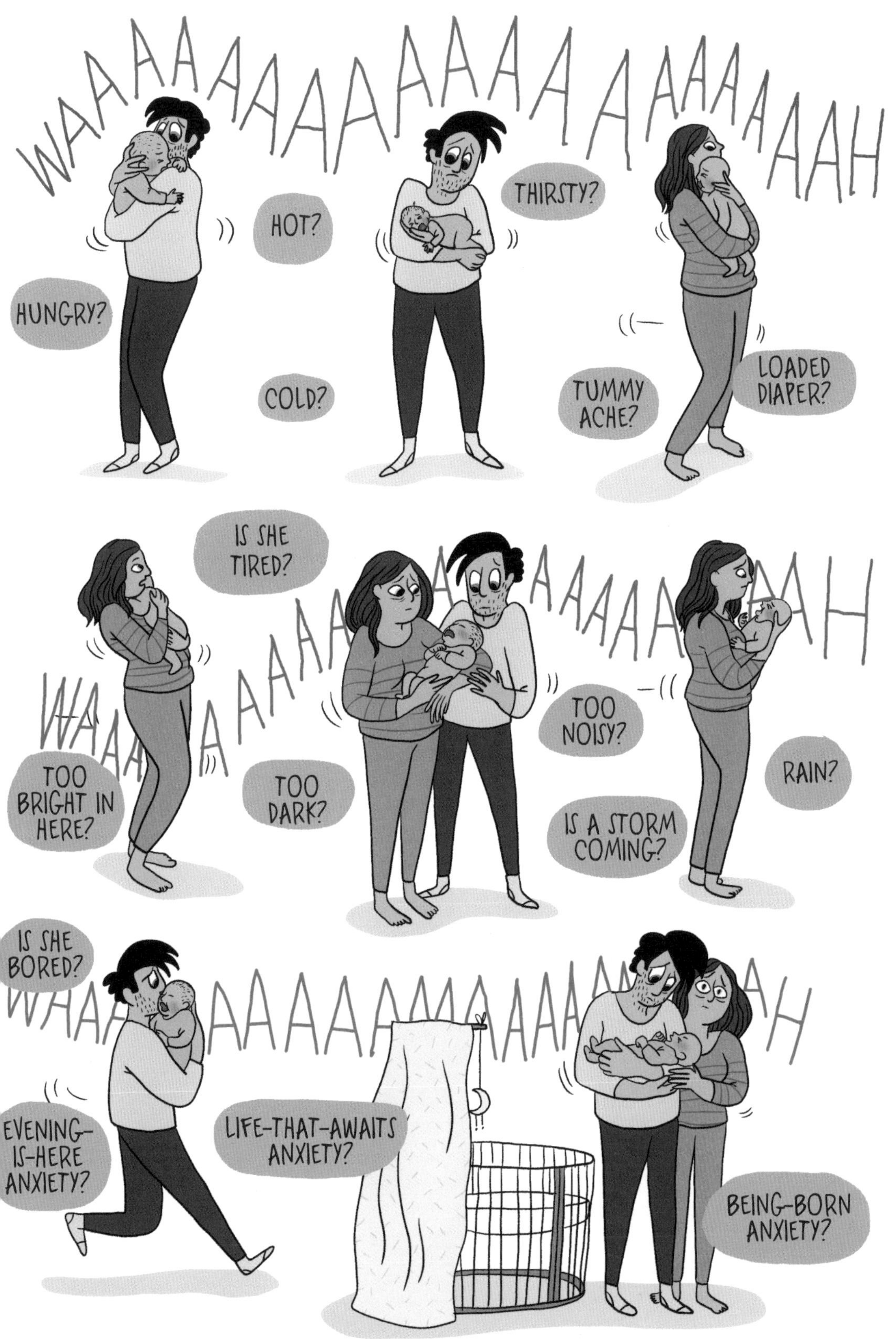
WAAAAAAAAAAAAAAAAAAAAAH
HOT?
THIRSTY?
HUNGRY?
COLD?
TUMMY ACHE?
LOADED DIAPER?
IS SHE TIRED?
WAAAAAAAAAAAAAAAAAH
TOO BRIGHT IN HERE?
TOO DARK?
TOO NOISY?
IS A STORM COMING?
RAIN?
IS SHE BORED?
WAAAAAAAAAAAAAAAAAH
EVENING-IS-HERE ANXIETY?
LIFE-THAT-AWAITS ANXIETY?
BEING-BORN ANXIETY?

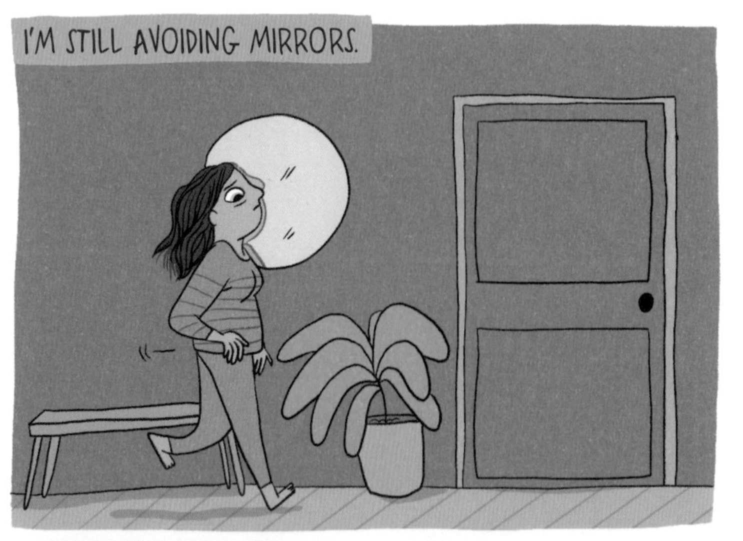

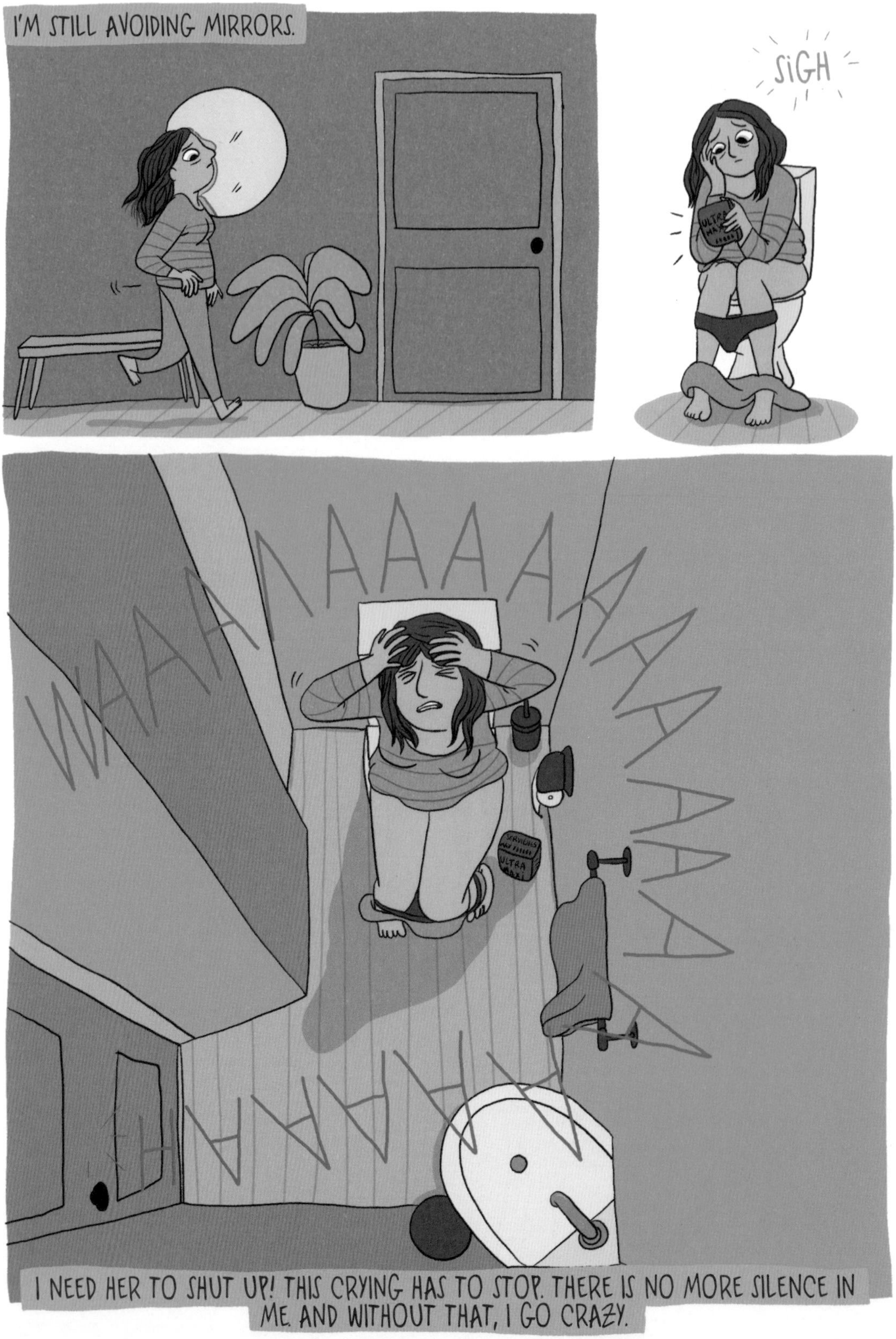

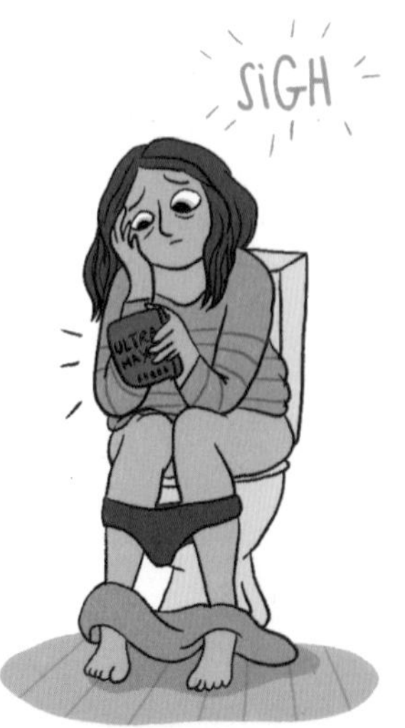

I NEED HER TO SHUT UP! THIS CRYING HAS TO STOP. THERE IS NO MORE SILENCE IN ME. AND WITHOUT THAT, I GO CRAZY.

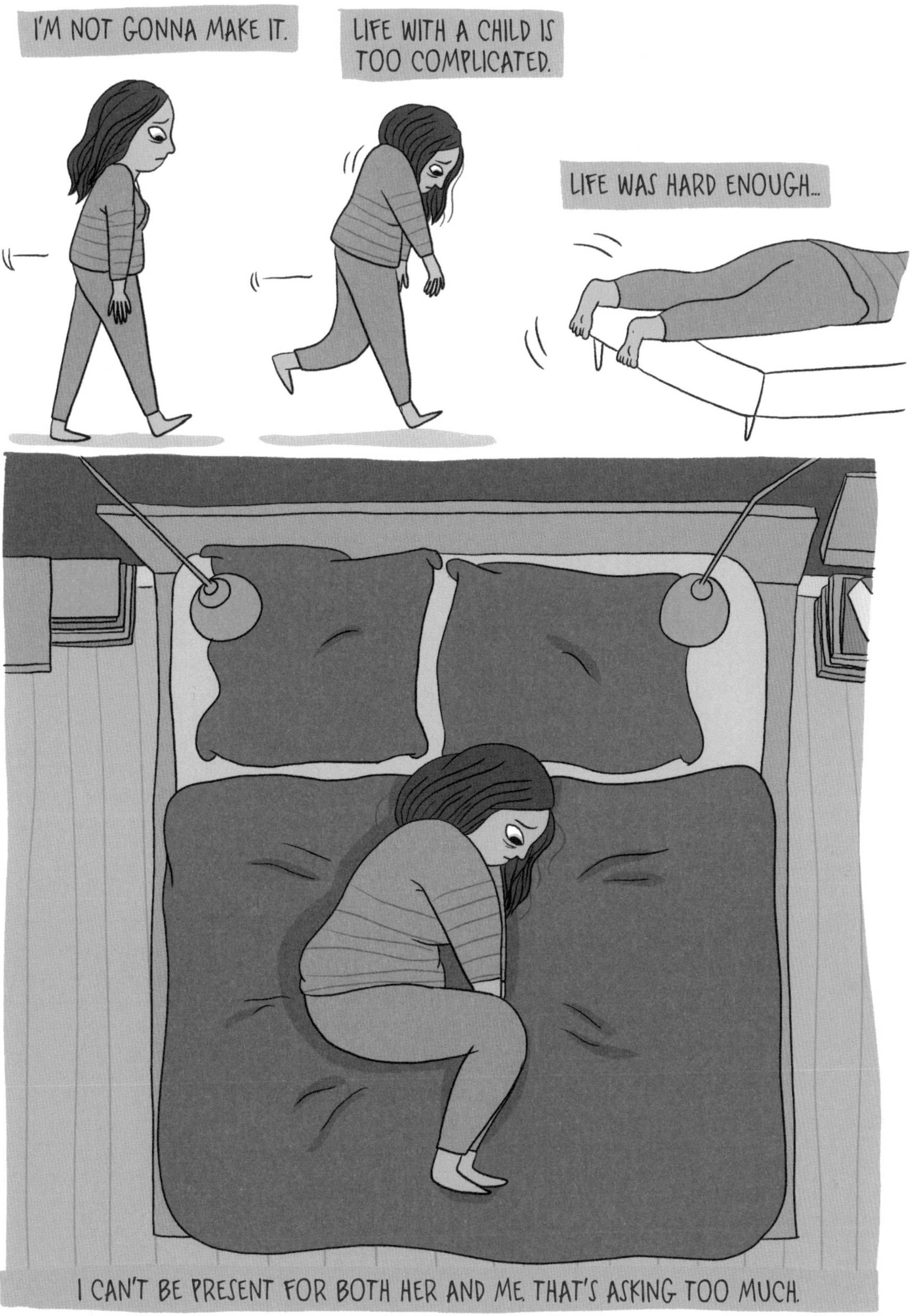

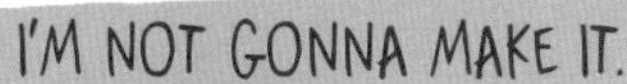

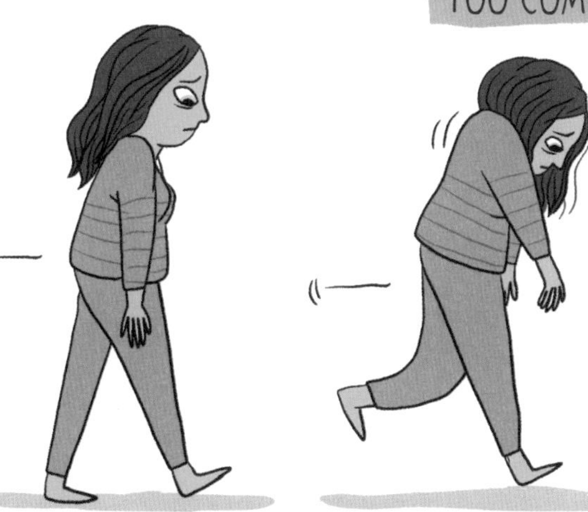

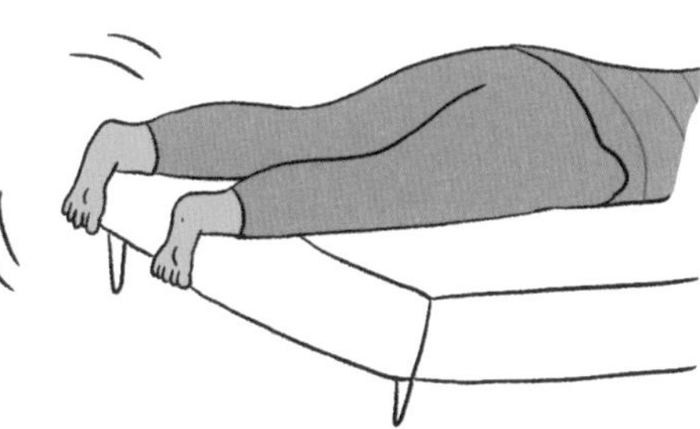

I CAN'T BE PRESENT FOR BOTH HER AND ME. THAT'S ASKING TOO MUCH.

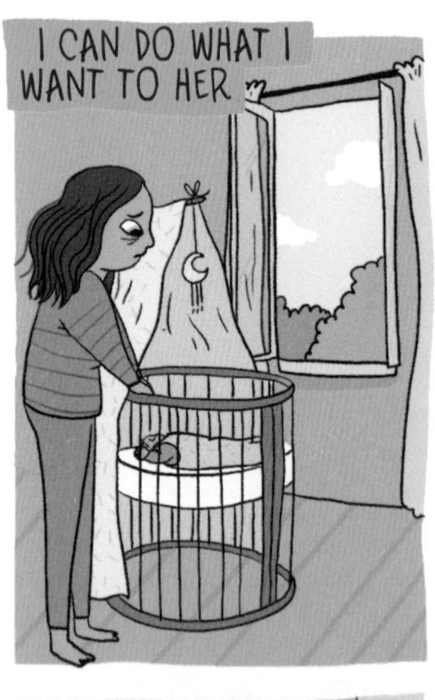
I CAN DO WHAT I WANT TO HER.
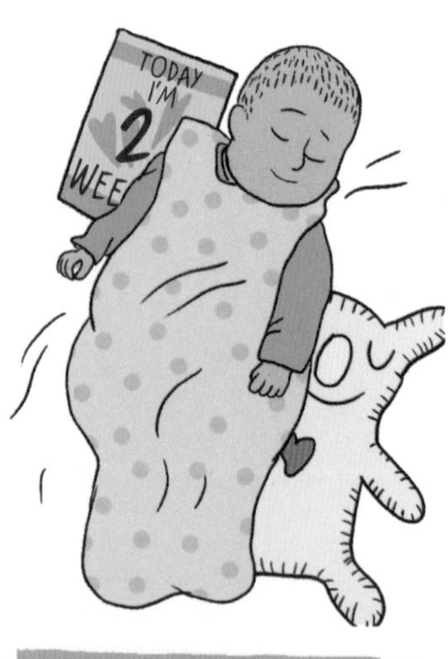
TODAY I'M 2 WEE
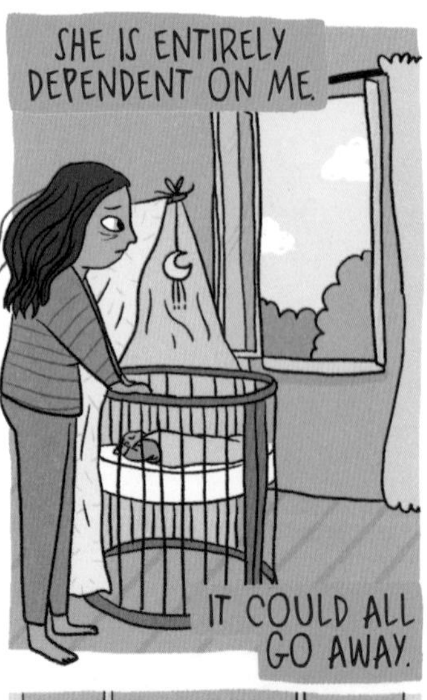
SHE IS ENTIRELY DEPENDENT ON ME.
IT COULD ALL GO AWAY.
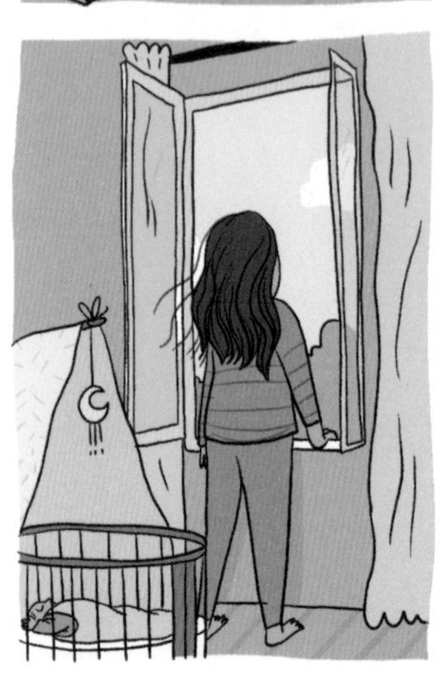
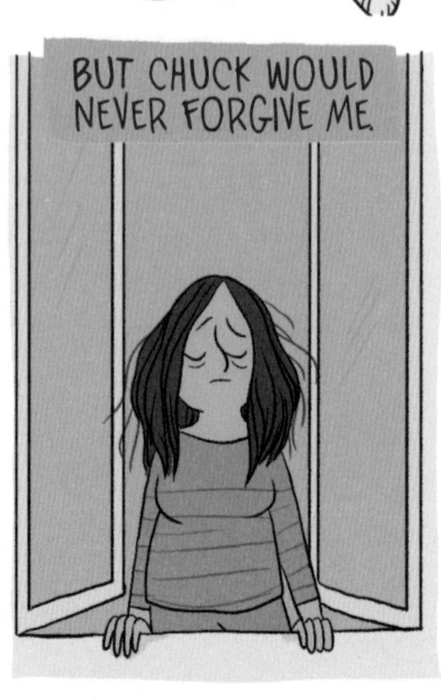
BUT CHUCK WOULD NEVER FORGIVE ME.
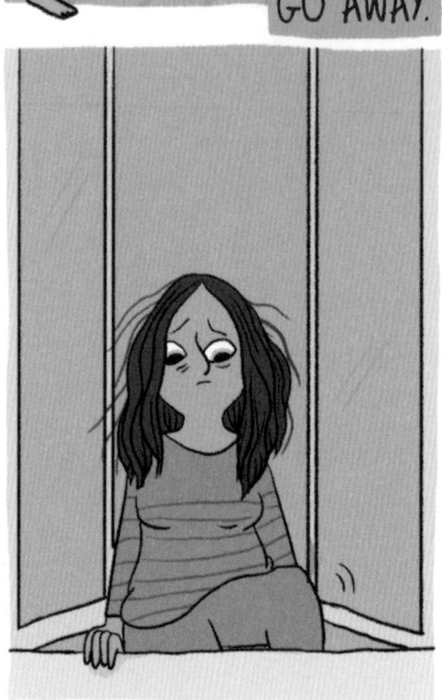
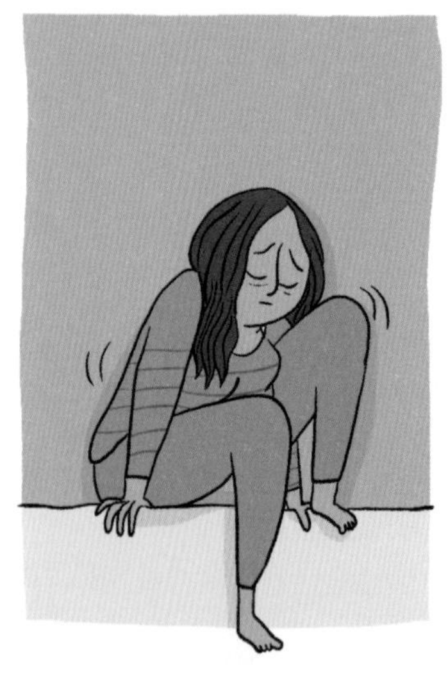
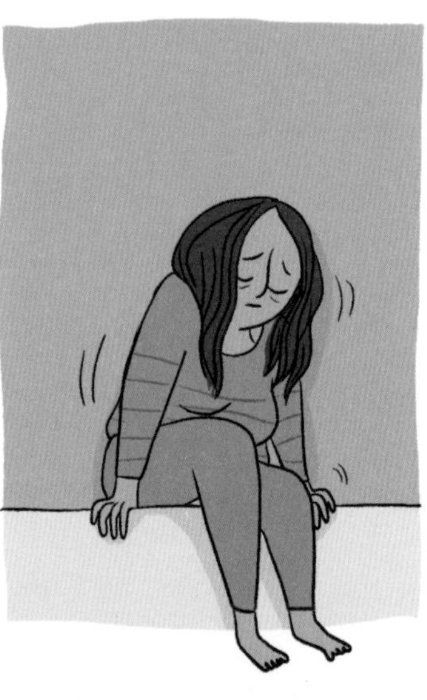
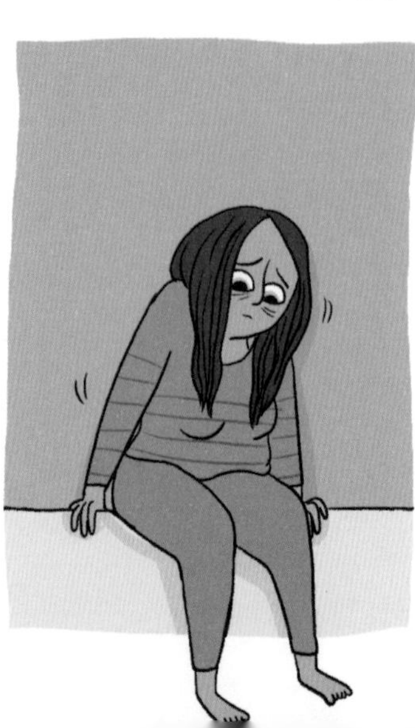

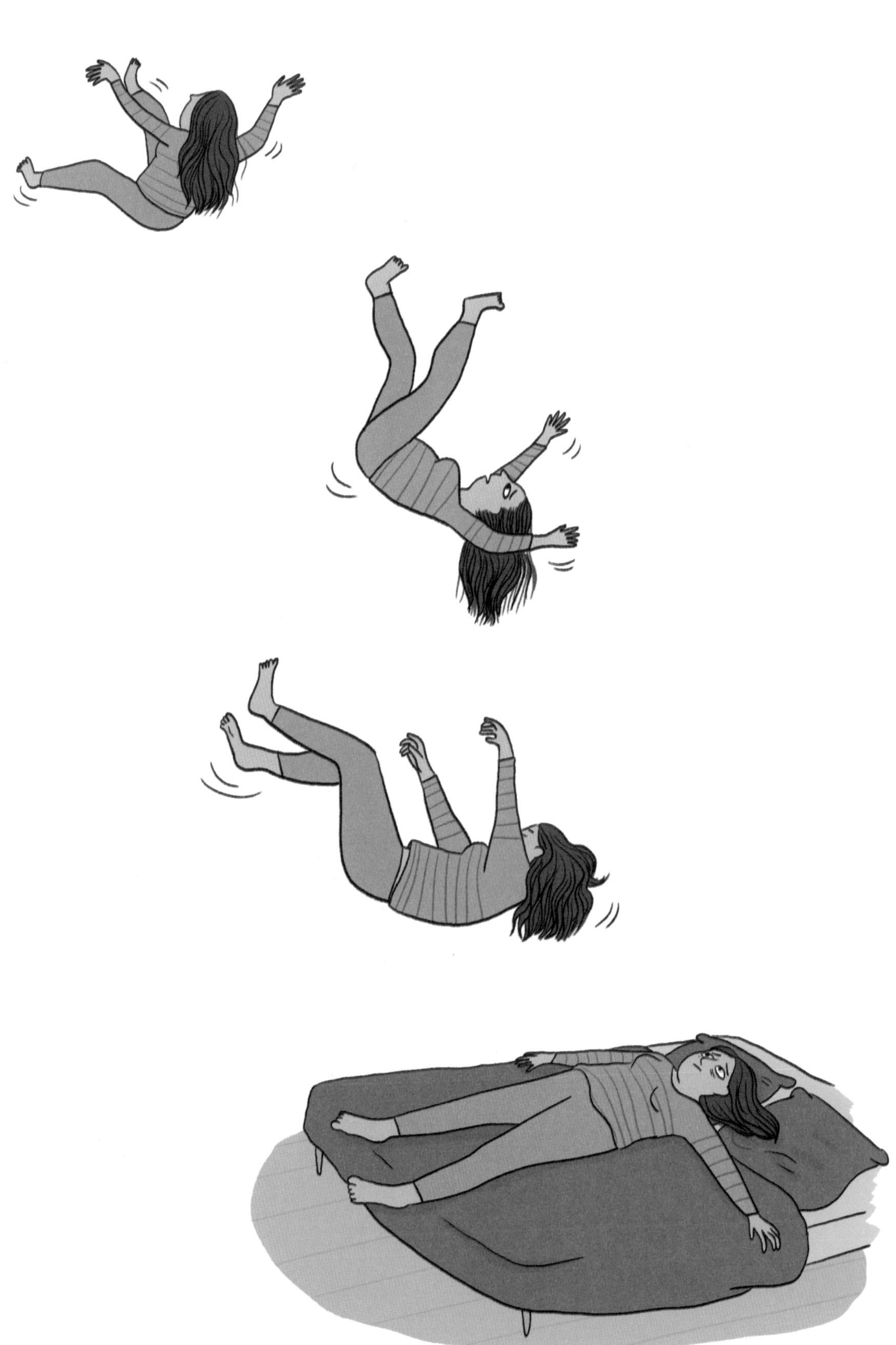

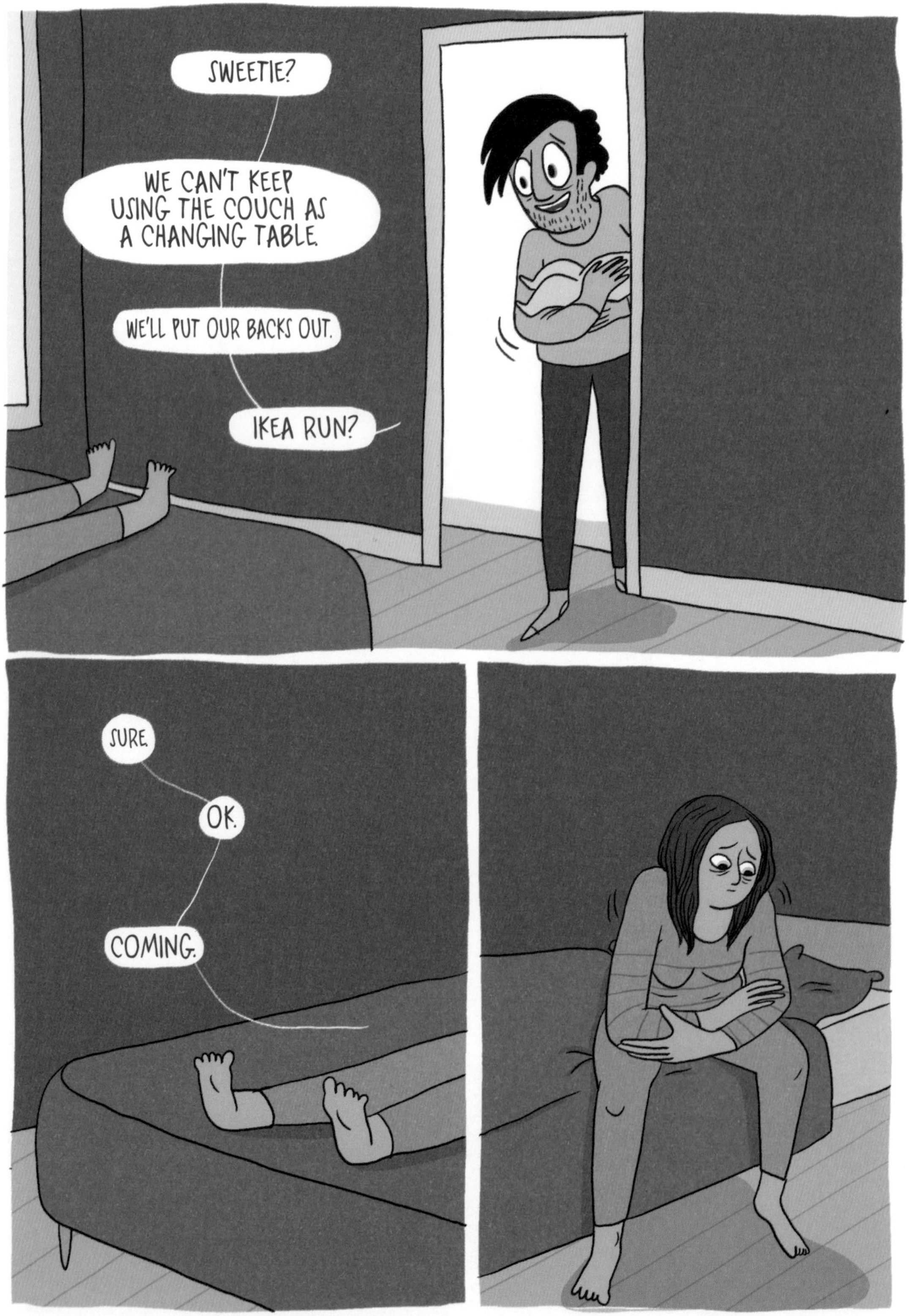

SWEETIE?
WE CAN'T KEEP USING THE COUCH AS A CHANGING TABLE.
WE'LL PUT OUR BACKS OUT.
IKEA RUN?

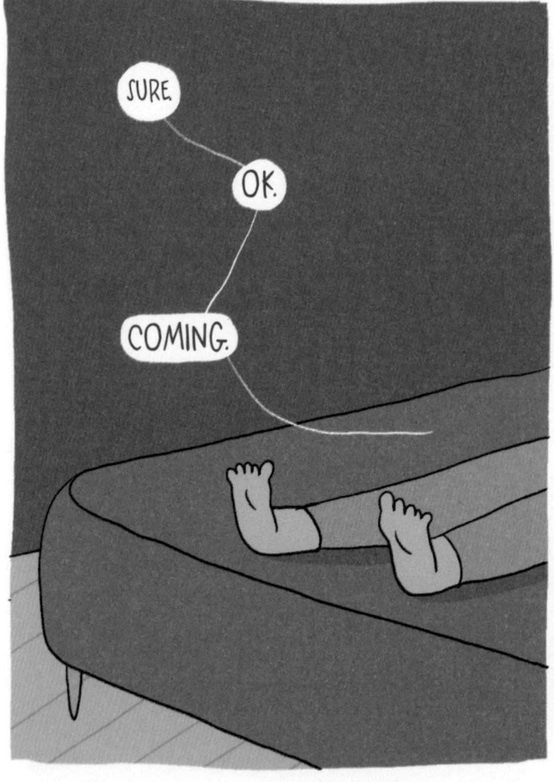
SURE.
OK.
COMING.

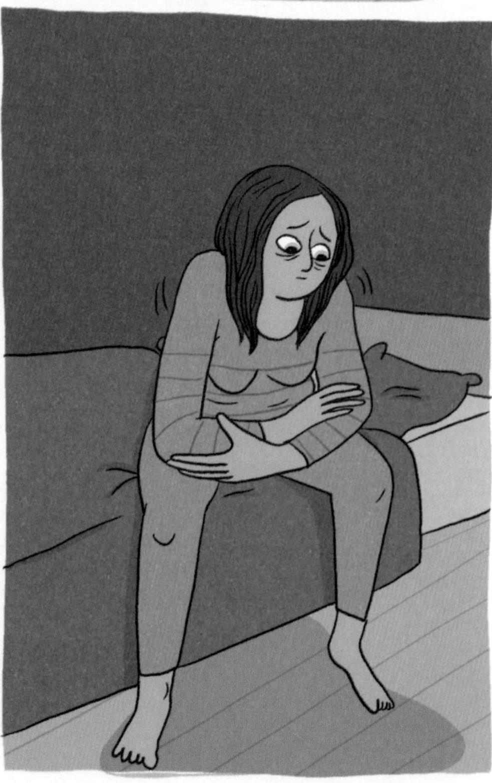

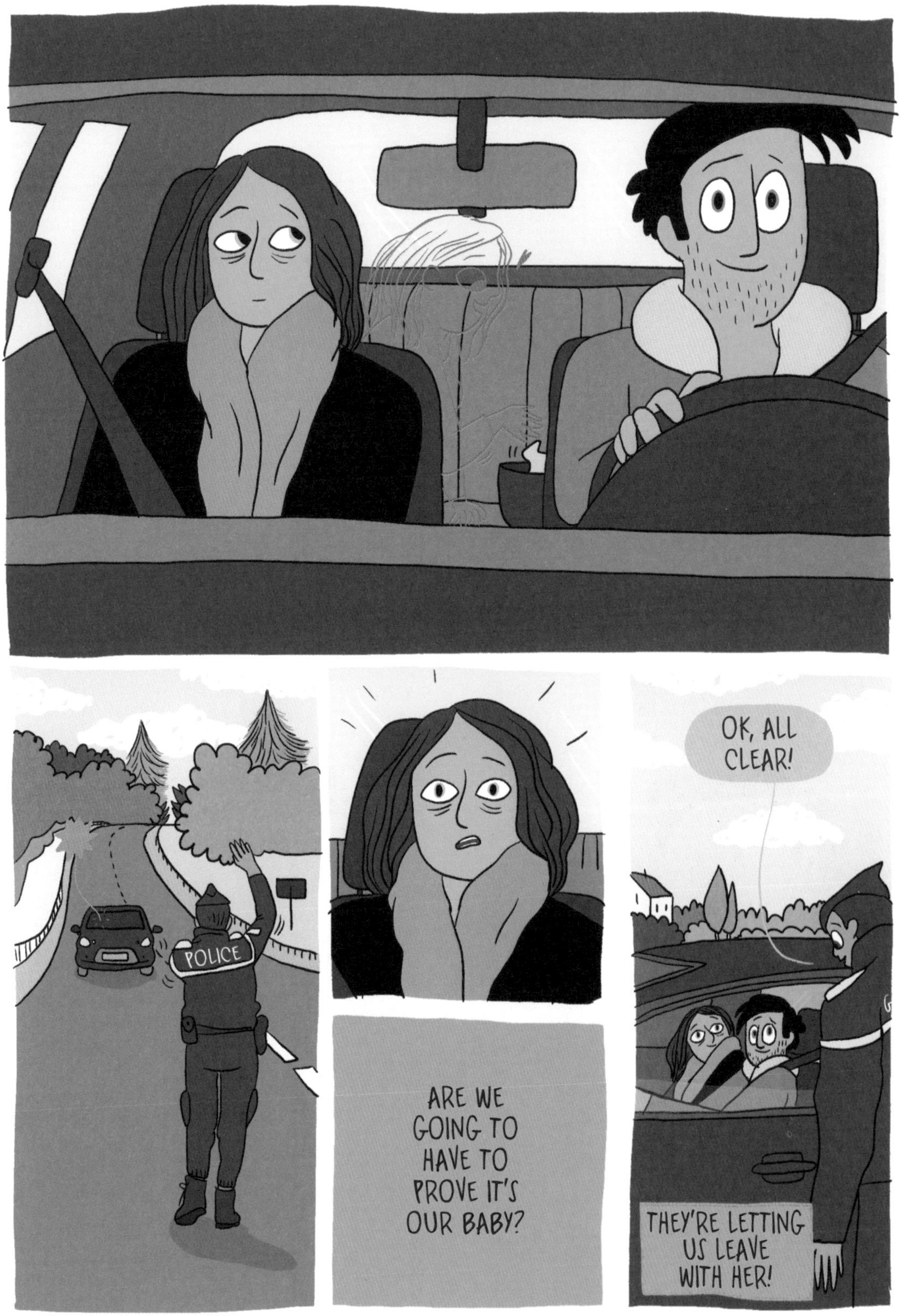

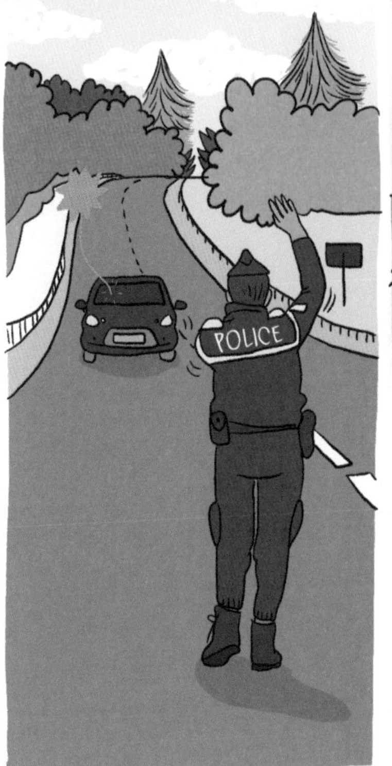
POLICE

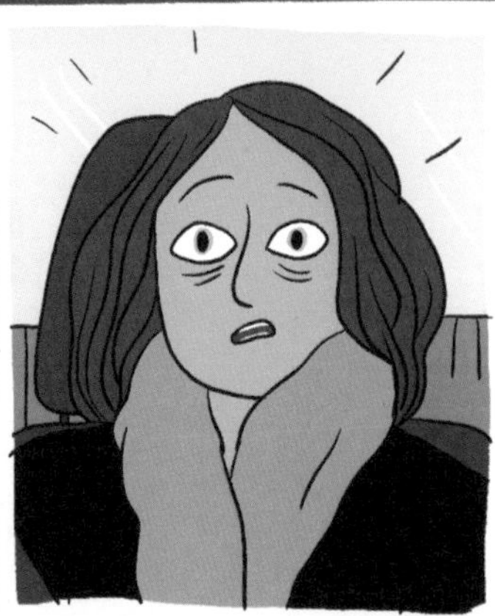

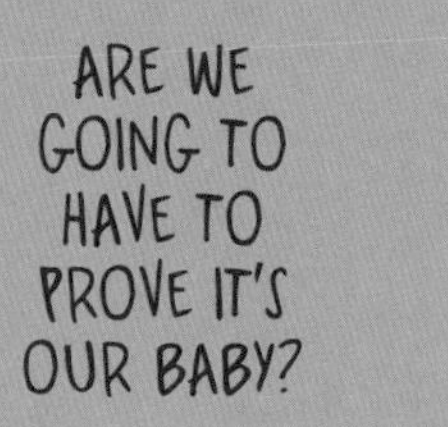
ARE WE GOING TO HAVE TO PROVE IT'S OUR BABY?

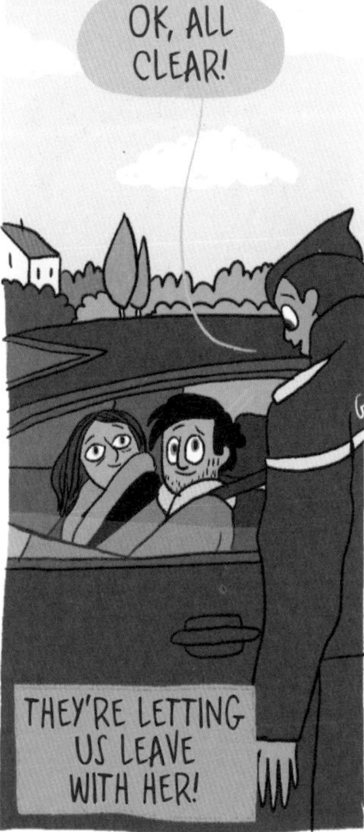
OK, ALL CLEAR!
THEY'RE LETTING US LEAVE WITH HER!

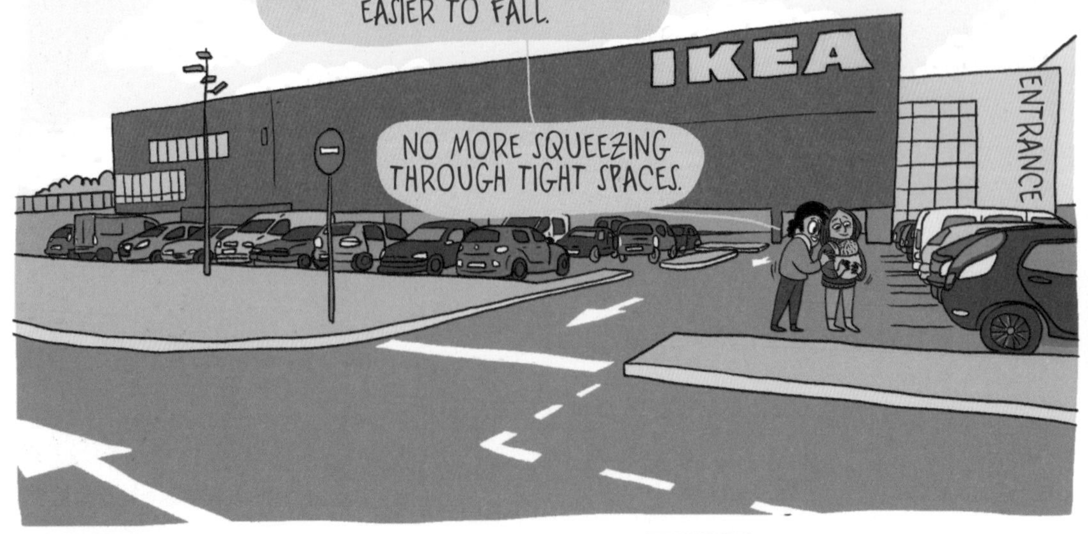
CAREFUL! WITH A BABY-CARRIER, YOU WON'T SEE YOUR FEET OR WHERE YOU'RE GOING.
YOUR CENTER OF GRAVITY IS PUSHED FORWARD, MAKING IT EASIER TO FALL.
IKEA
ENTRANCE
NO MORE SQUEEZING THROUGH TIGHT SPACES.

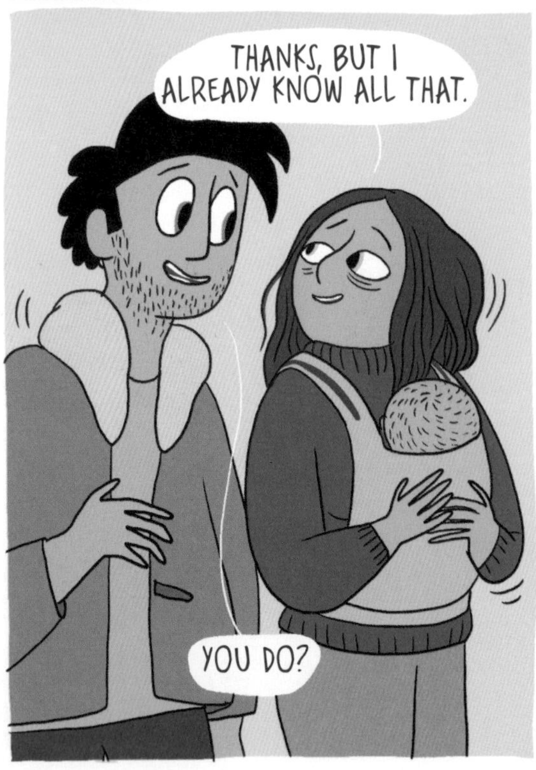
THANKS, BUT I ALREADY KNOW ALL THAT.
YOU DO?

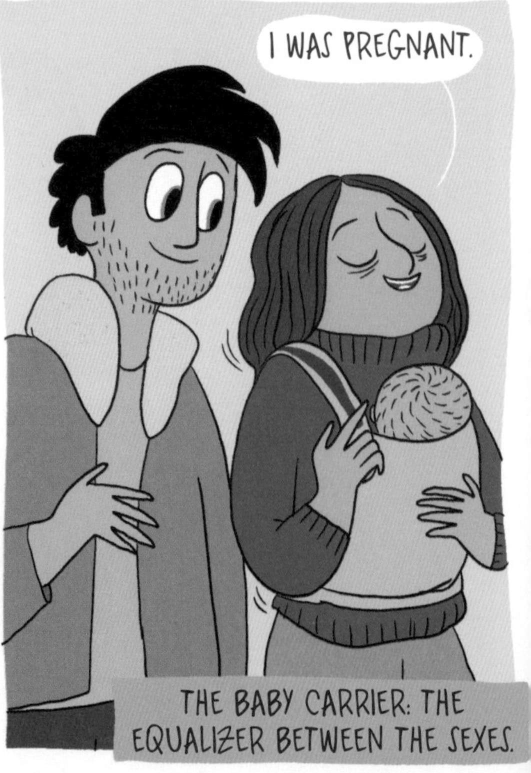
I WAS PREGNANT.
THE BABY CARRIER: THE EQUALIZER BETWEEN THE SEXES.

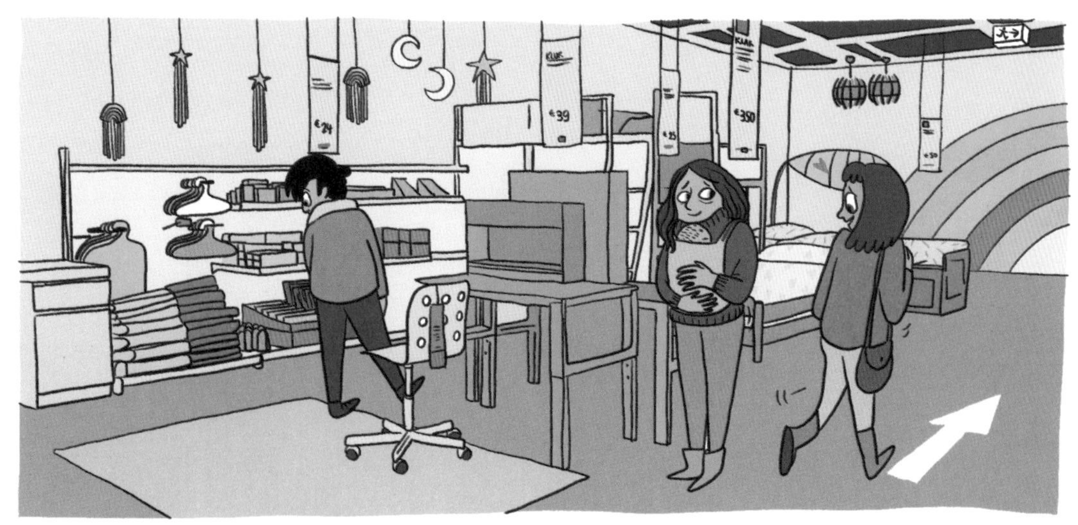
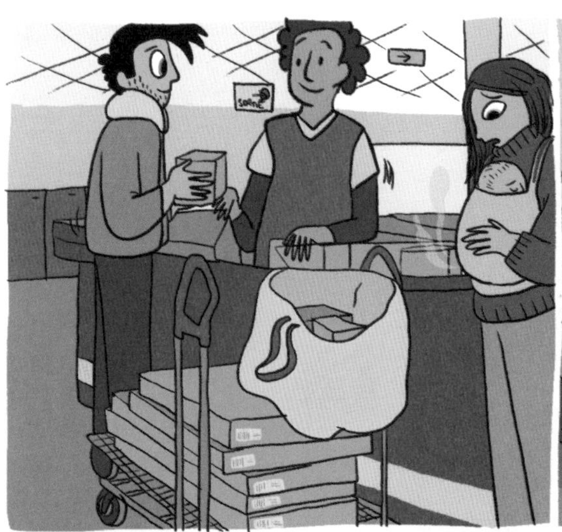
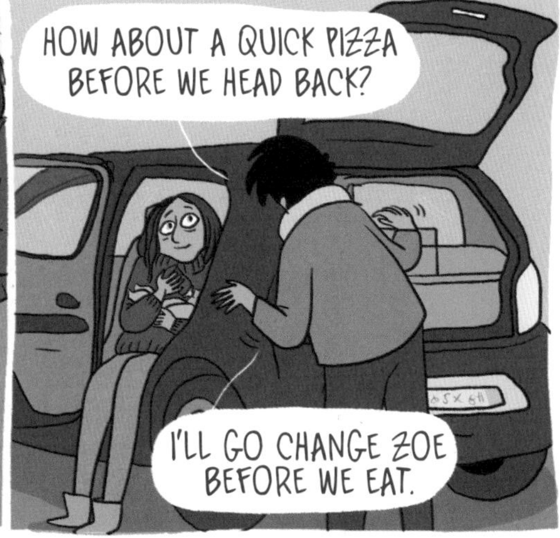
HOW ABOUT A QUICK PIZZA BEFORE WE HEAD BACK?
I'LL GO CHANGE ZOE BEFORE WE EAT.
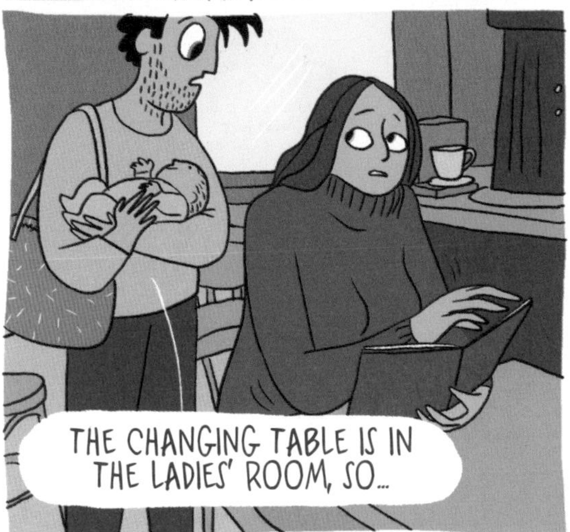
THE CHANGING TABLE IS IN THE LADIES' ROOM, SO...
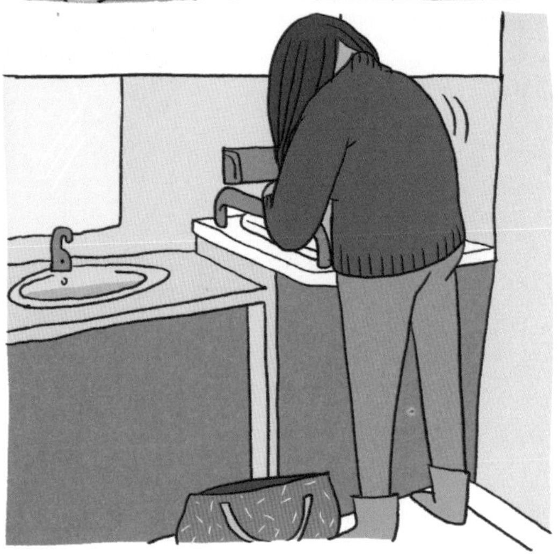

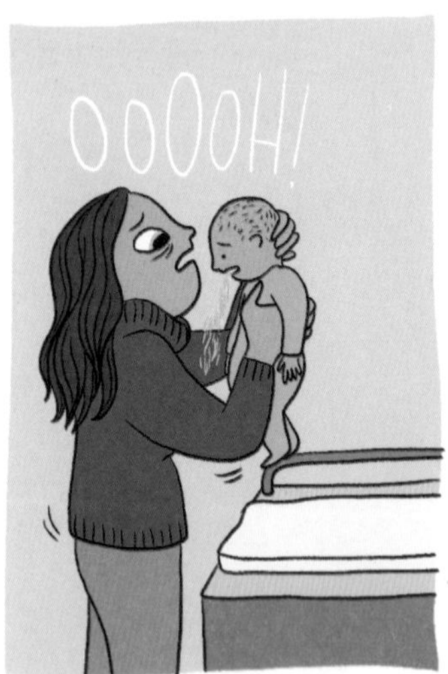
OOOOH!

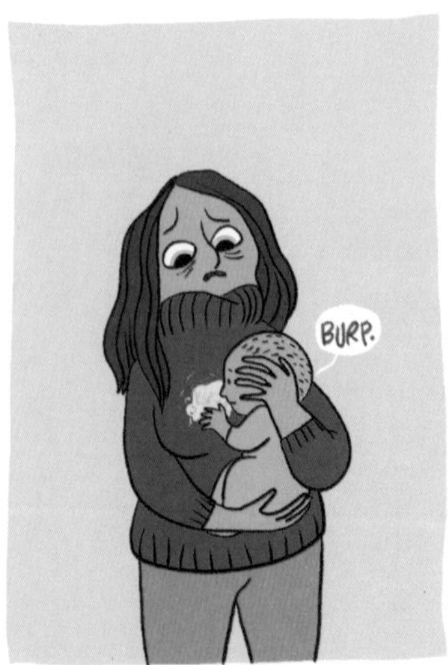
BURP.

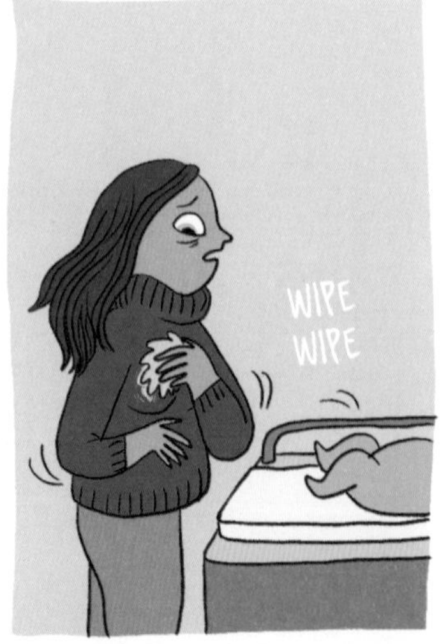
WIPE
WIPE

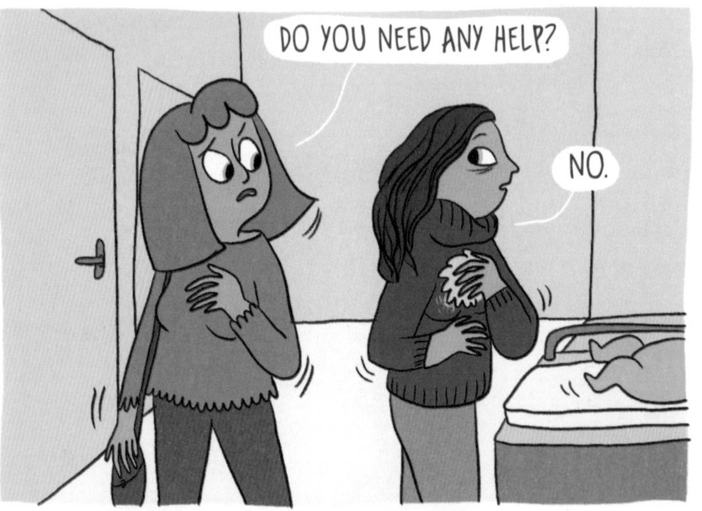
DO YOU NEED ANY HELP?
NO.

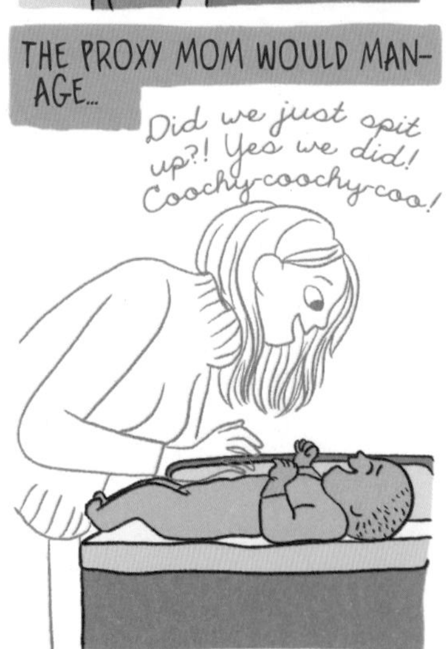
THE PROXY MOM WOULD MAN-
AGE...
Did we just spit up?! Yes we did! Coochy-coochy-coo!

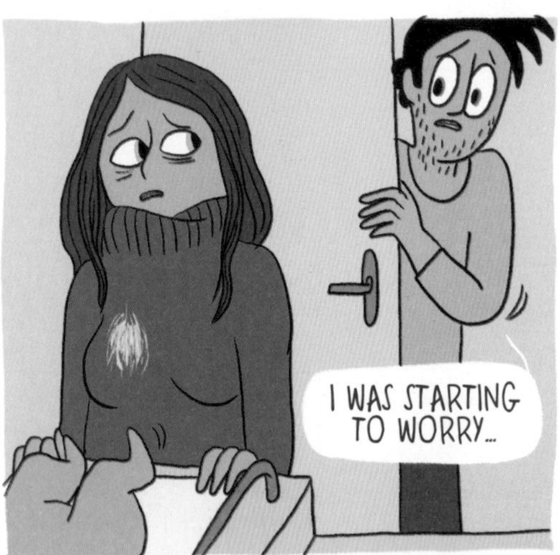
I WAS STARTING TO WORRY...

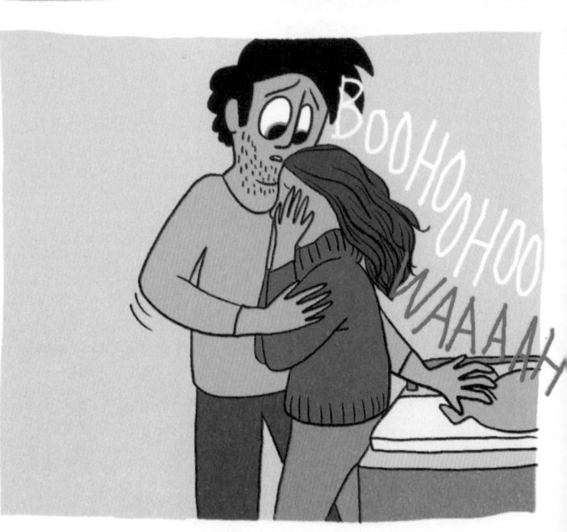
BOOHOOHOOHOO
WAAAAH

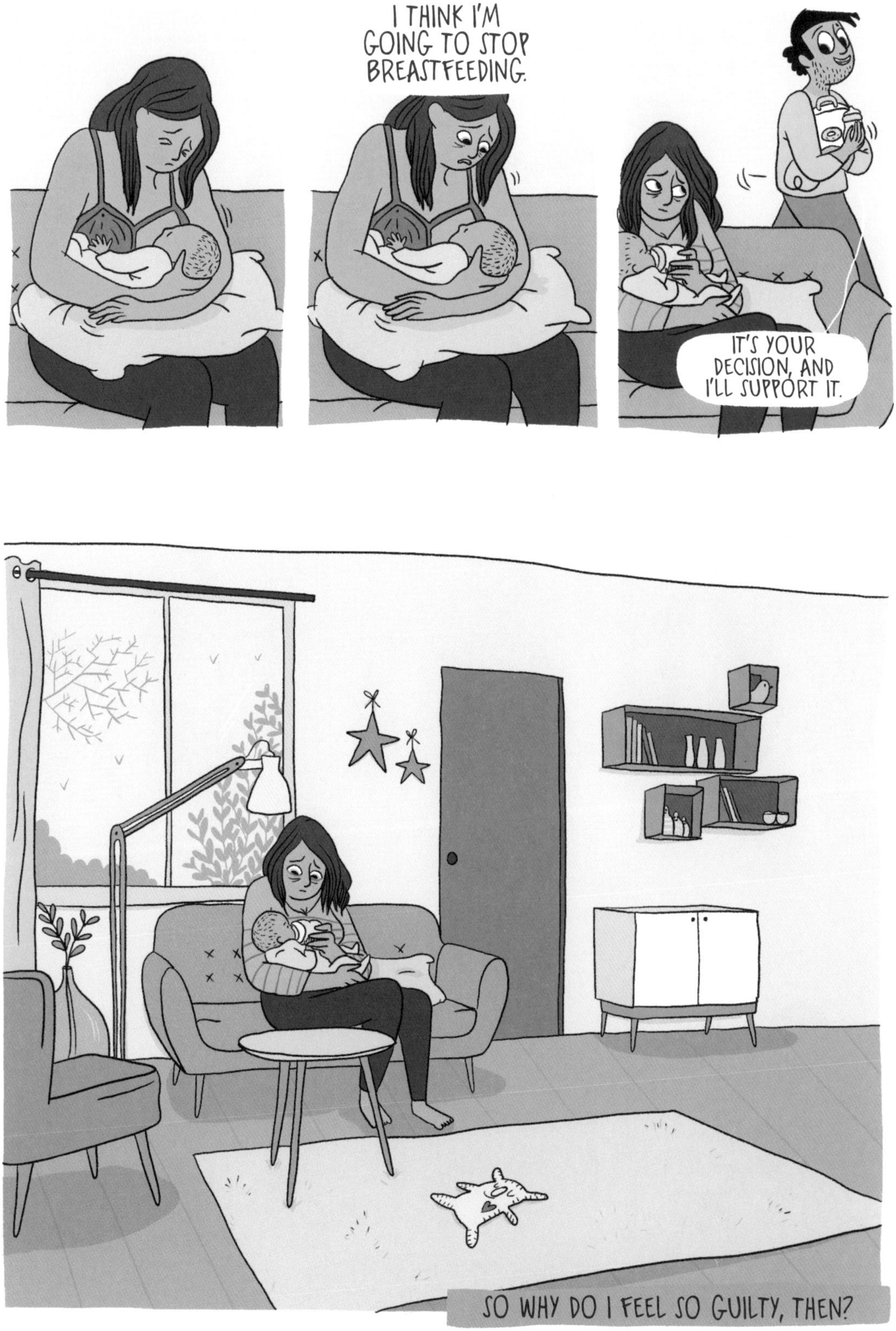

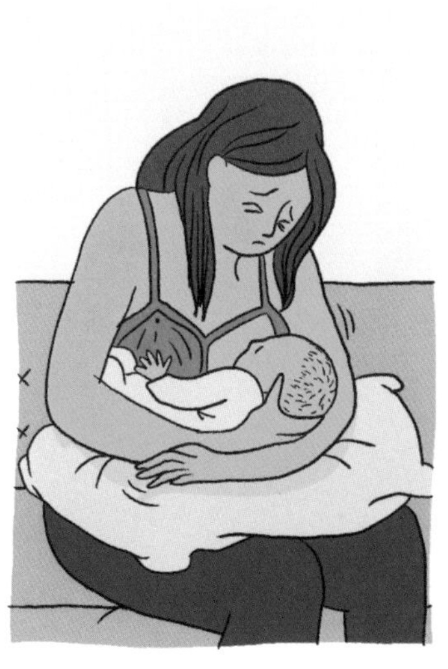

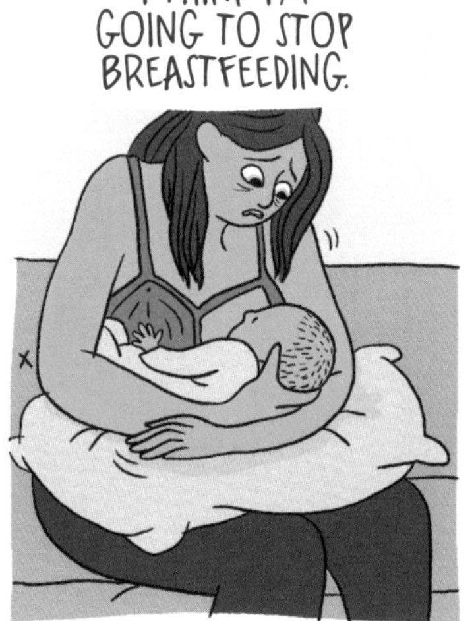

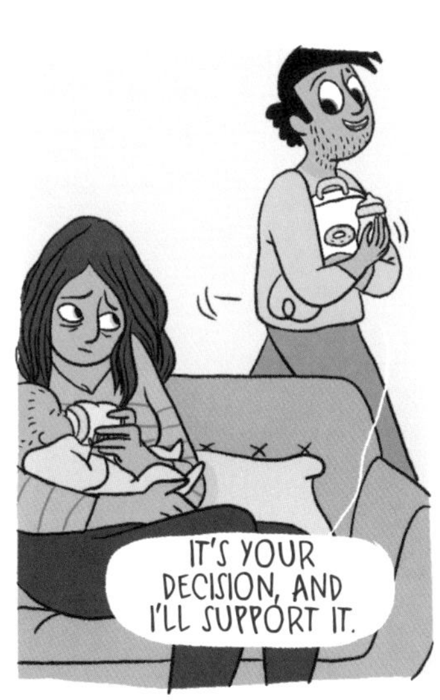

SO WHY DO I FEEL SO GUILTY, THEN?

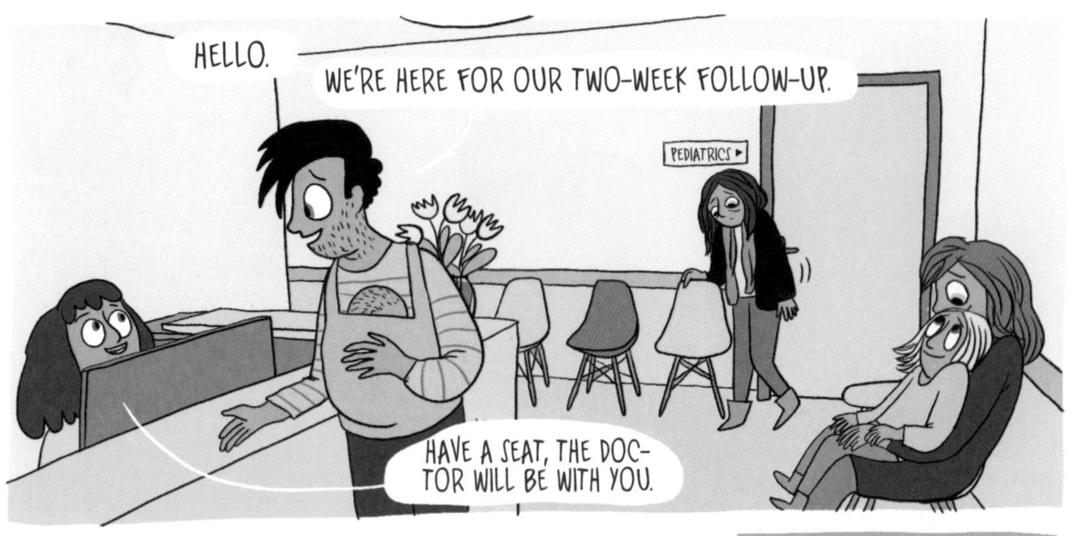
HELLO.
WE'RE HERE FOR OUR TWO-WEEK FOLLOW-UP.
PEDIATRICS ▶
HAVE A SEAT, THE DOCTOR WILL BE WITH YOU.

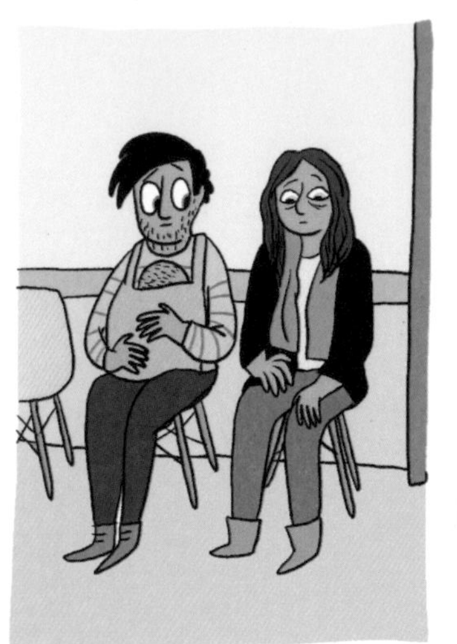

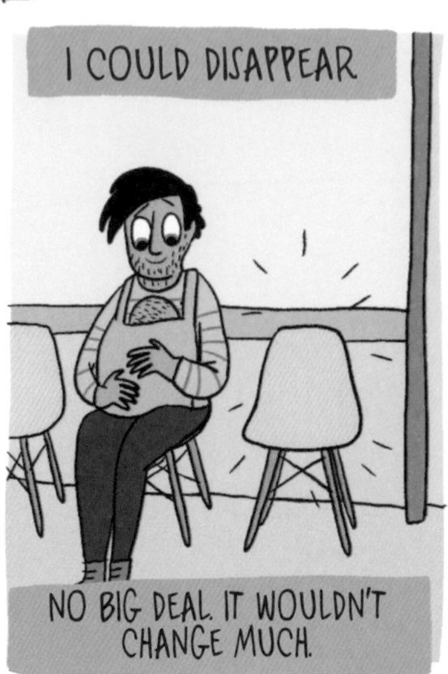
I COULD DISAPPEAR
NO BIG DEAL. IT WOULDN'T CHANGE MUCH.

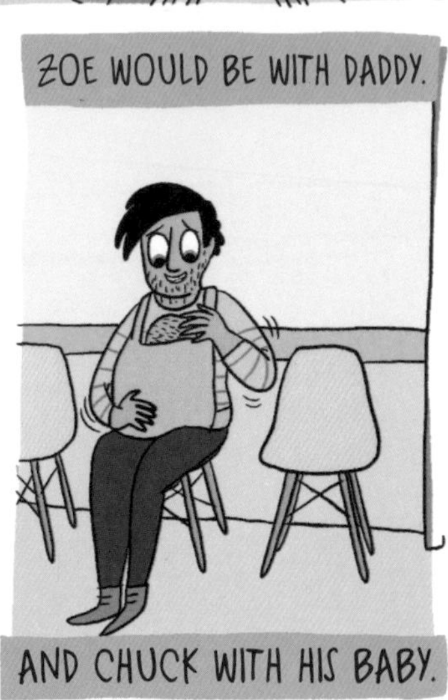
ZOE WOULD BE WITH DADDY.
AND CHUCK WITH HIS BABY.

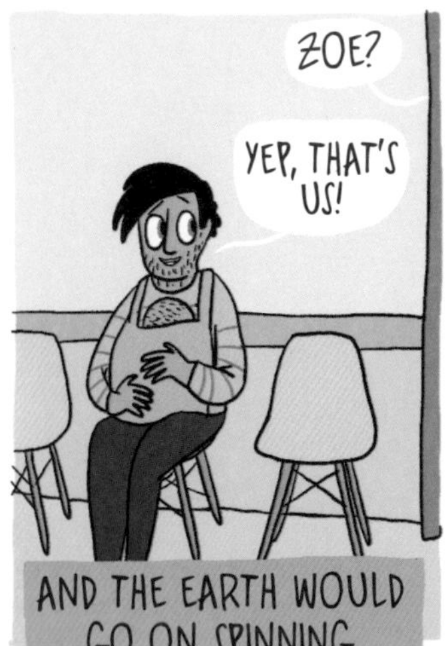
ZOE?
YEP, THAT'S US!
AND THE EARTH WOULD GO ON SPINNING.

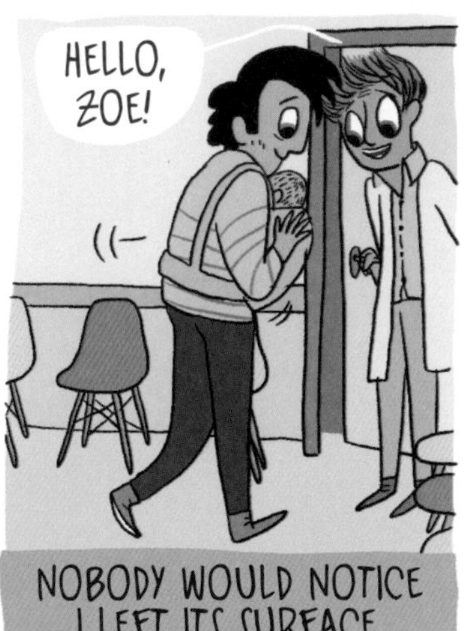
HELLO, ZOE!
NOBODY WOULD NOTICE I LEFT ITS SURFACE.

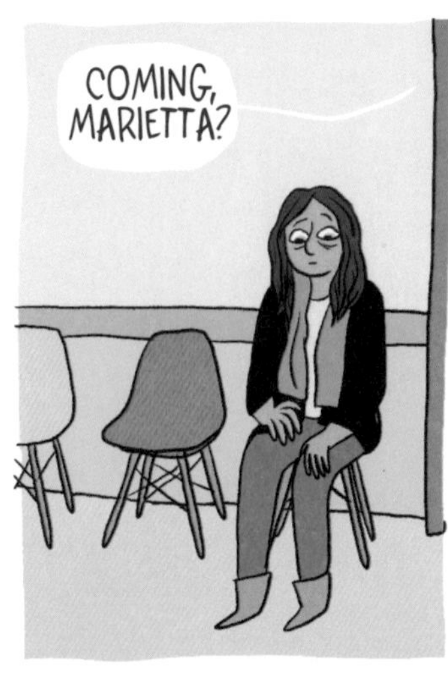
COMING, MARIETTA?

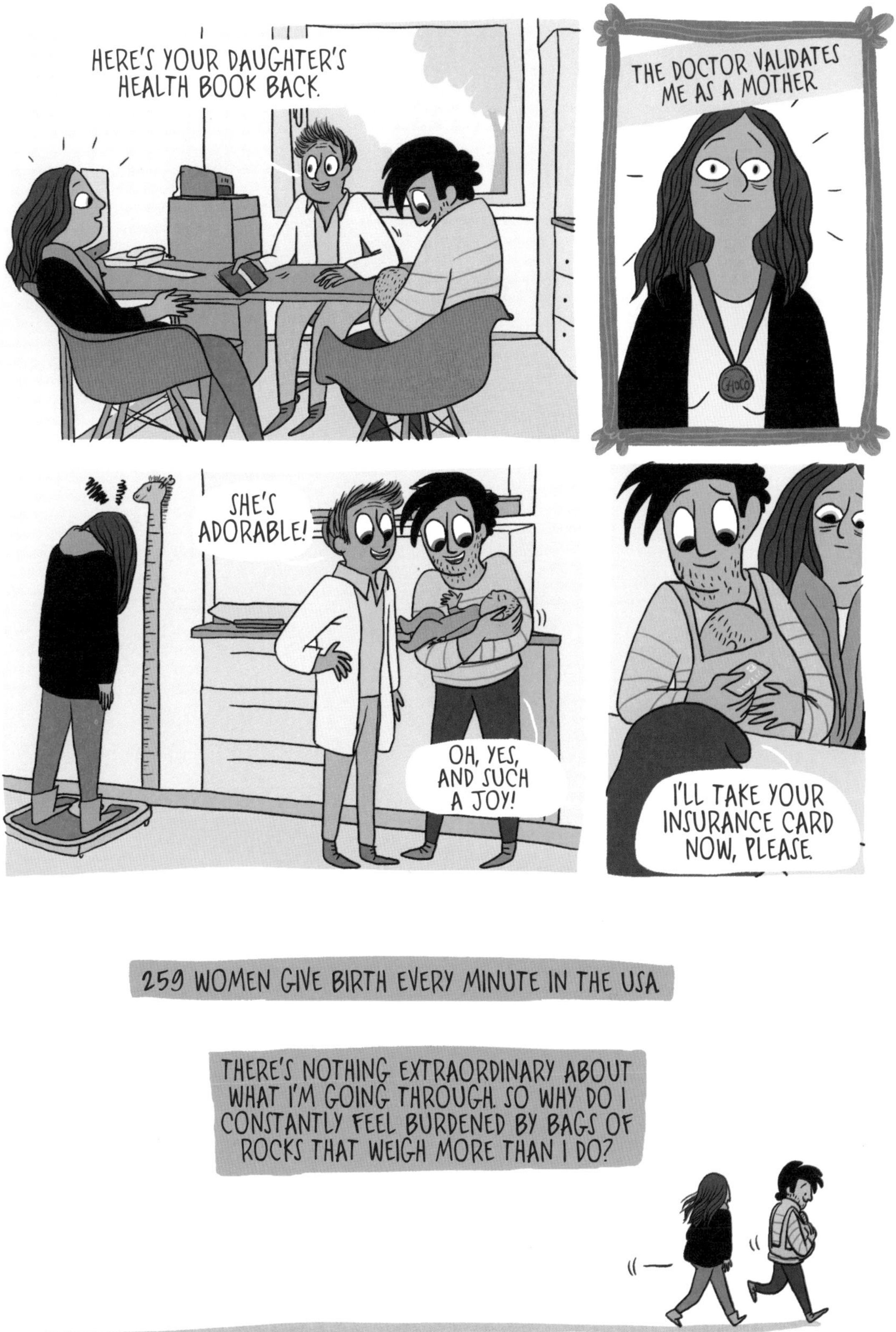

HERE'S YOUR DAUGHTER'S HEALTH BOOK BACK.

THE DOCTOR VALIDATES ME AS A MOTHER

SHE'S ADORABLE!

OH, YES, AND SUCH A JOY!

I'LL TAKE YOUR INSURANCE CARD NOW, PLEASE.

259 WOMEN GIVE BIRTH EVERY MINUTE IN THE USA

THERE'S NOTHING EXTRAORDINARY ABOUT WHAT I'M GOING THROUGH. SO WHY DO I CONSTANTLY FEEL BURDENED BY BAGS OF ROCKS THAT WEIGH MORE THAN I DO?

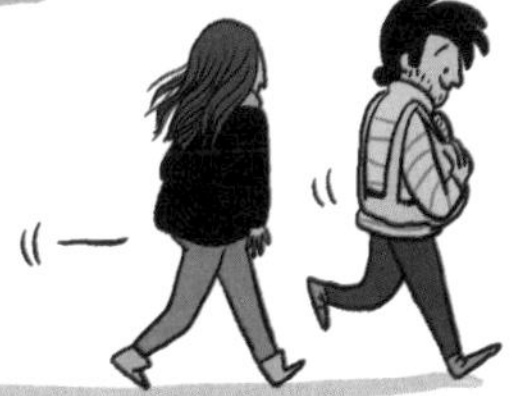

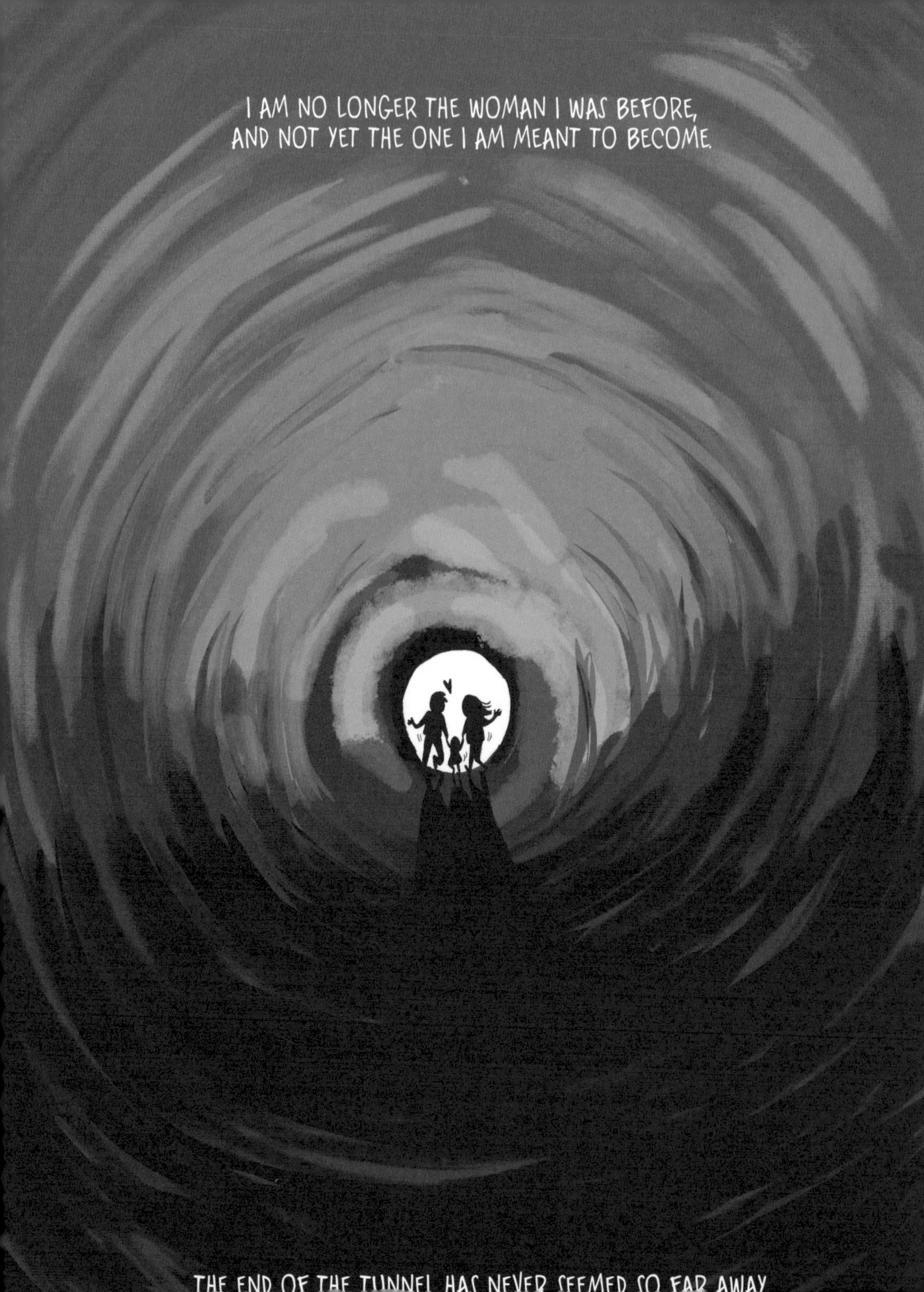
I AM NO LONGER THE WOMAN I WAS BEFORE,
AND NOT YET THE ONE I AM MEANT TO BECOME.
THE END OF THE TUNNEL HAS NEVER SEEMED SO FAR AWAY

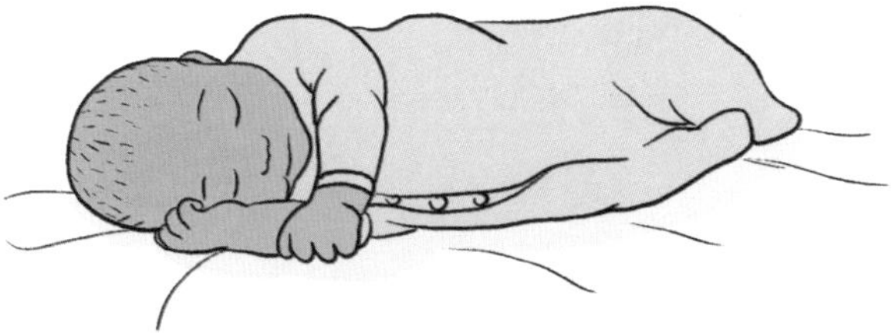

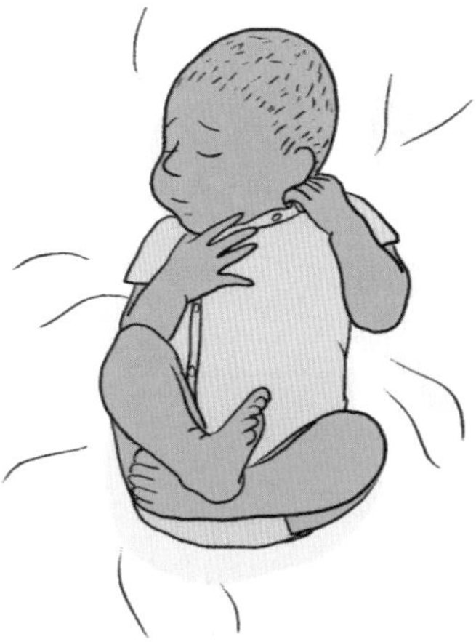

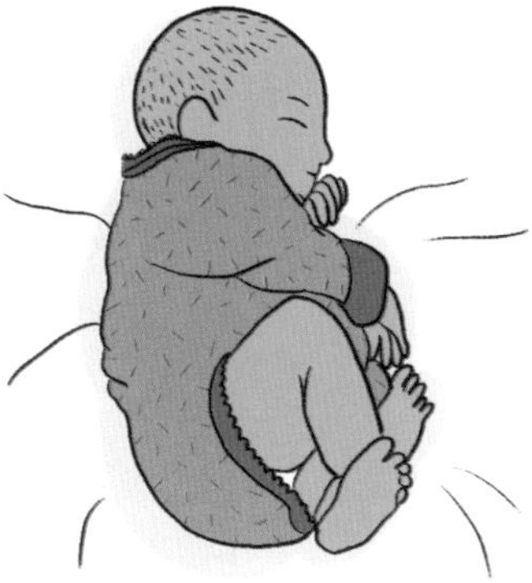

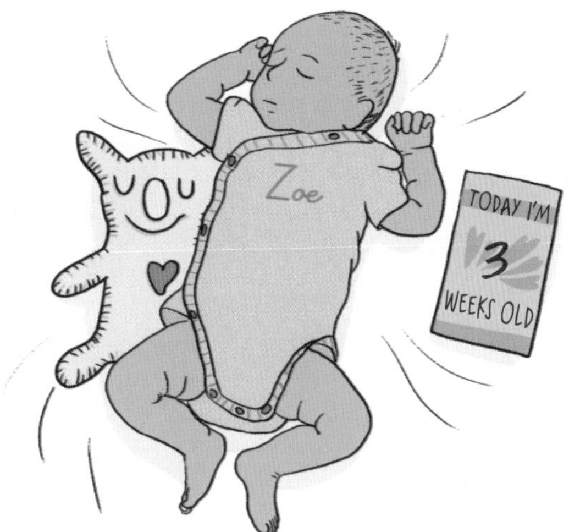
Zoe
TODAY I'M
3
WEEKS OLD

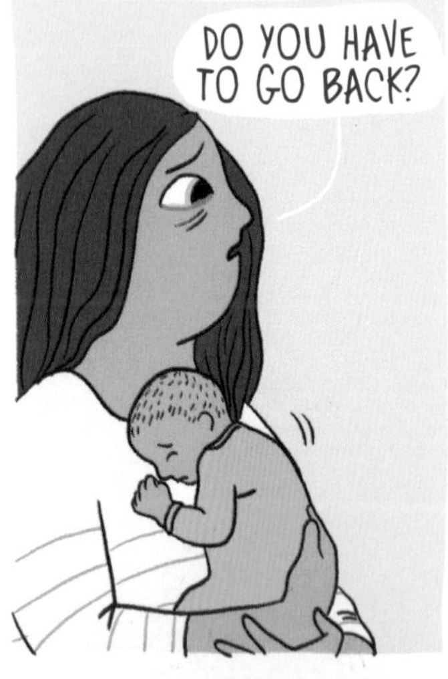
DO YOU HAVE TO GO BACK?

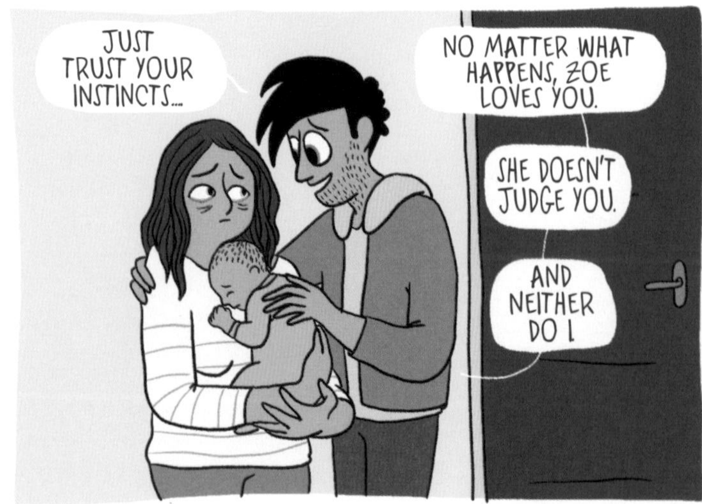
JUST TRUST YOUR INSTINCTS...
NO MATTER WHAT HAPPENS, ZOE LOVES YOU.
SHE DOESN'T JUDGE YOU.
AND NEITHER DO I.

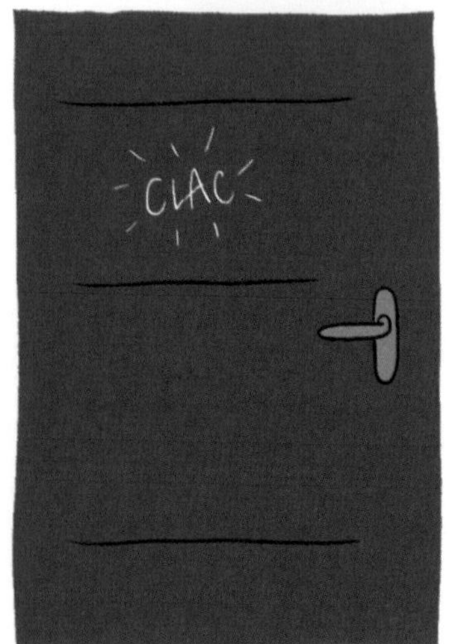
CLAC

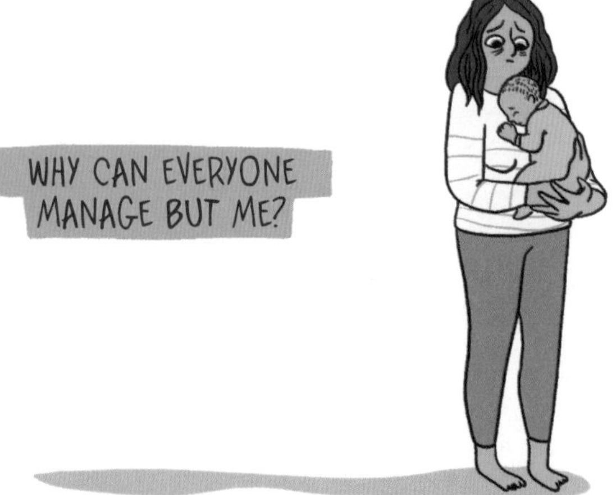
WHY CAN EVERYONE MANAGE BUT ME?

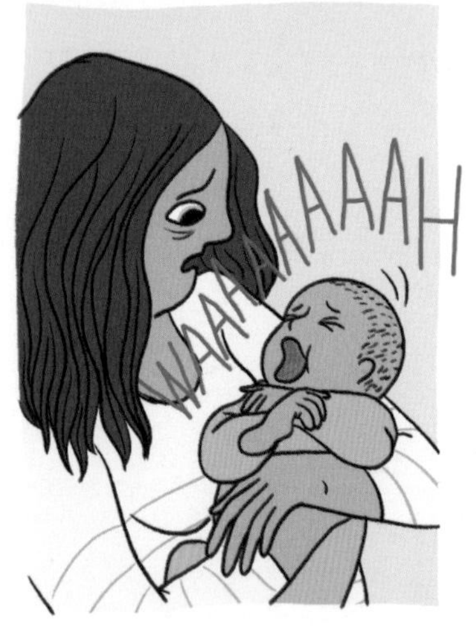
WAAAAAAAAH

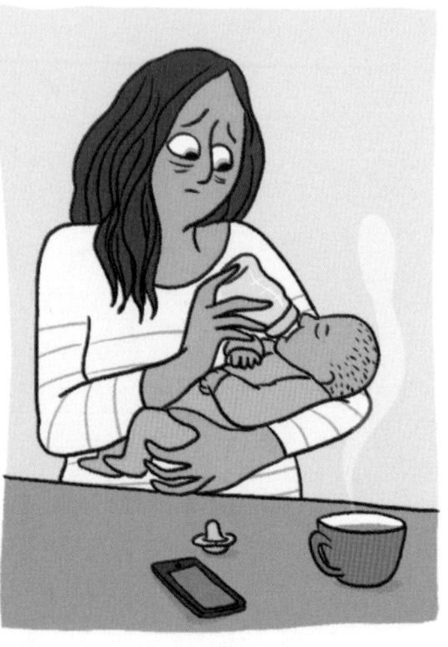

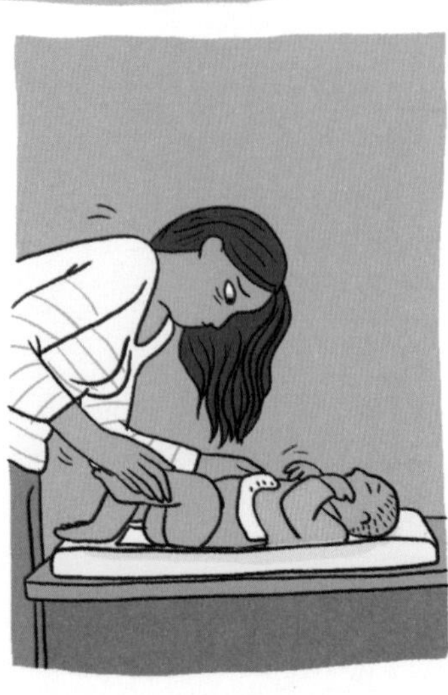

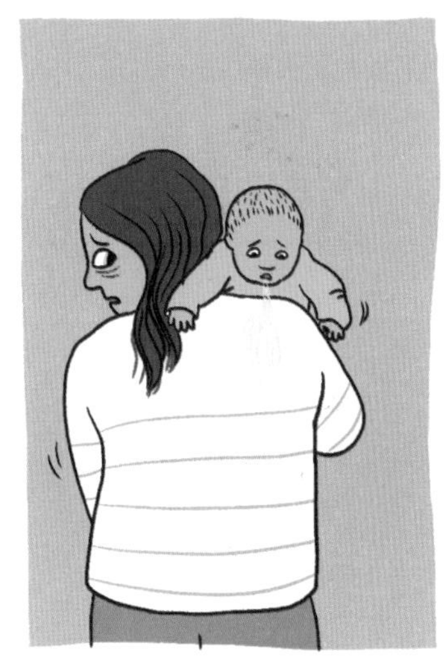
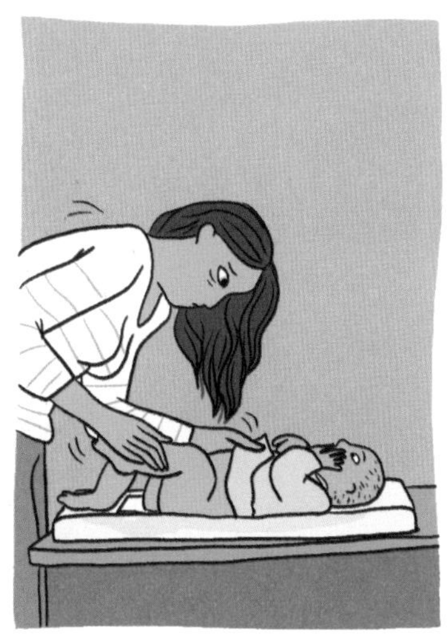
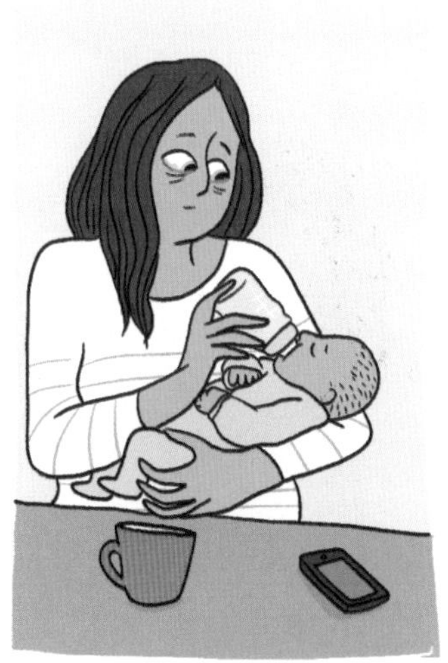
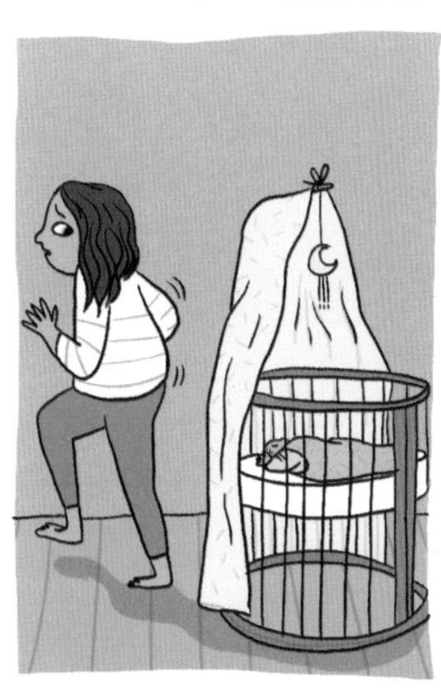
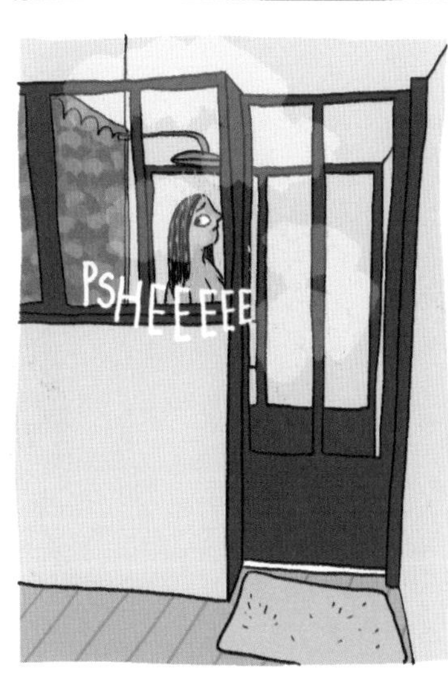
PSHEEEEEE
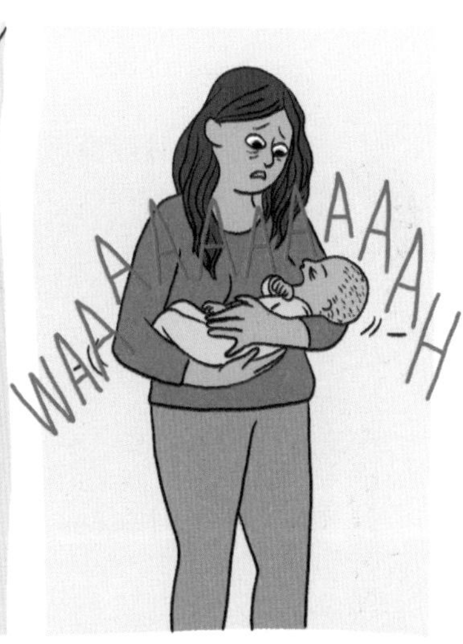
WAAAAAAAAA-H
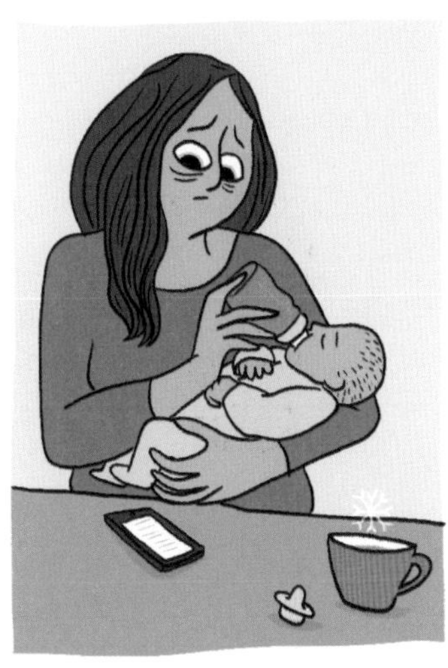
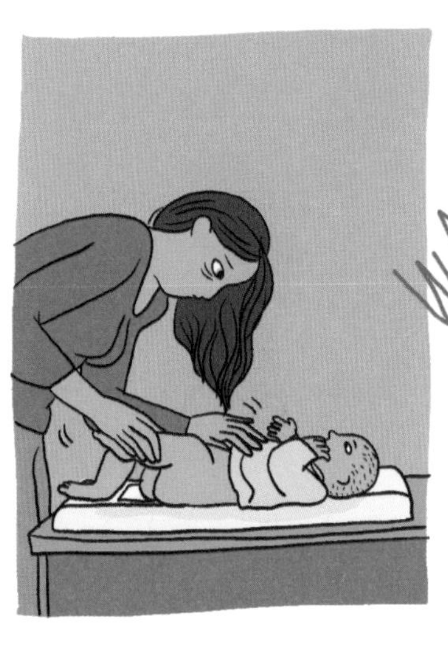
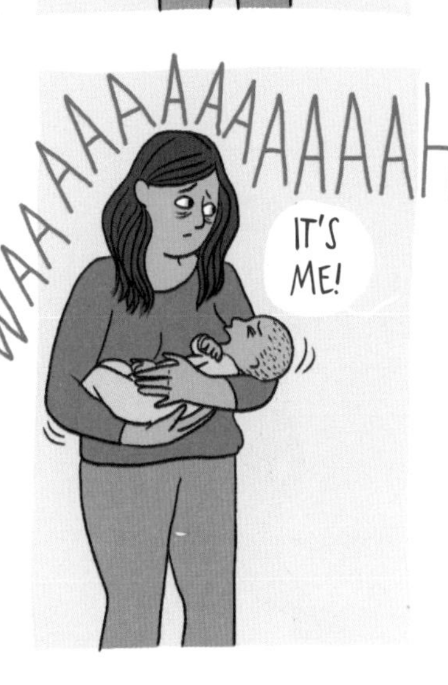
WAAAAAAAAAAAAH
IT'S ME!

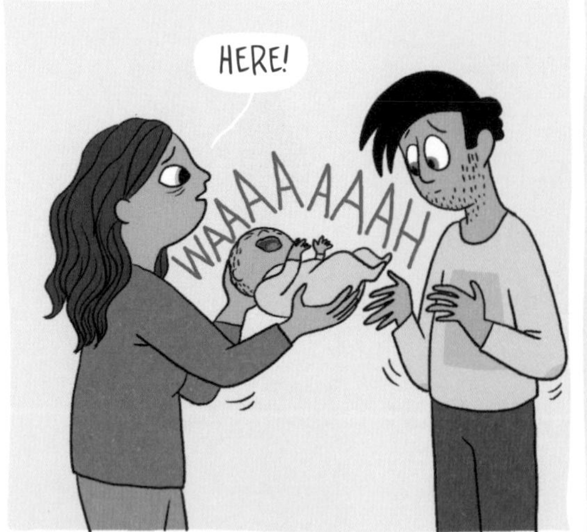
HERE!
WAAAAAAAAH

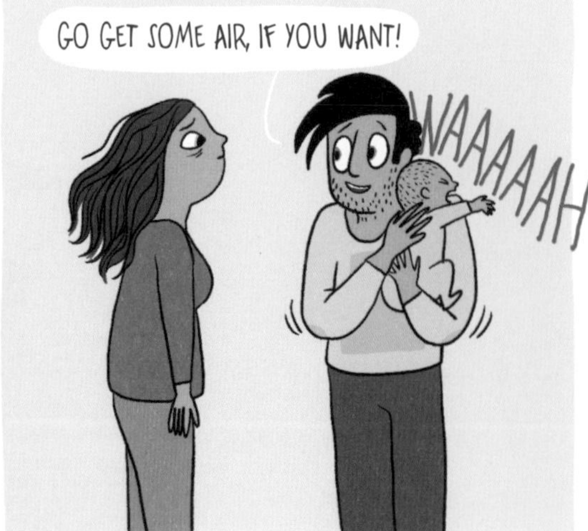
GO GET SOME AIR, IF YOU WANT!
WAAAAAAH

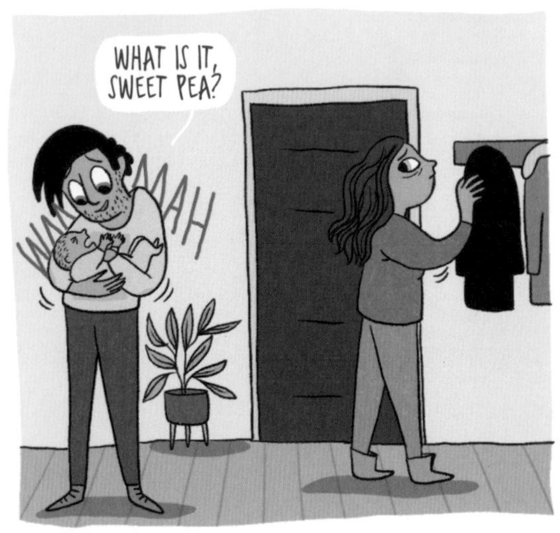
WHAT IS IT, SWEET PEA?

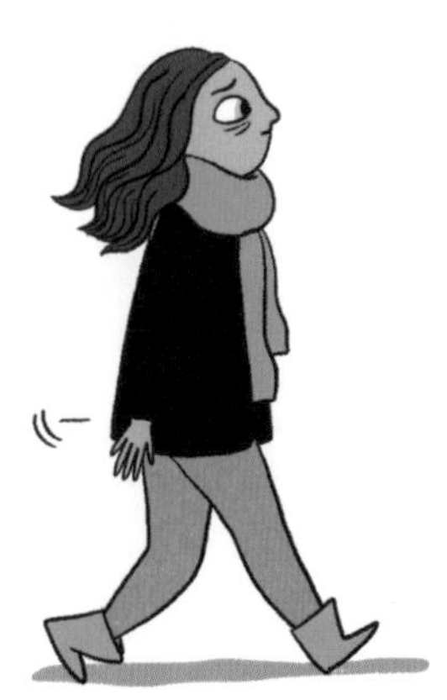

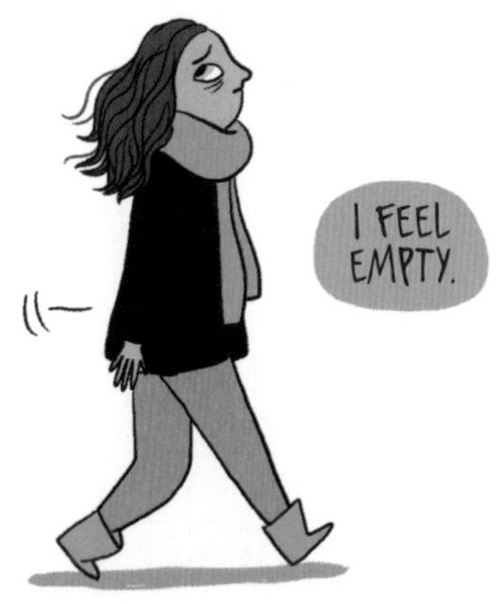
I FEEL EMPTY.

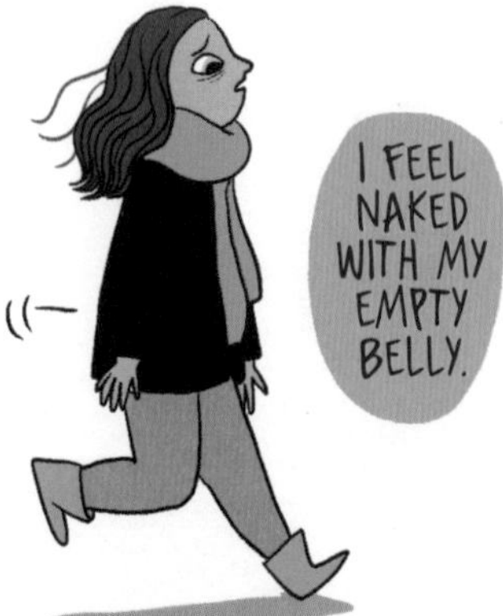
I FEEL NAKED WITH MY EMPTY BELLY.

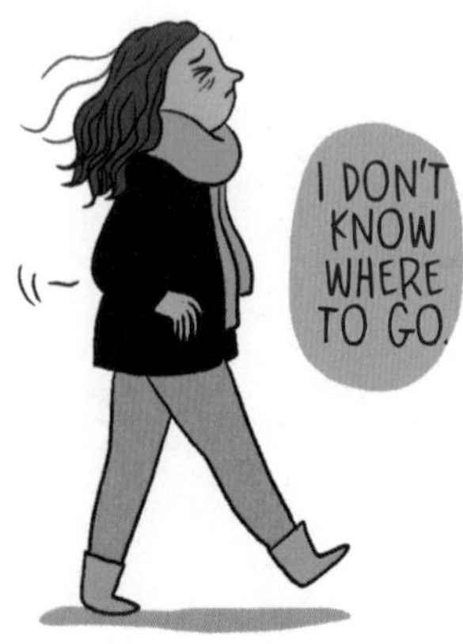
I DON'T KNOW WHERE TO GO.

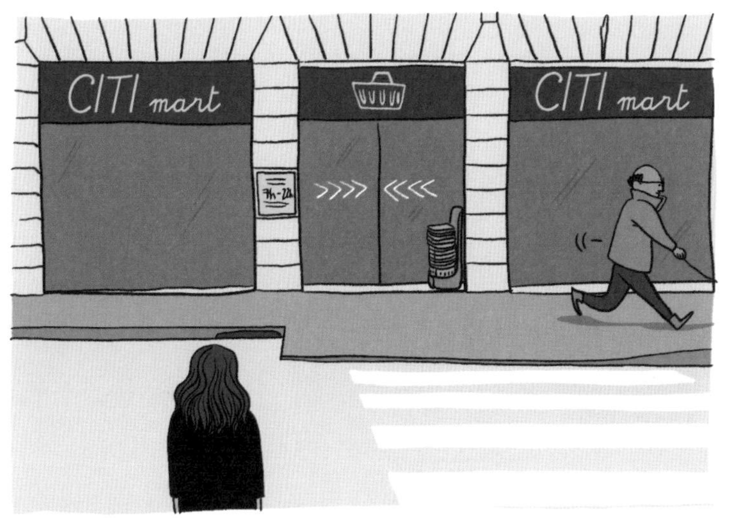
CITI mart
CITI mart

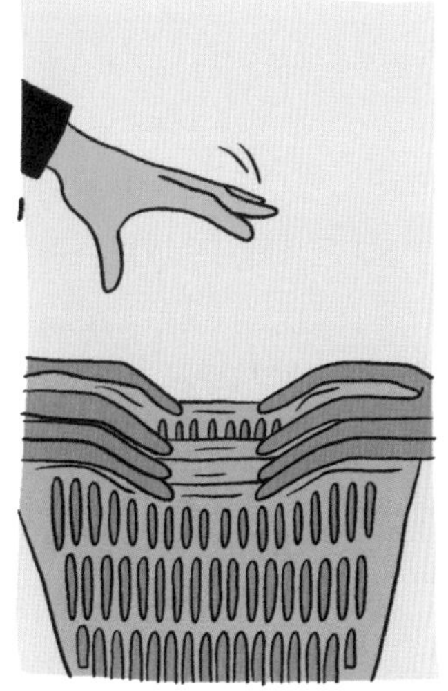

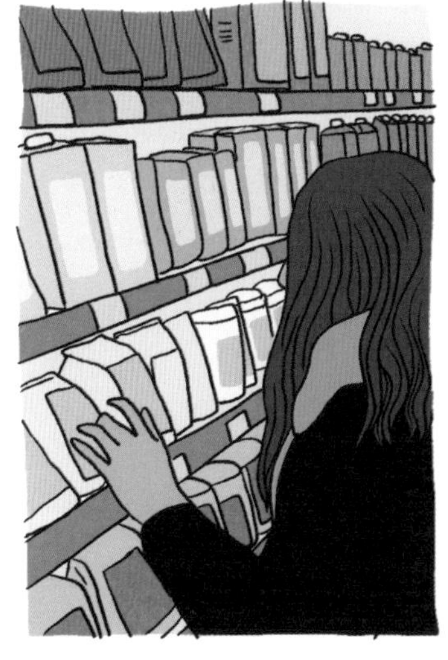

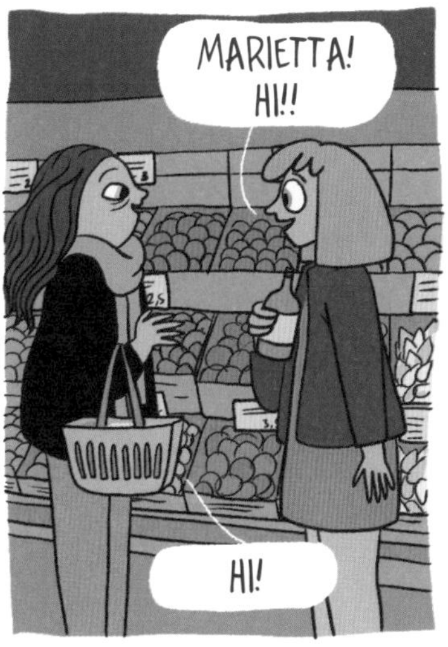
MARIETTA! HI!!
HI!

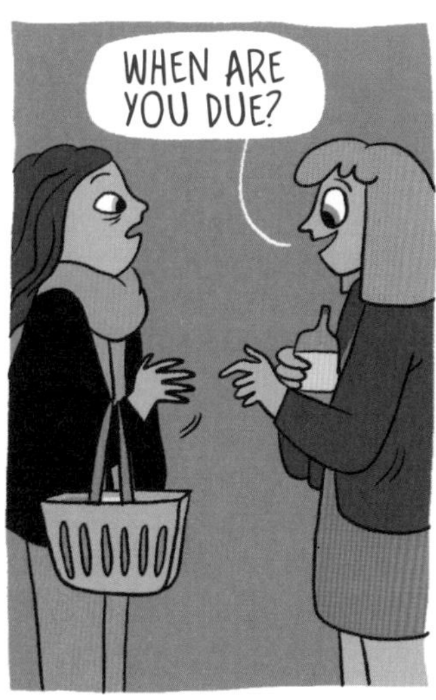
WHEN ARE YOU DUE?

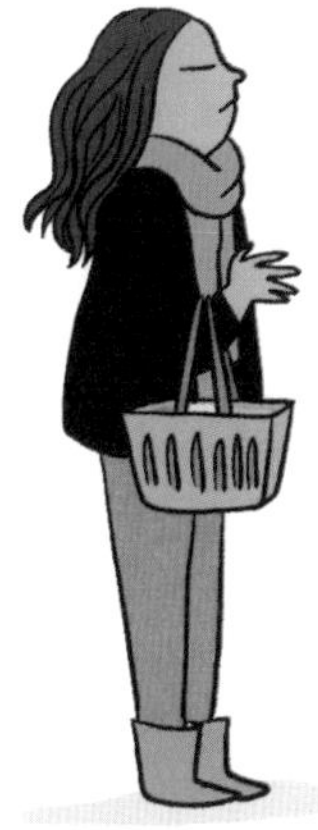

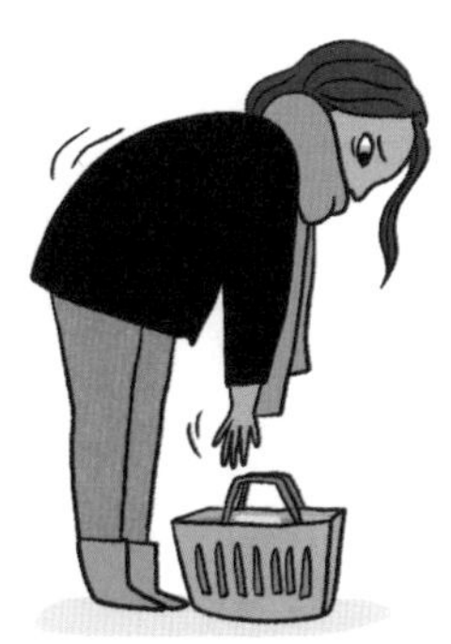

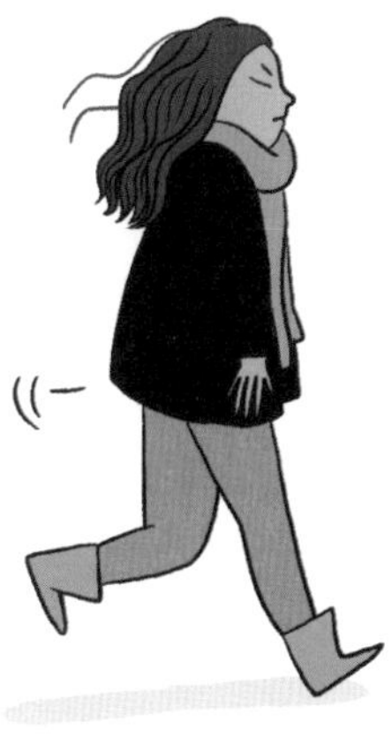

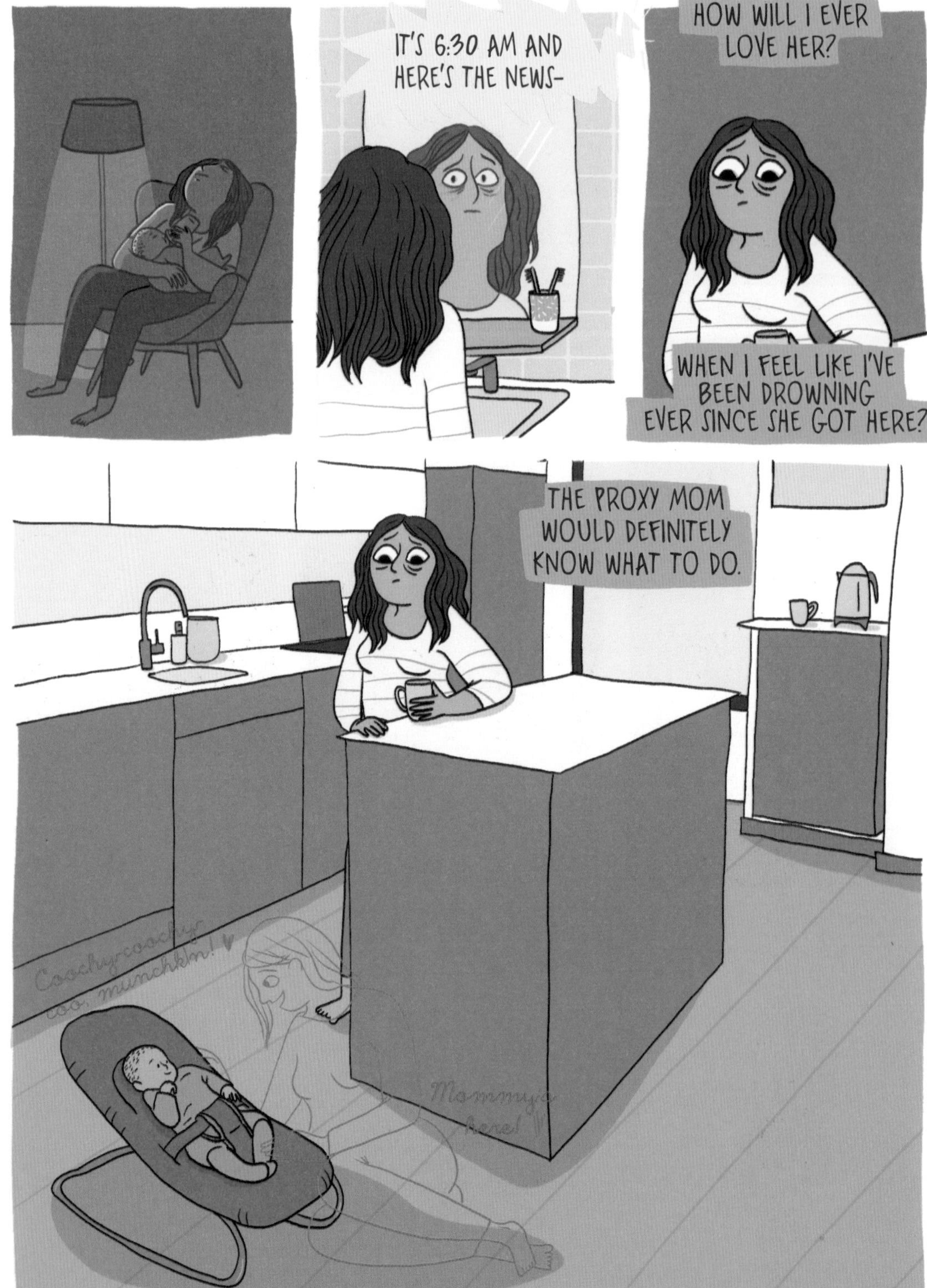
IT'S 6:30 AM AND HERE'S THE NEWS-
HOW WILL I EVER LOVE HER?
WHEN I FEEL LIKE I'VE BEEN DROWNING EVER SINCE SHE GOT HERE?
THE PROXY MOM WOULD DEFINITELY KNOW WHAT TO DO.
Coochy-coochy-coo, munchkin!
Mommy's here!

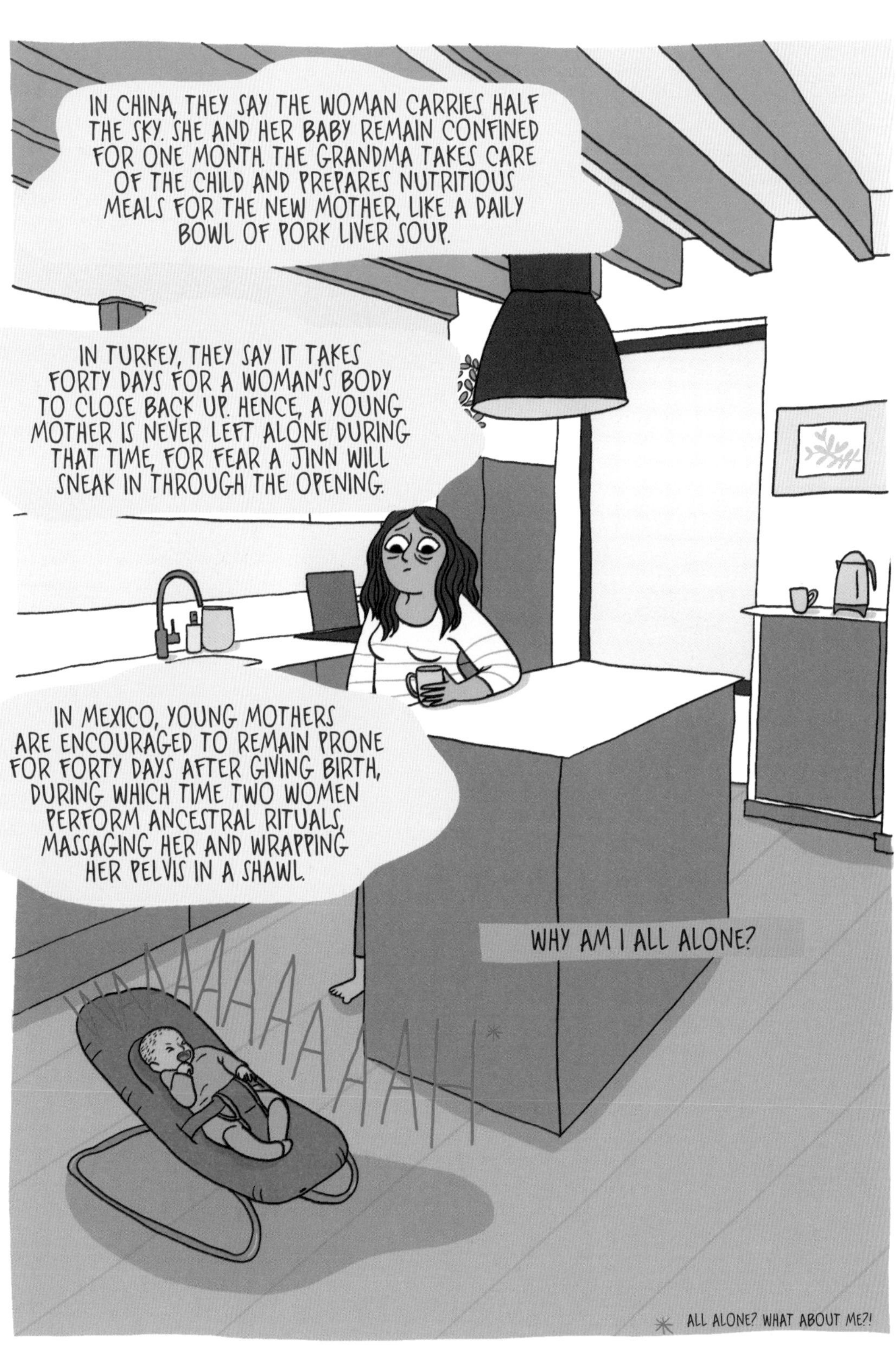
IN CHINA, THEY SAY THE WOMAN CARRIES HALF THE SKY. SHE AND HER BABY REMAIN CONFINED FOR ONE MONTH. THE GRANDMA TAKES CARE OF THE CHILD AND PREPARES NUTRITIOUS MEALS FOR THE NEW MOTHER, LIKE A DAILY BOWL OF PORK LIVER SOUP.
IN TURKEY, THEY SAY IT TAKES FORTY DAYS FOR A WOMAN'S BODY TO CLOSE BACK UP. HENCE, A YOUNG MOTHER IS NEVER LEFT ALONE DURING THAT TIME, FOR FEAR A JINN WILL SNEAK IN THROUGH THE OPENING.
IN MEXICO, YOUNG MOTHERS ARE ENCOURAGED TO REMAIN PRONE FOR FORTY DAYS AFTER GIVING BIRTH, DURING WHICH TIME TWO WOMEN PERFORM ANCESTRAL RITUALS, MASSAGING HER AND WRAPPING HER PELVIS IN A SHAWL.
WHY AM I ALL ALONE?
WAAAAAAAAAH*
* ALL ALONE? WHAT ABOUT ME?!

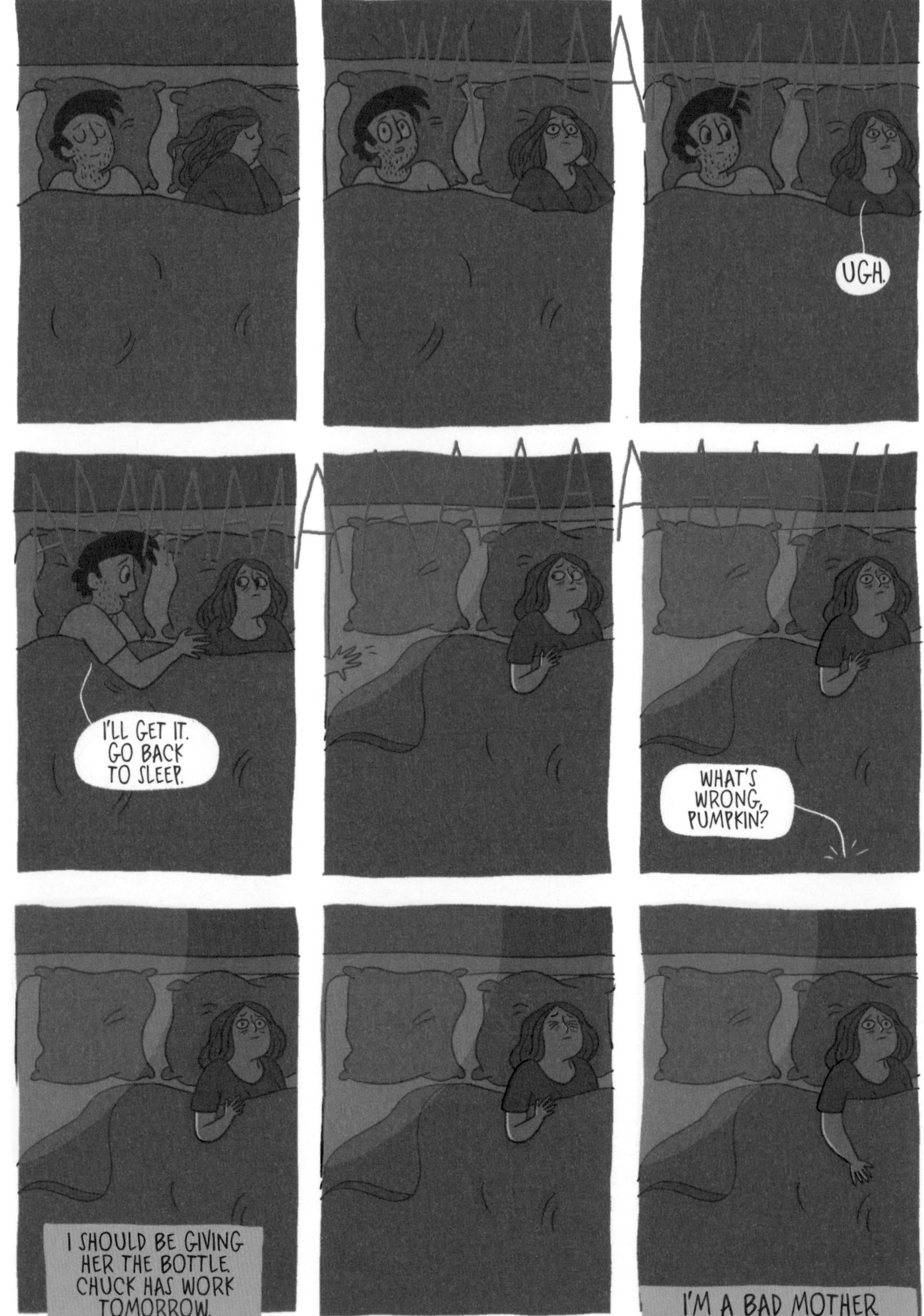
UGH.
I'LL GET IT. GO BACK TO SLEEP.
WHAT'S WRONG, PUMPKIN?
I SHOULD BE GIVING HER THE BOTTLE. CHUCK HAS WORK TOMORROW.
I'M A BAD MOTHER

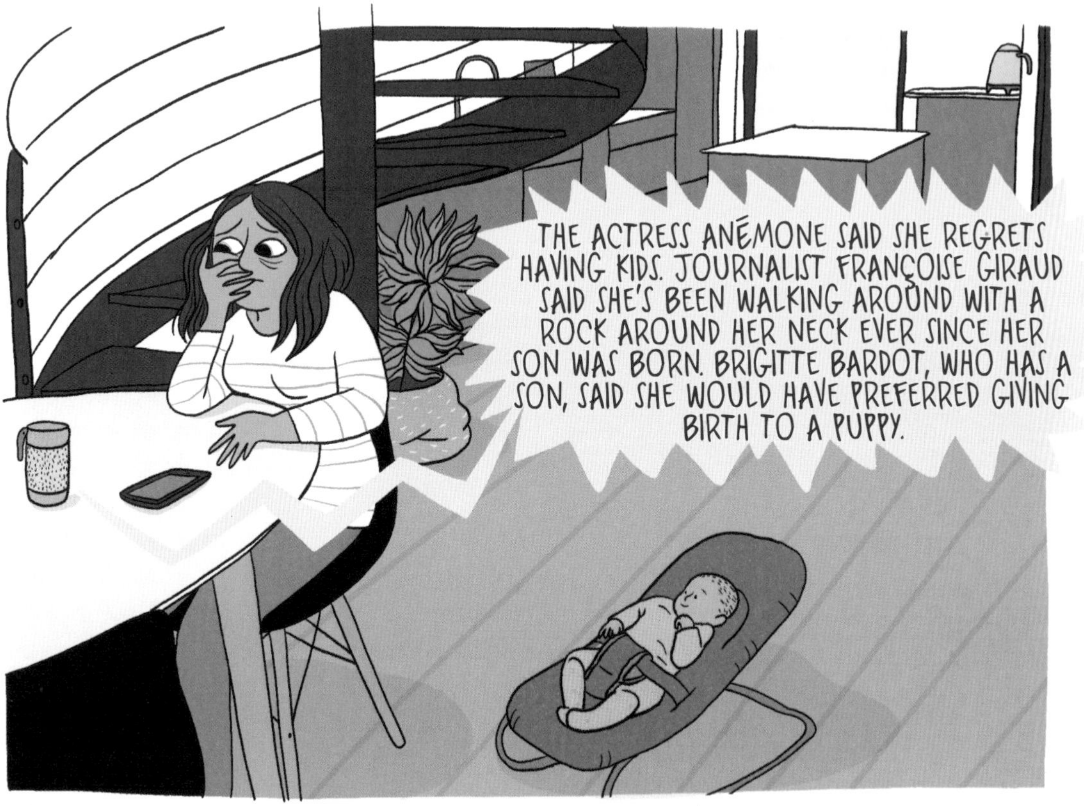

THE ACTRESS ANÉMONE SAID SHE REGRETS HAVING KIDS. JOURNALIST FRANÇOISE GIRAUD SAID SHE'S BEEN WALKING AROUND WITH A ROCK AROUND HER NECK EVER SINCE HER SON WAS BORN. BRIGITTE BARDOT, WHO HAS A SON, SAID SHE WOULD HAVE PREFERRED GIVING BIRTH TO A PUPPY.

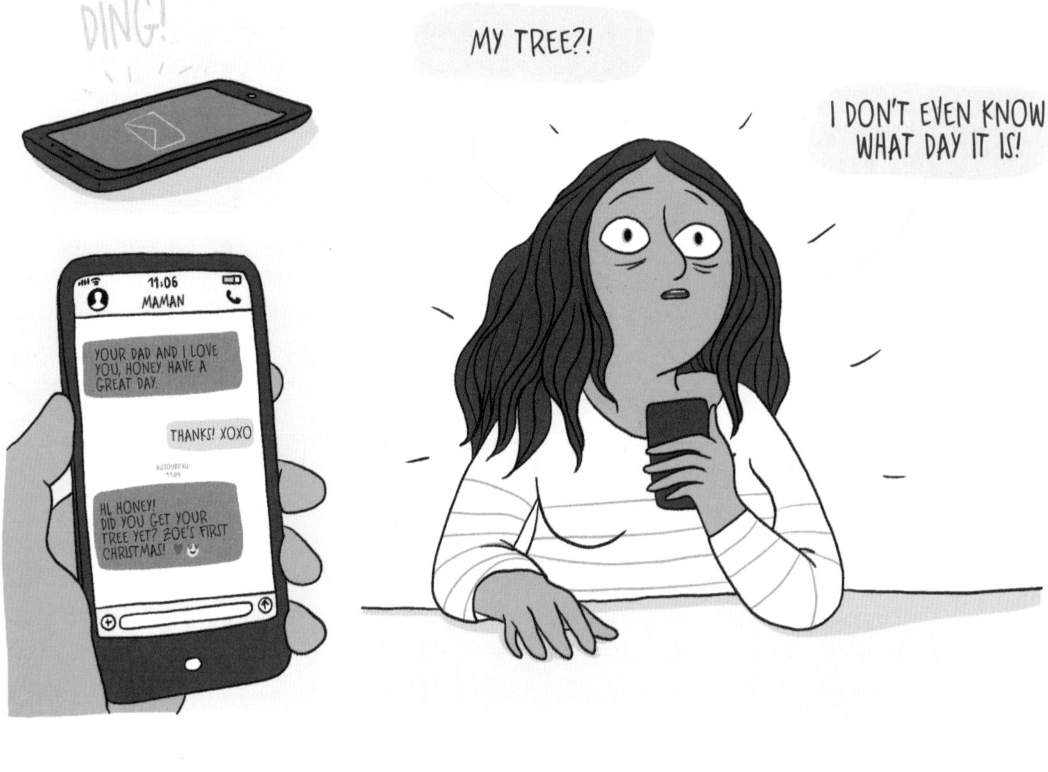

DING!

11:06
MAMAN

YOUR DAD AND I LOVE YOU, HONEY. HAVE A GREAT DAY.

THANKS! XOXO

AUJOURD'HUI
11:05

HI, HONEY!
DID YOU GET YOUR TREE YET? ZOE'S FIRST CHRISTMAS!

MY TREE?!

I DON'T EVEN KNOW WHAT DAY IT IS!

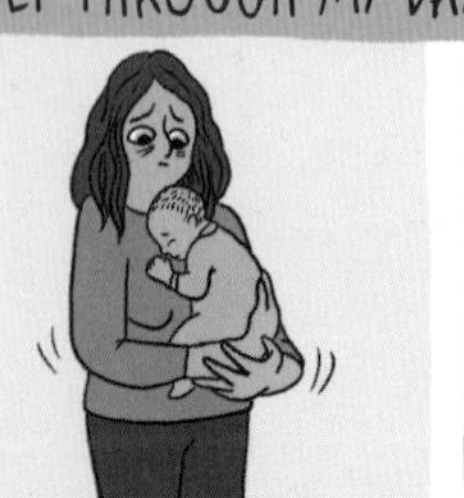
I GET THROUGH MY DAY

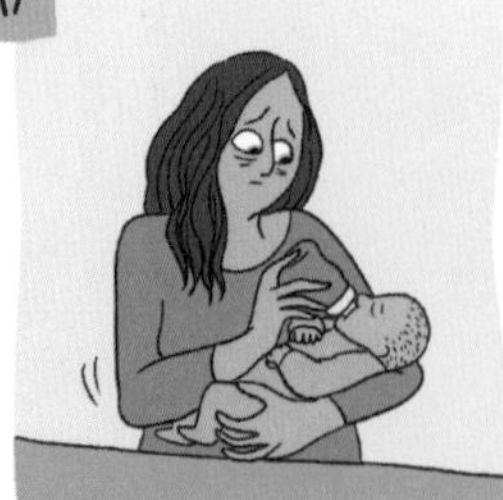

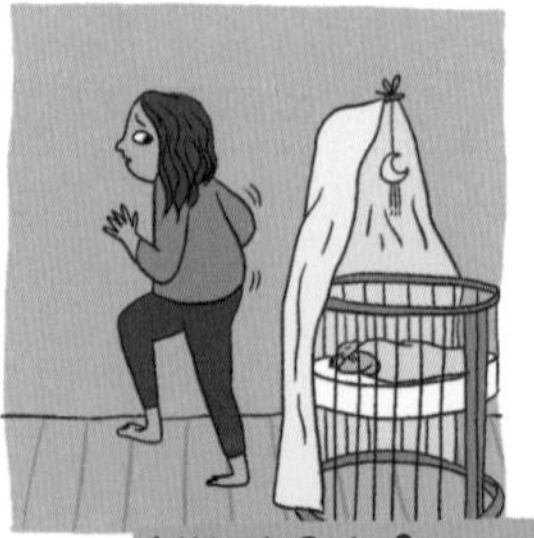

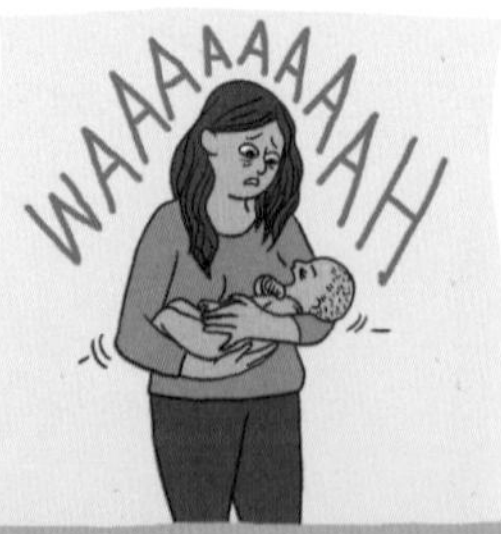
WAAAAAAAAH

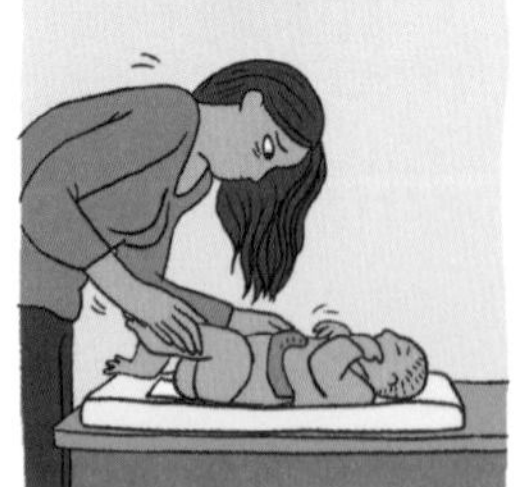

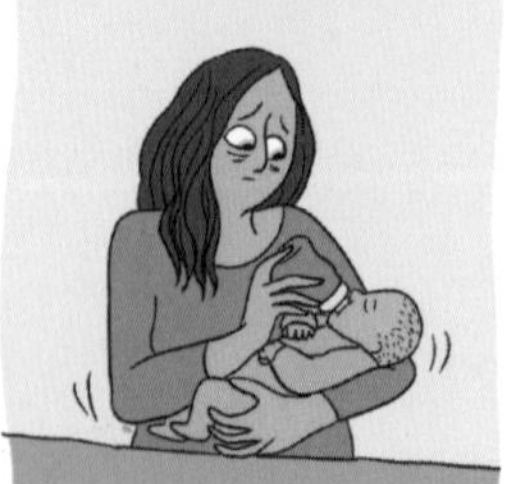

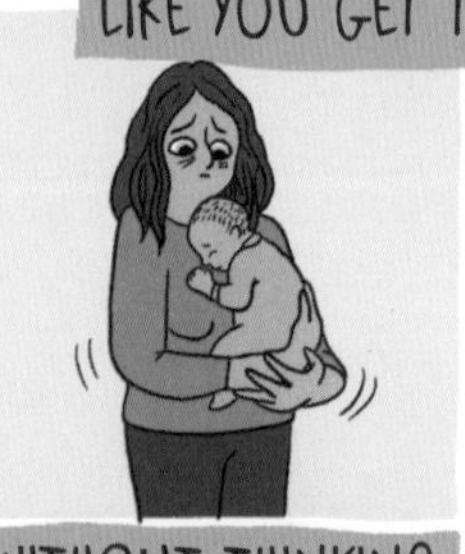
LIKE YOU GET THROUGH A MINEFIELD.

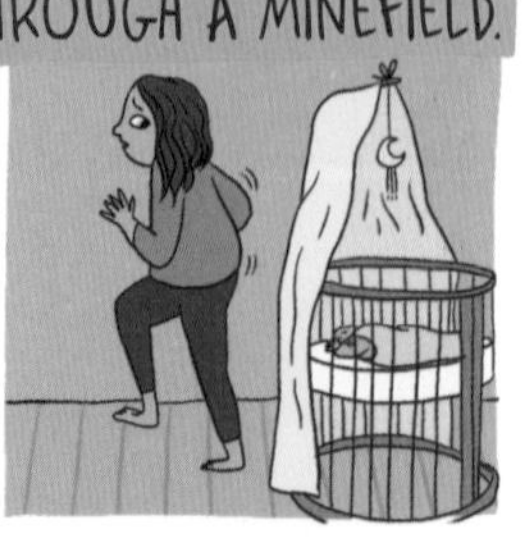

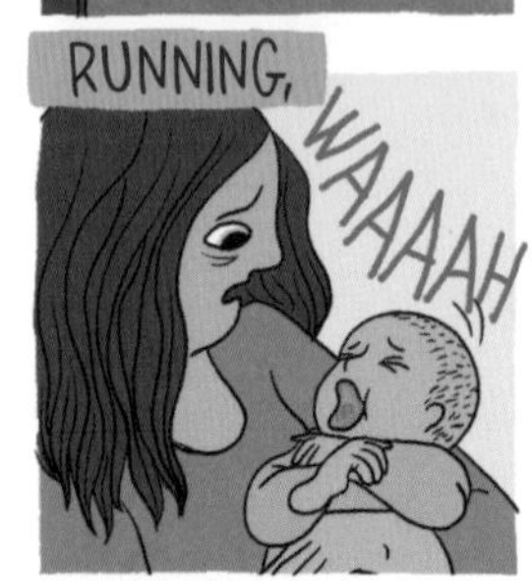
RUNNING,
WAAAAAH

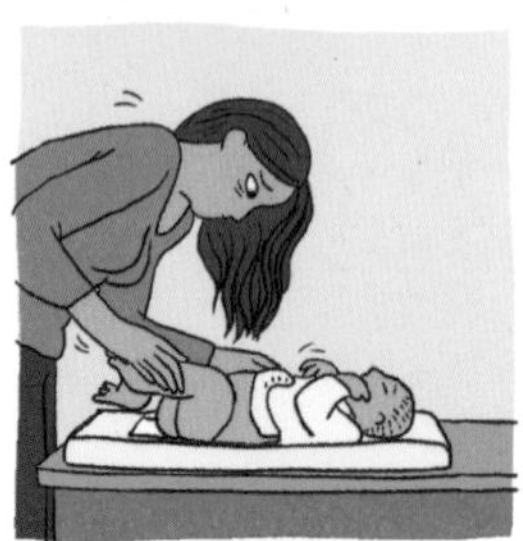

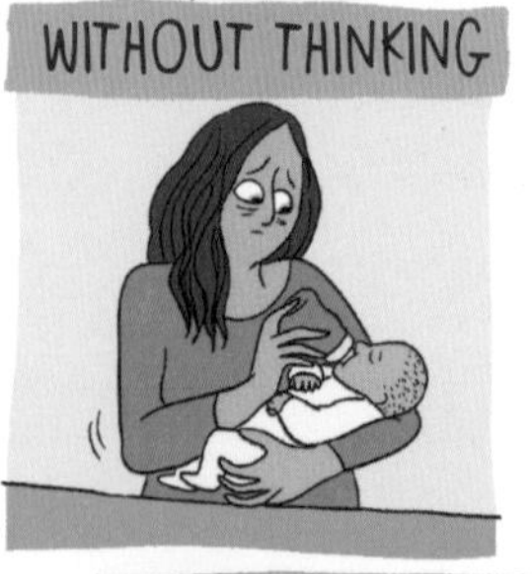
WITHOUT THINKING

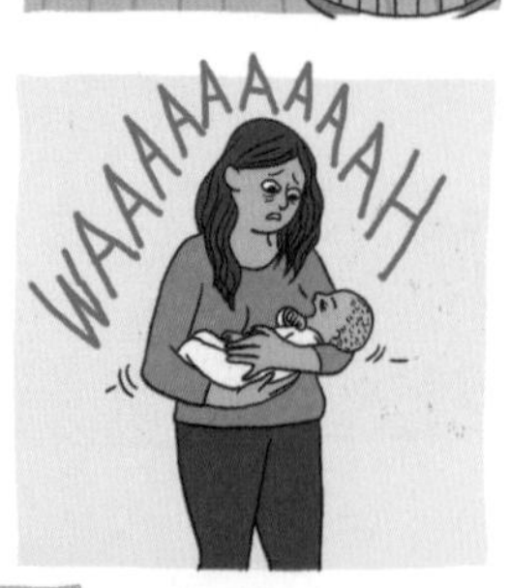
WAAAAAAAAH

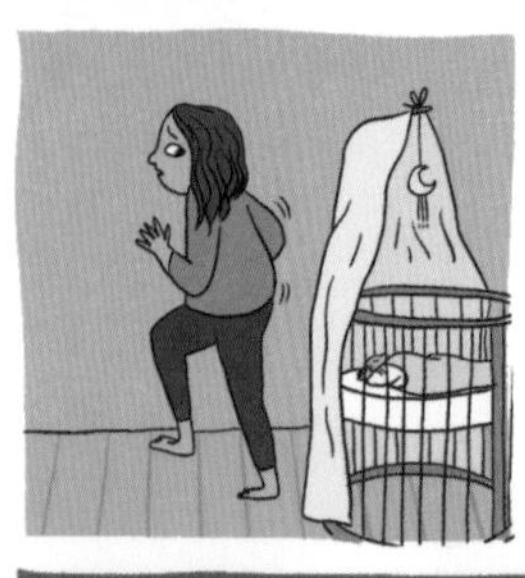

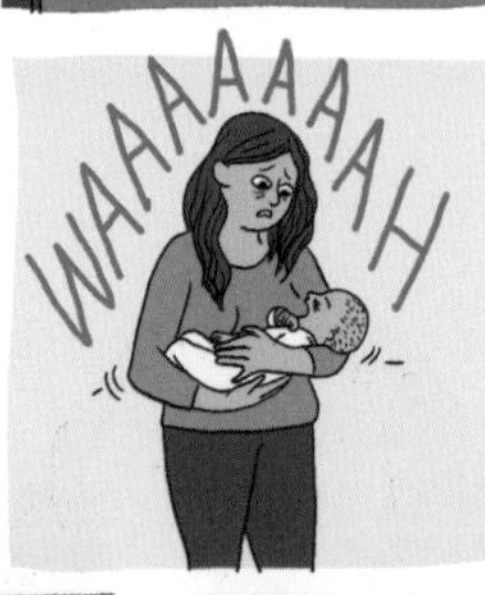
WAAAAAAAH

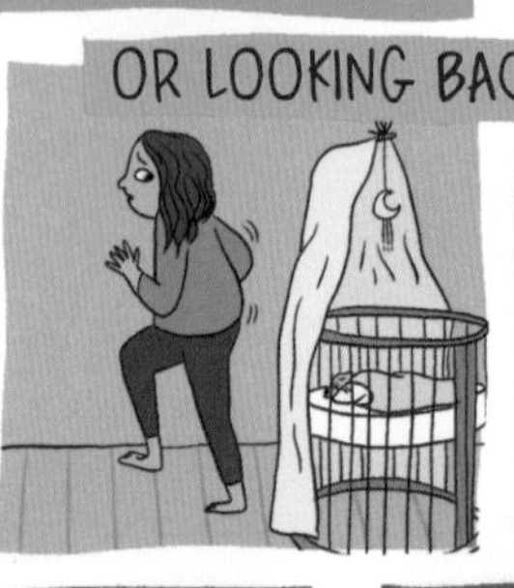
OR LOOKING BACK.

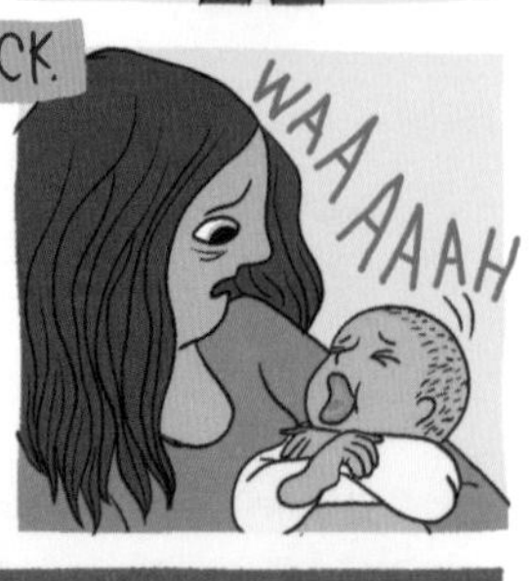
WAAAAAH

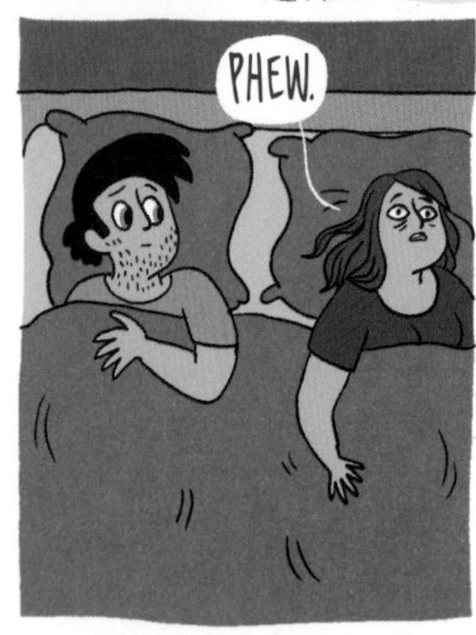
PHEW.

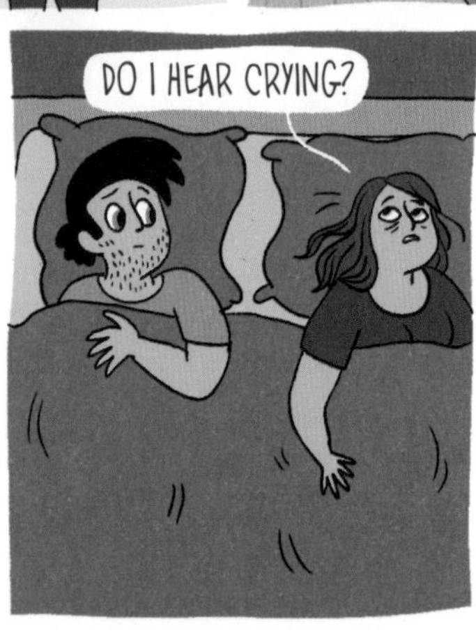
DO I HEAR CRYING?

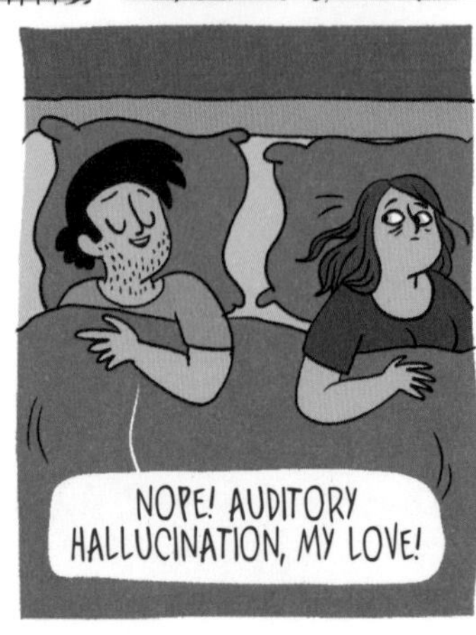
NOPE! AUDITORY HALLUCINATION, MY LOVE!

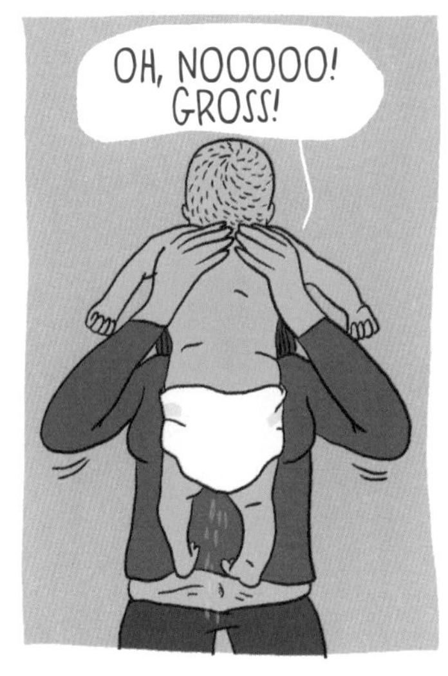
OH, NOOOOO! GROSS!

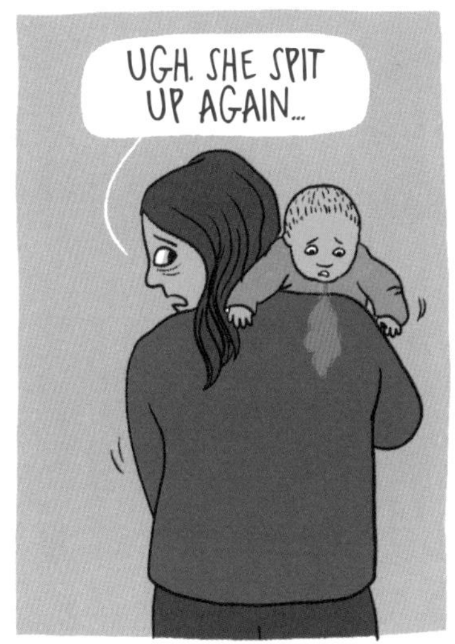
UGH. SHE SPIT UP AGAIN...

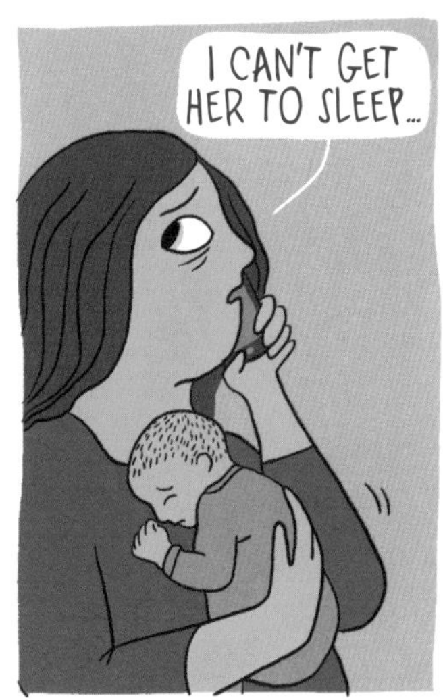
I CAN'T GET HER TO SLEEP...

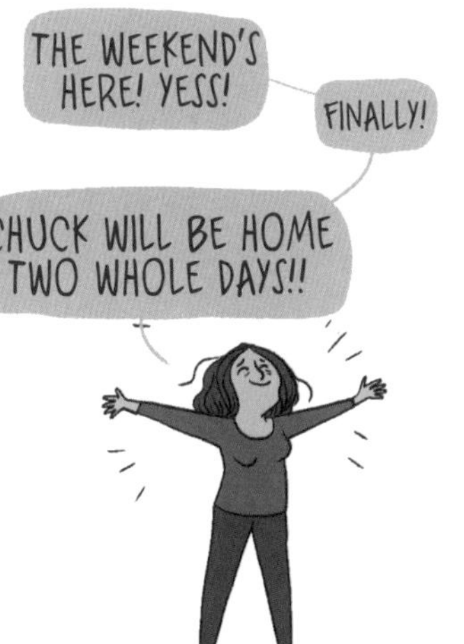
THE WEEKEND'S HERE! YESS!
FINALLY!
CHUCK WILL BE HOME TWO WHOLE DAYS!!

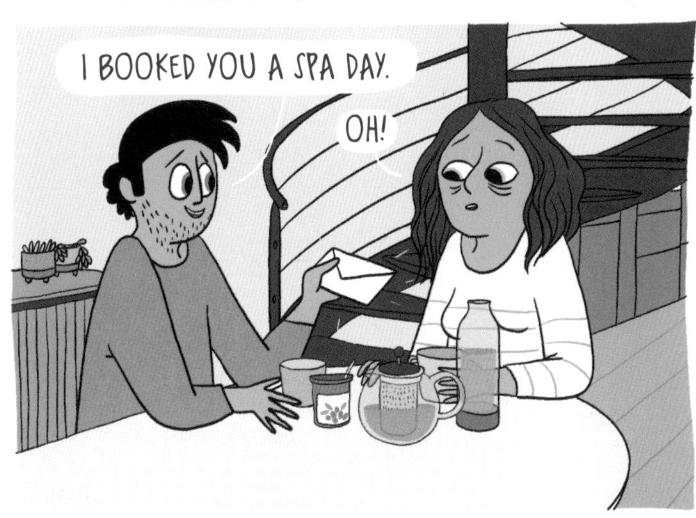
I BOOKED YOU A SPA DAY.
OH!

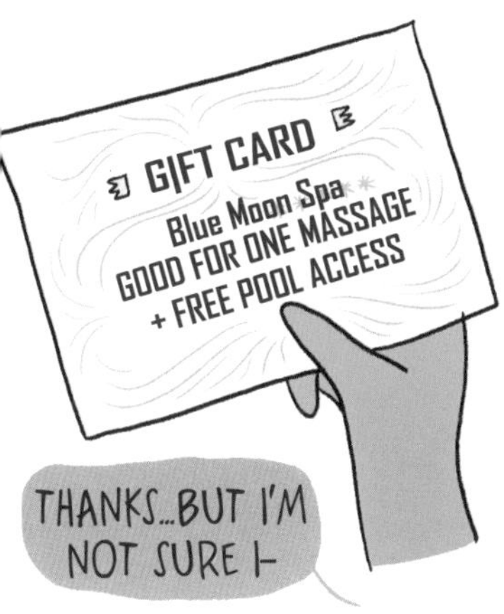
GIFT CARD
Blue Moon Spa
GOOD FOR ONE MASSAGE
+ FREE POOL ACCESS
THANKS...BUT I'M NOT SURE I-

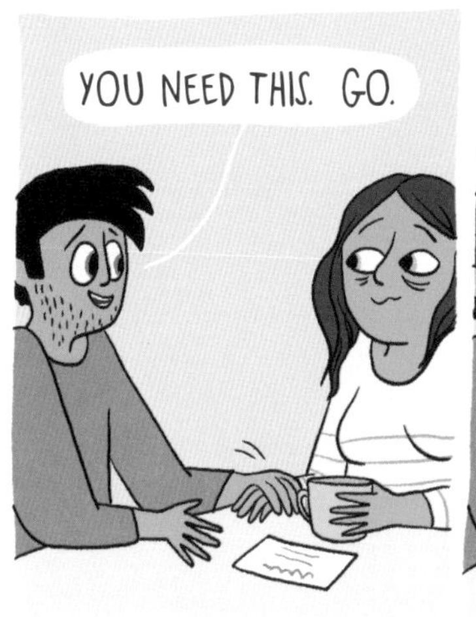
YOU NEED THIS. GO.

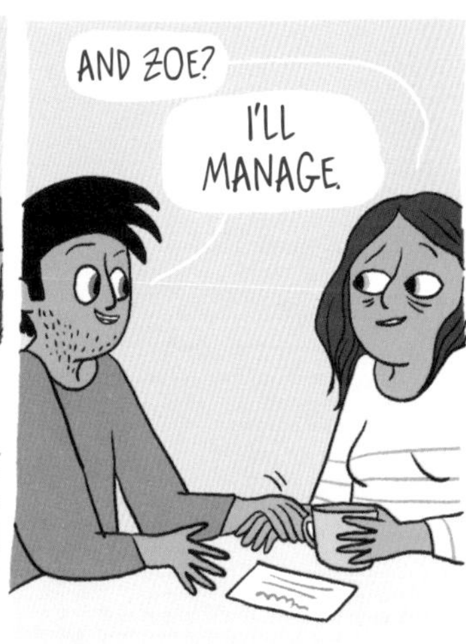
AND ZOE?
I'LL MANAGE.

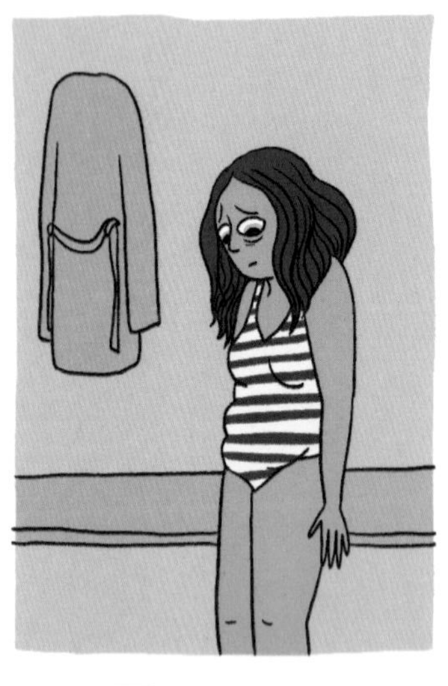

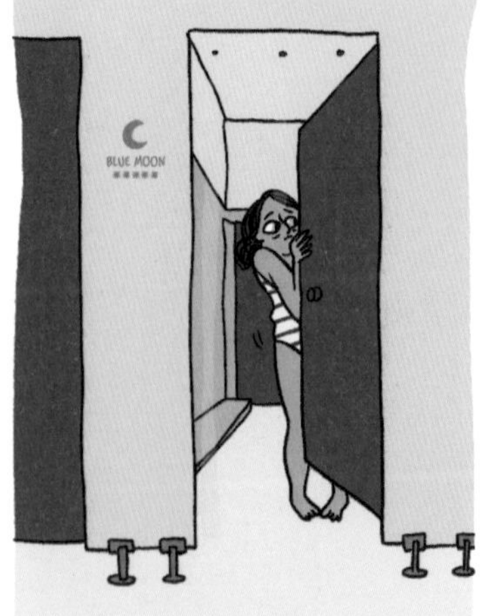
BLUE MOON

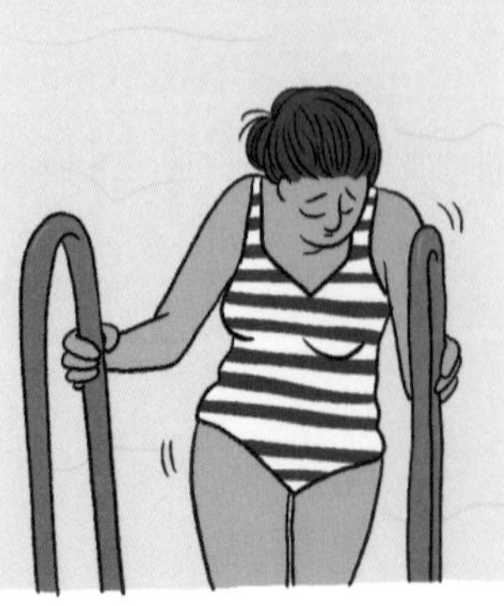

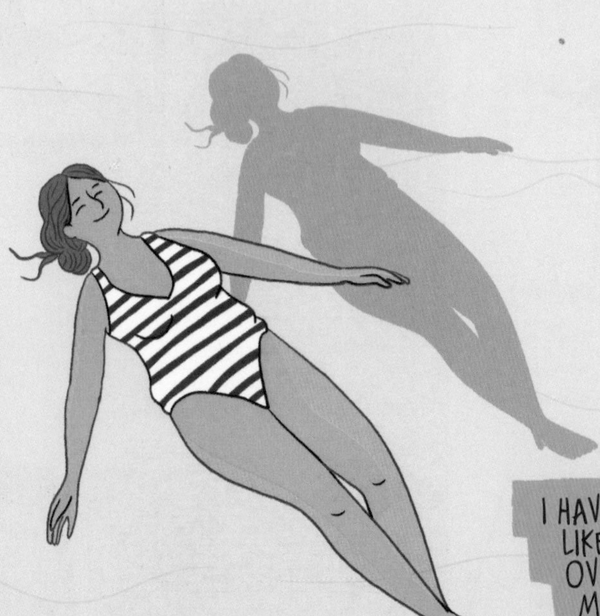
IT ALL FADES.
EVEN ZOE.
IT'S JUST ME NOW.
I HAVEN'T FELT LIKE THIS IN OVER NINE MONTHS.
IT FEELS AMAZING.

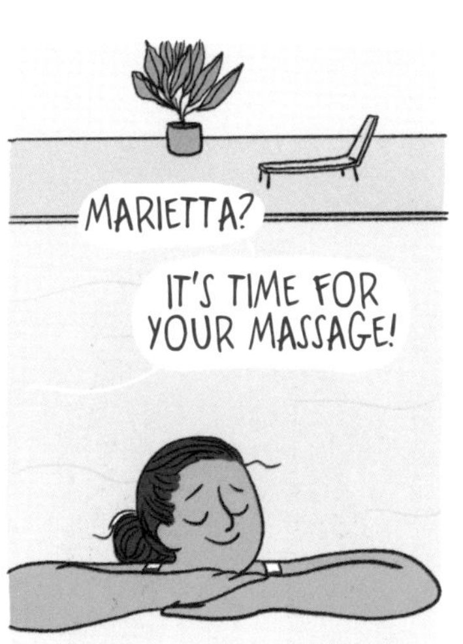
MARIETTA?
IT'S TIME FOR YOUR MASSAGE!

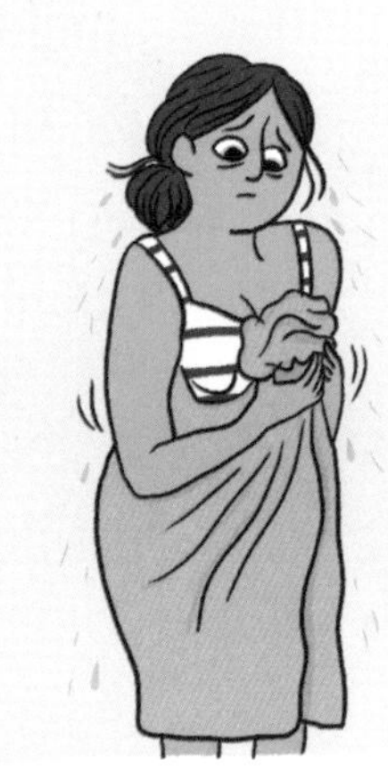

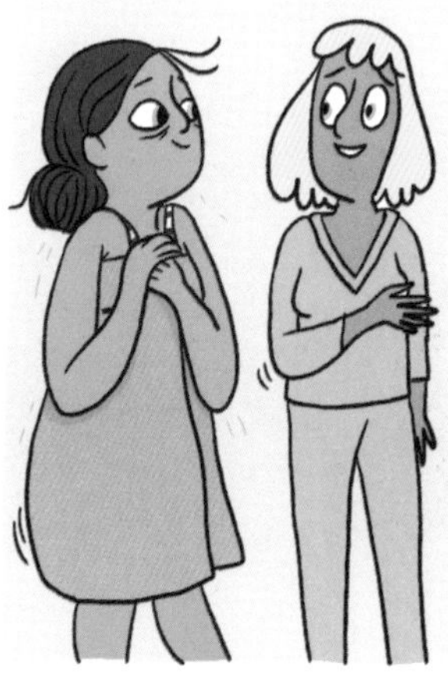
THIS WAY.

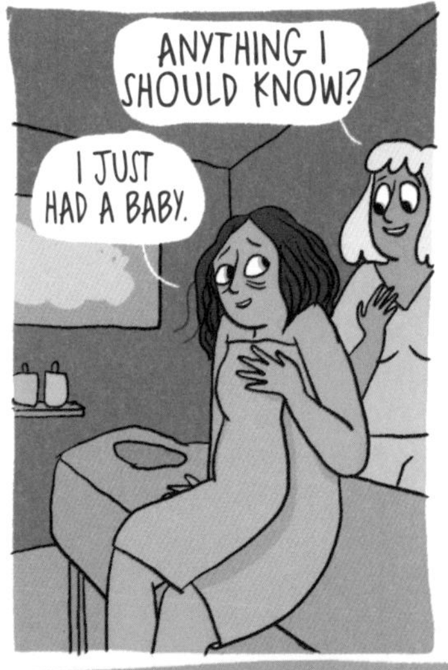
ANYTHING I SHOULD KNOW?
I JUST HAD A BABY.

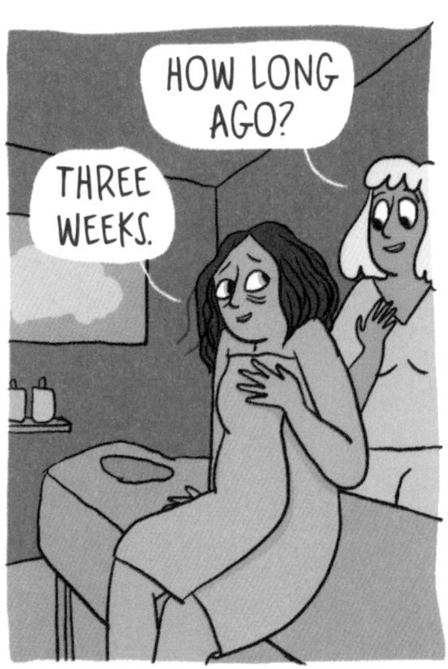
HOW LONG AGO?
THREE WEEKS.

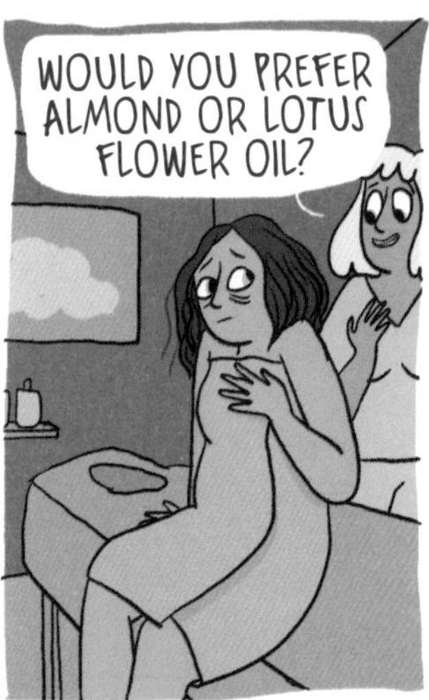
WOULD YOU PREFER ALMOND OR LOTUS FLOWER OIL?

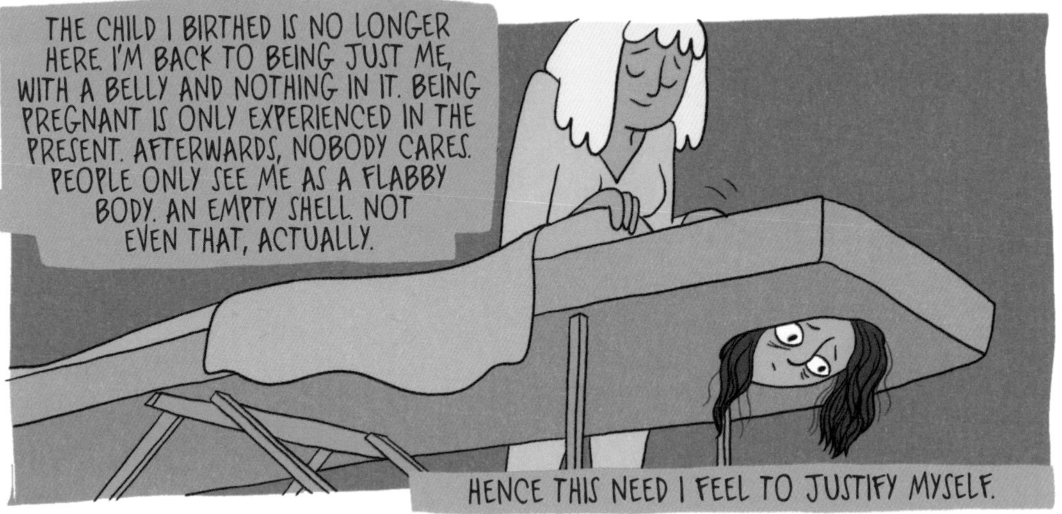
THE CHILD I BIRTHED IS NO LONGER HERE. I'M BACK TO BEING JUST ME, WITH A BELLY AND NOTHING IN IT. BEING PREGNANT IS ONLY EXPERIENCED IN THE PRESENT. AFTERWARDS, NOBODY CARES. PEOPLE ONLY SEE ME AS A FLABBY BODY. AN EMPTY SHELL. NOT EVEN THAT, ACTUALLY.
HENCE THIS NEED I FEEL TO JUSTIFY MYSELF.

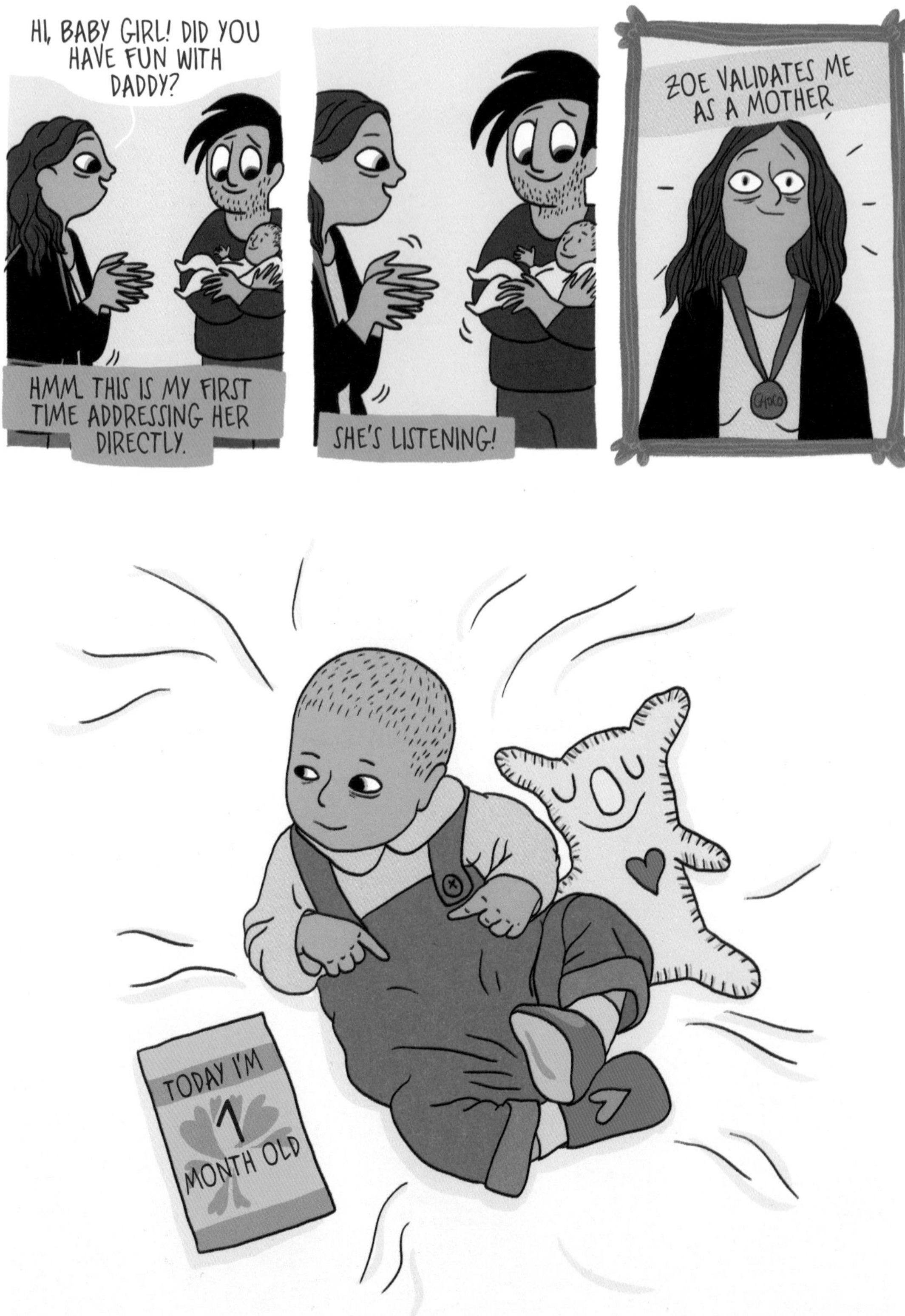

HI, BABY GIRL! DID YOU HAVE FUN WITH DADDY?
HMM. THIS IS MY FIRST TIME ADDRESSING HER DIRECTLY.

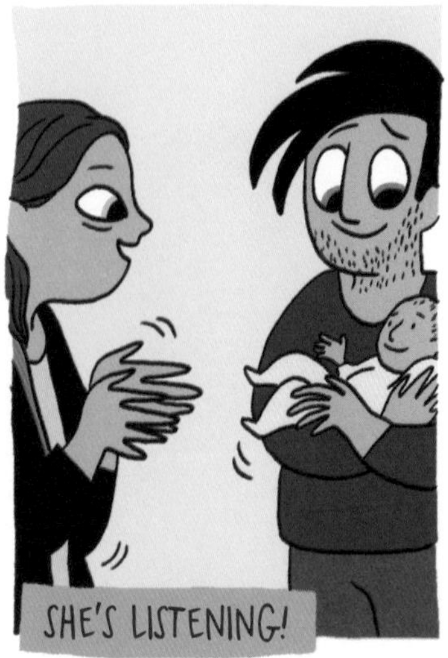

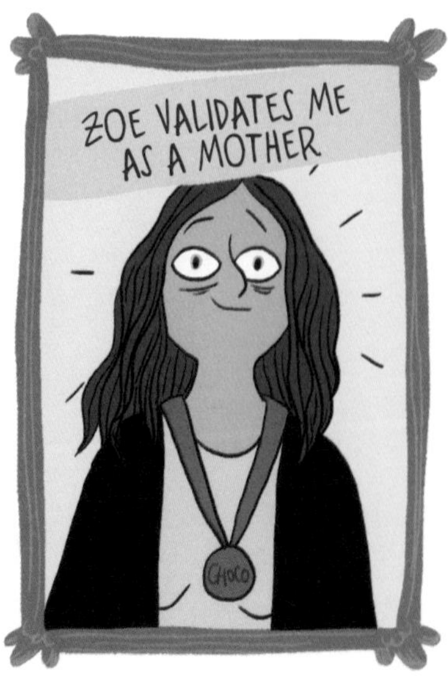

TODAY I'M
1
MONTH OLD

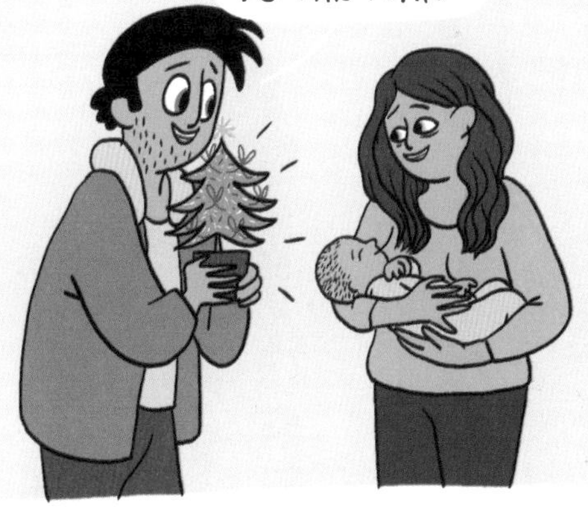
IT'S PLASTIC, BUT IT'S READY TO GO. IT'LL JUST HAVE TO DO THIS YEAR!

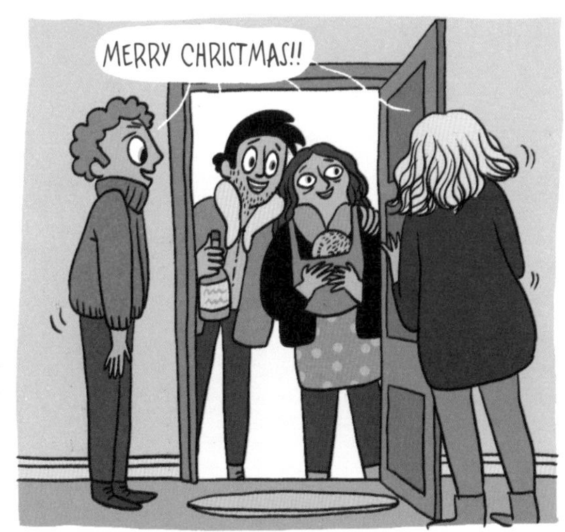
MERRY CHRISTMAS!!

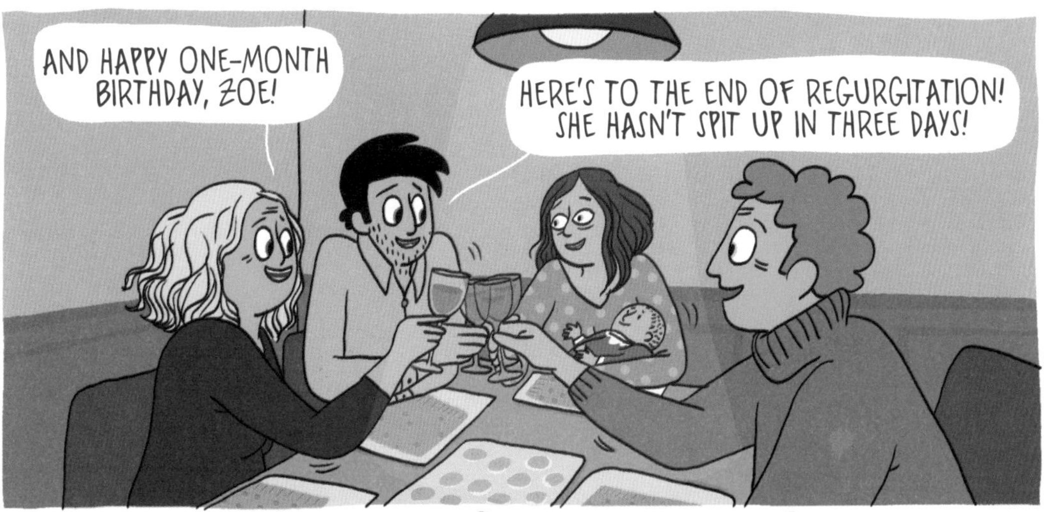
AND HAPPY ONE-MONTH BIRTHDAY, ZOE!
HERE'S TO THE END OF REGURGITATION! SHE HASN'T SPIT UP IN THREE DAYS!

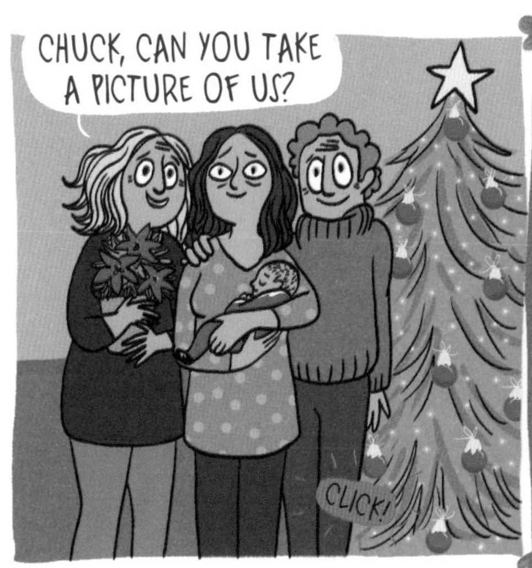
CHUCK, CAN YOU TAKE A PICTURE OF US?
CLICK!

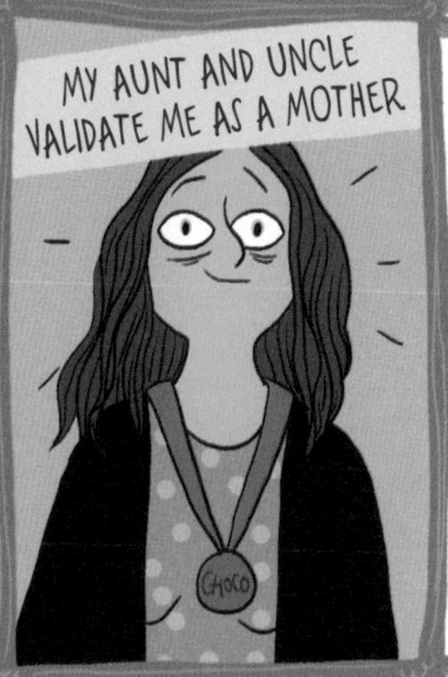
MY AUNT AND UNCLE VALIDATE ME AS A MOTHER
CHOCO

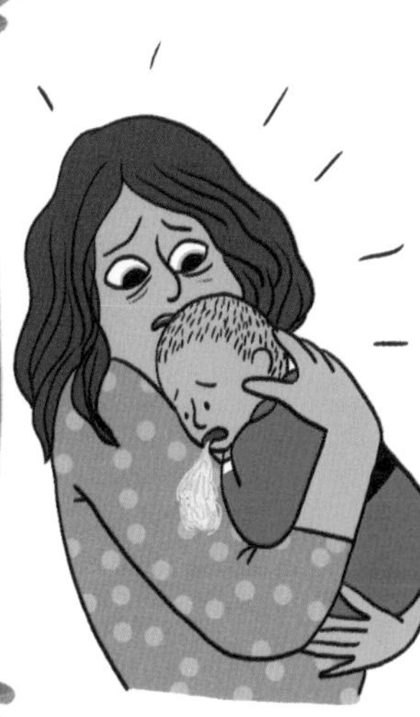

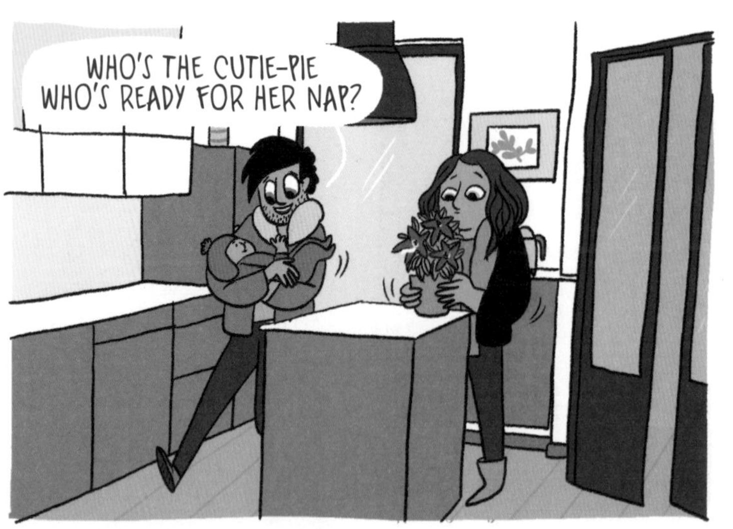
WHO'S THE CUTIE-PIE WHO'S READY FOR HER NAP?

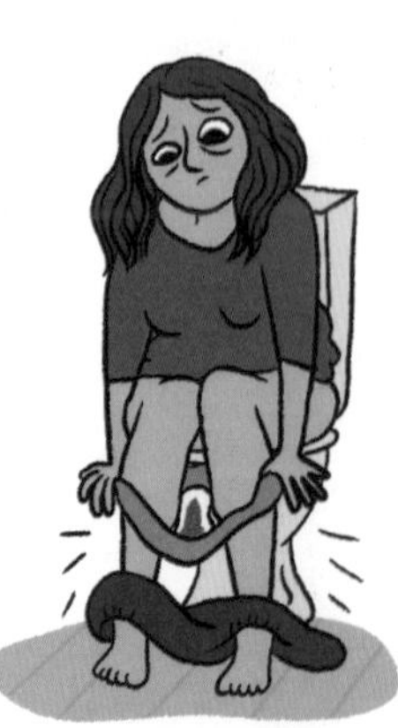
I'VE BEEN BLEEDING FOR A MONTH.

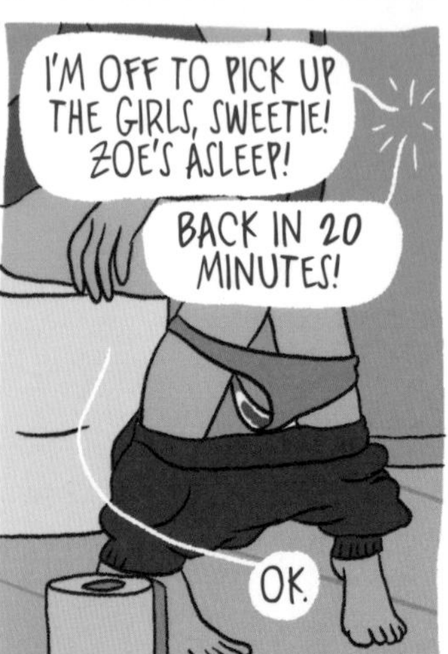
I'M OFF TO PICK UP THE GIRLS, SWEETIE! ZOE'S ASLEEP!
BACK IN 20 MINUTES!
OK.

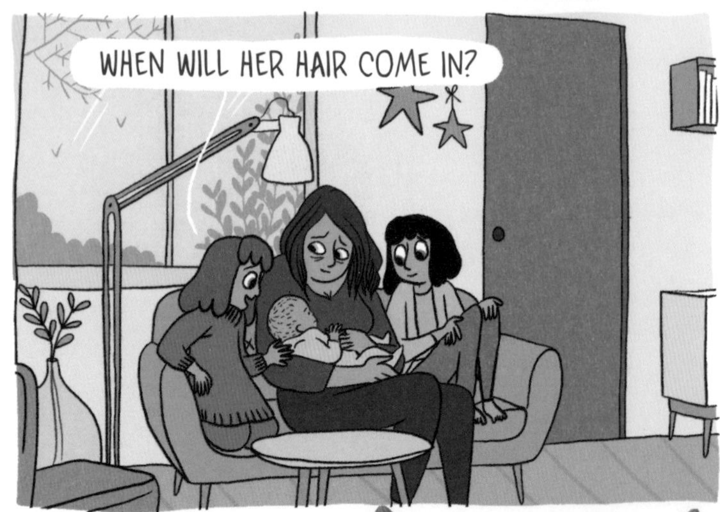
WHEN WILL HER HAIR COME IN?

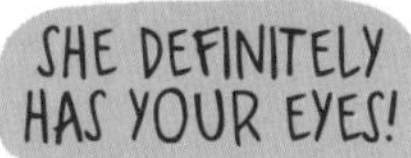
SHE DEFINITELY HAS YOUR EYES!

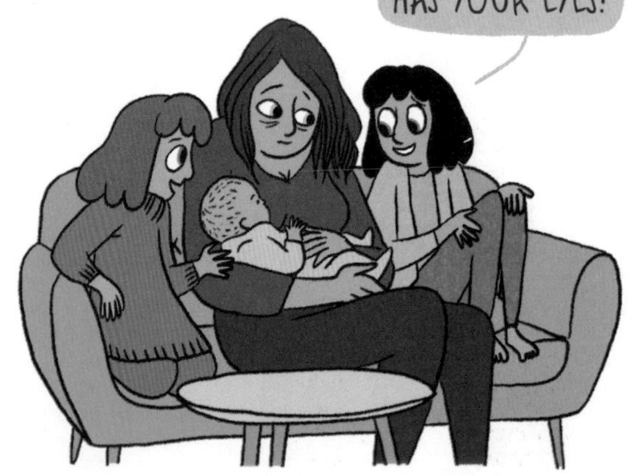

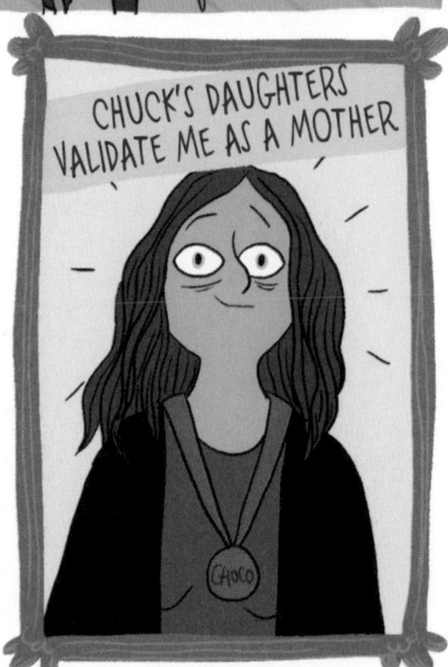
CHUCK'S DAUGHTERS VALIDATE ME AS A MOTHER
CHOCO

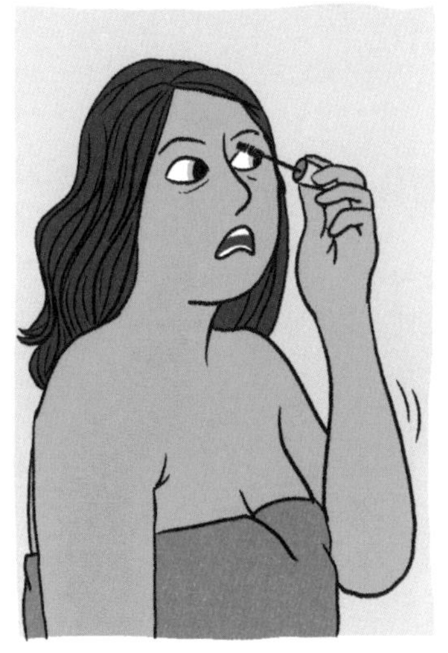
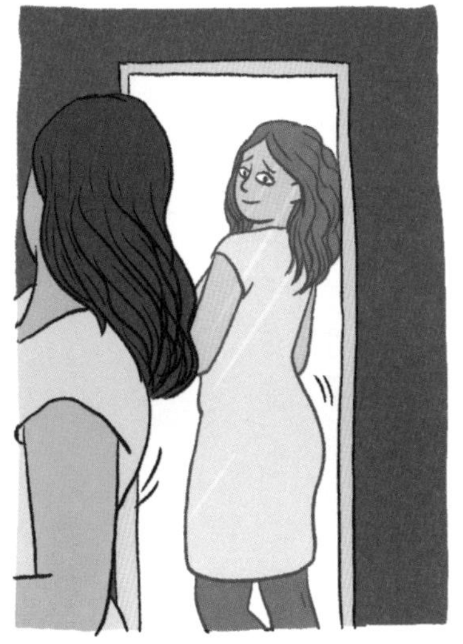
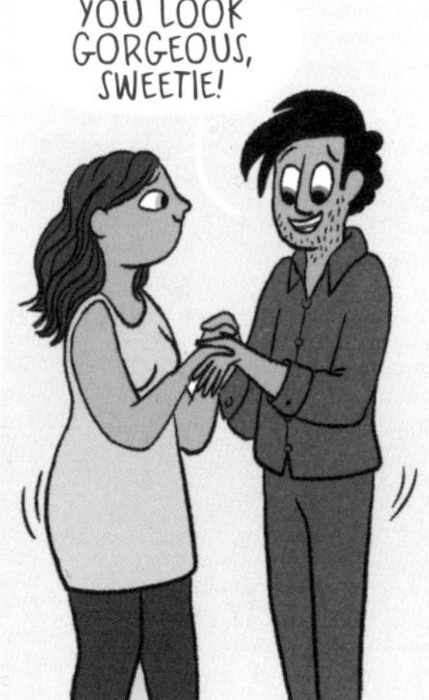
YOU LOOK GORGEOUS, SWEETIE!
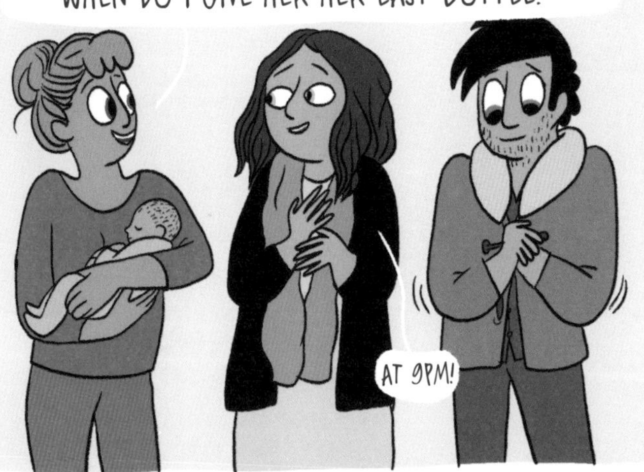
WHEN DO I GIVE HER HER LAST BOTTLE?
AT 9PM!
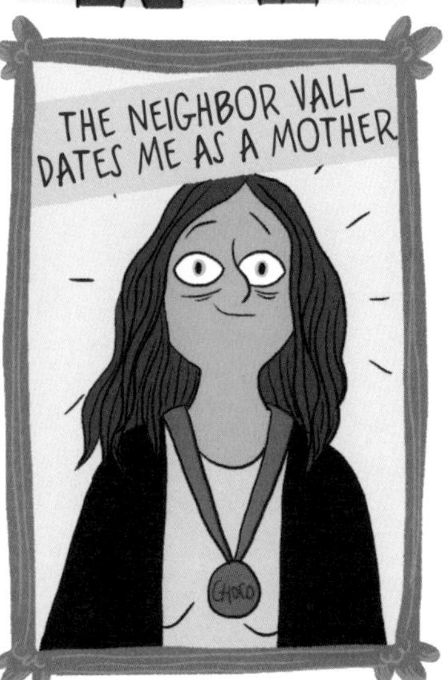
THE NEIGHBOR VALI-DATES ME AS A MOTHER
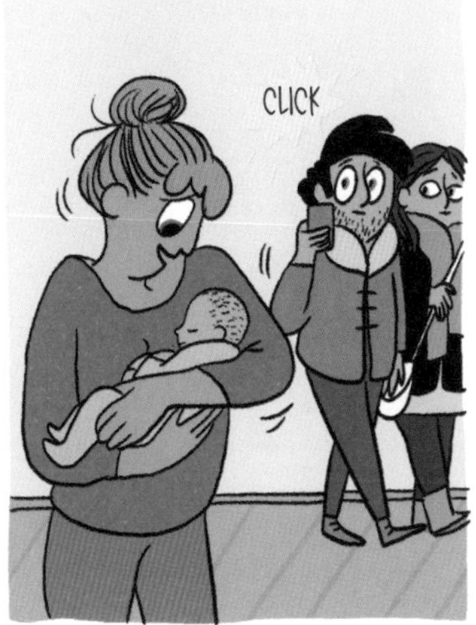
CLICK
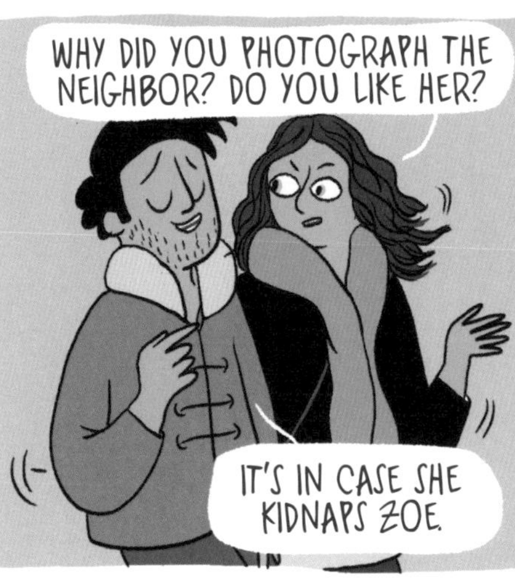
WHY DID YOU PHOTOGRAPH THE NEIGHBOR? DO YOU LIKE HER?
IT'S IN CASE SHE KIDNAPS ZOE.
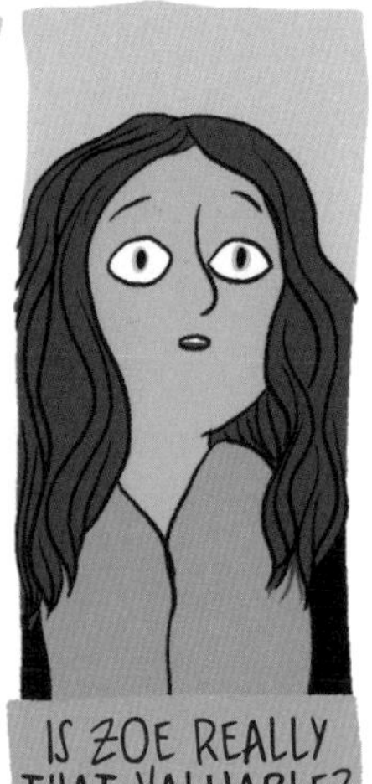
IS ZOE REALLY THAT VALUABLE?

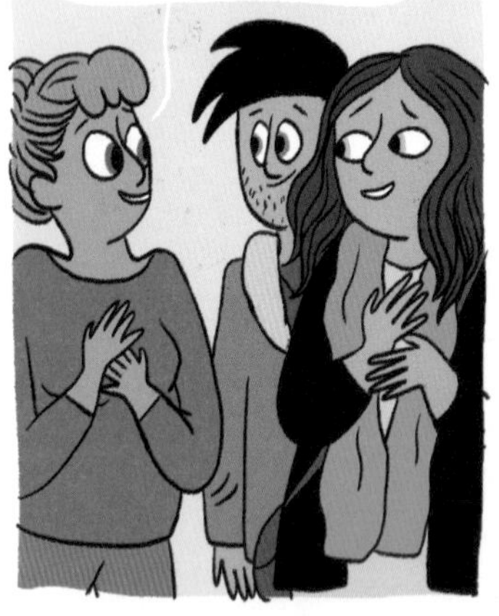
IT WENT GREAT! SHE'S ADORABLE!

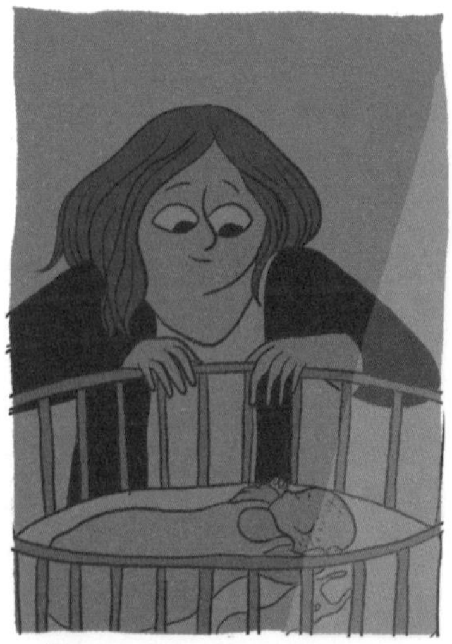

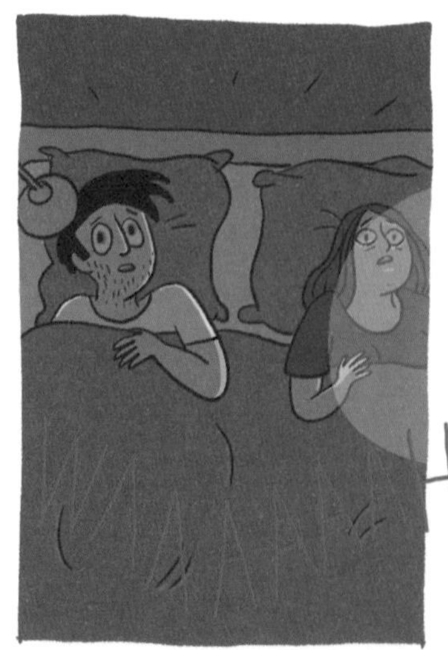
WAAAAAH

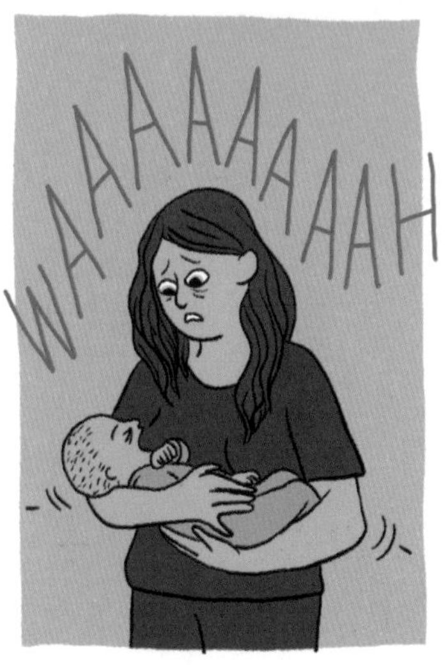
WAAAAAAAAH

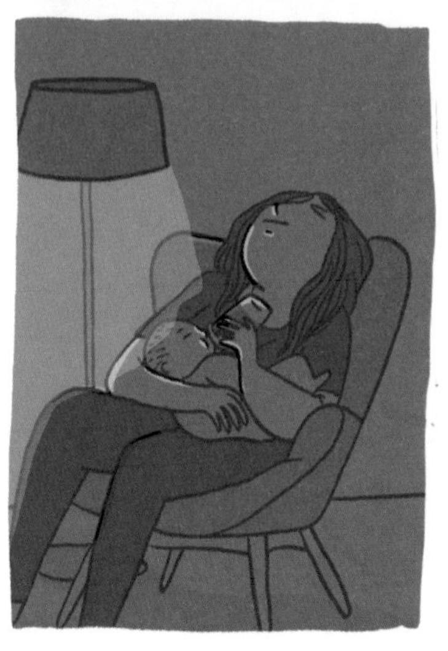

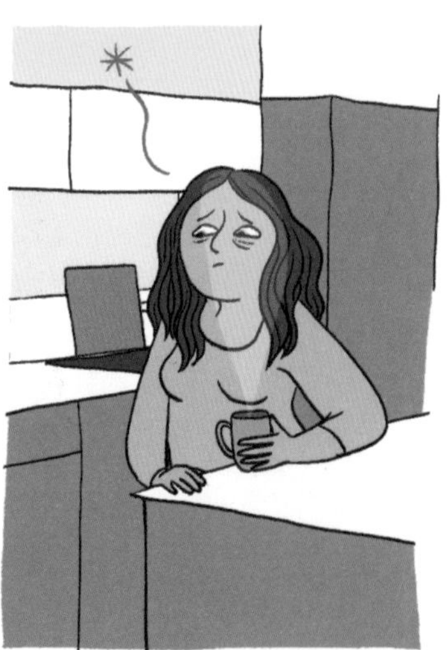

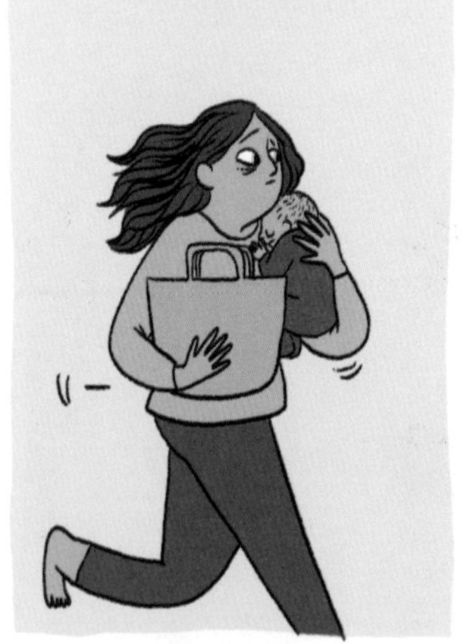

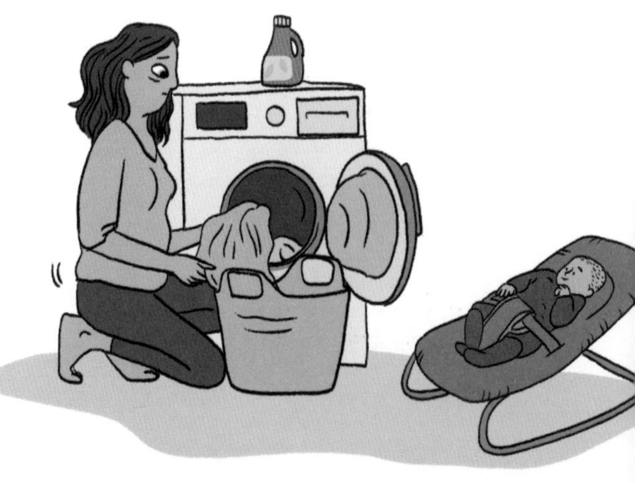

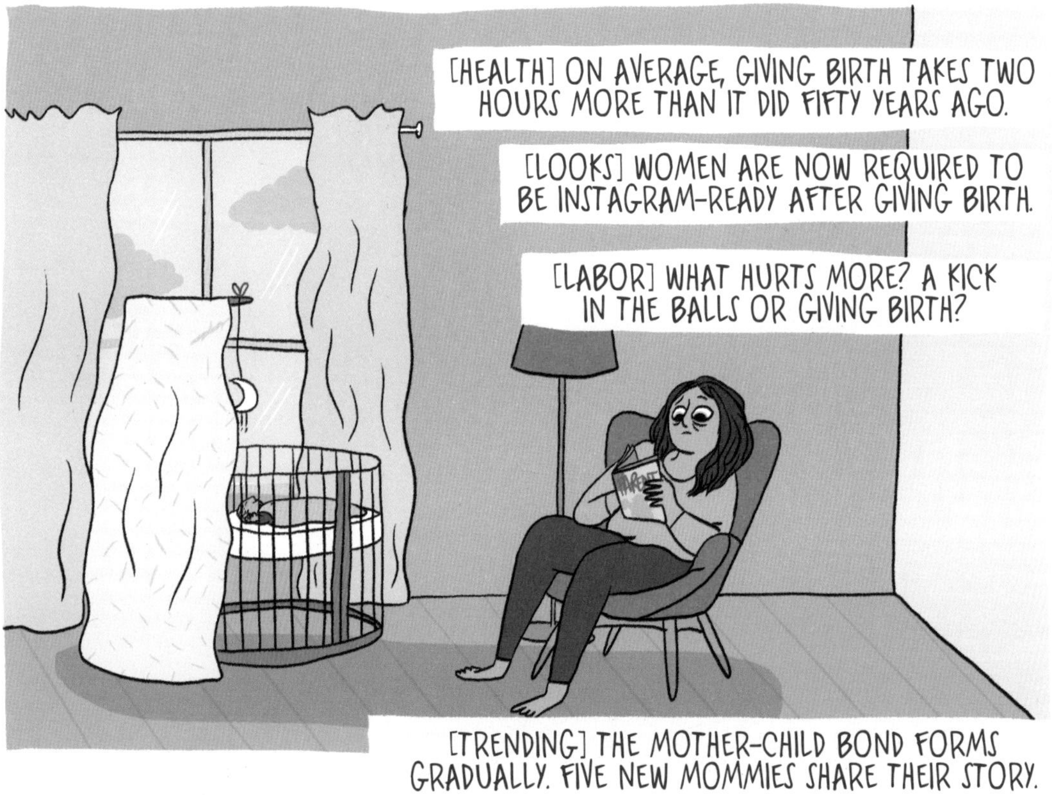

[HEALTH] ON AVERAGE, GIVING BIRTH TAKES TWO HOURS MORE THAN IT DID FIFTY YEARS AGO.

[LOOKS] WOMEN ARE NOW REQUIRED TO BE INSTAGRAM-READY AFTER GIVING BIRTH.

[LABOR] WHAT HURTS MORE? A KICK IN THE BALLS OR GIVING BIRTH?

[TRENDING] THE MOTHER-CHILD BOND FORMS GRADUALLY. FIVE NEW MOMMIES SHARE THEIR STORY.

WHEN WILL I START TO BOND?
I WANT TO BE A GOOD MOTHER. A WONDER-MOM. THAT'S HOW I ALWAYS PICTURED MYSELF. BUT REALITY IS A WHOLE DIFFERENT STORY. I DON'T FEEL ANYTHING EVEN REMOTELY CLOSE TO A MATERNAL INSTINCT, AT LEAST NOT AS I UNDERSTAND IT. I DON'T FEEL THE NEED TO BREASTFEED HER. I DON'T THINK I COULD SACRIFICE EVERYTHING FOR HER EXISTENCE AND HER CRYING DOESN'T BREAK MY HEART.

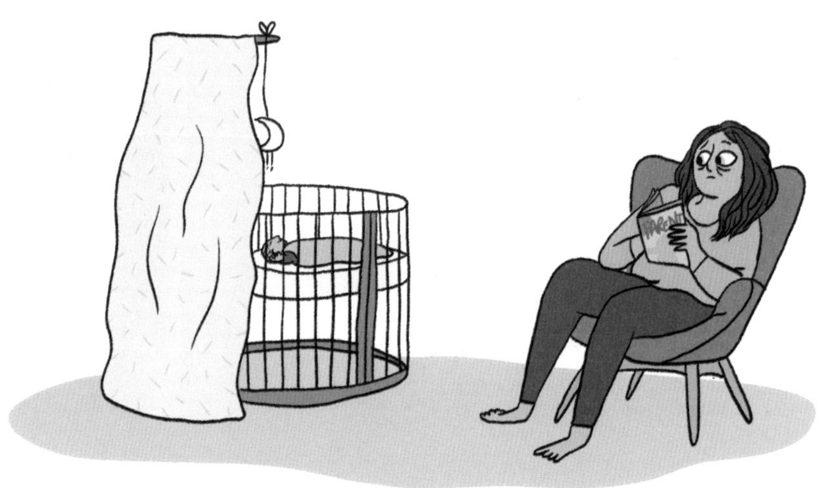

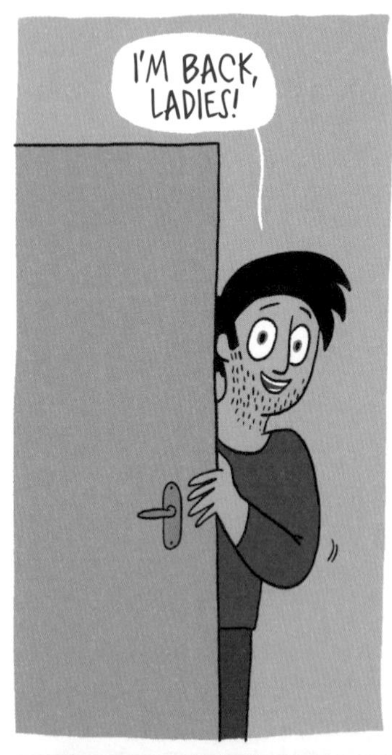
I'M BACK, LADIES!

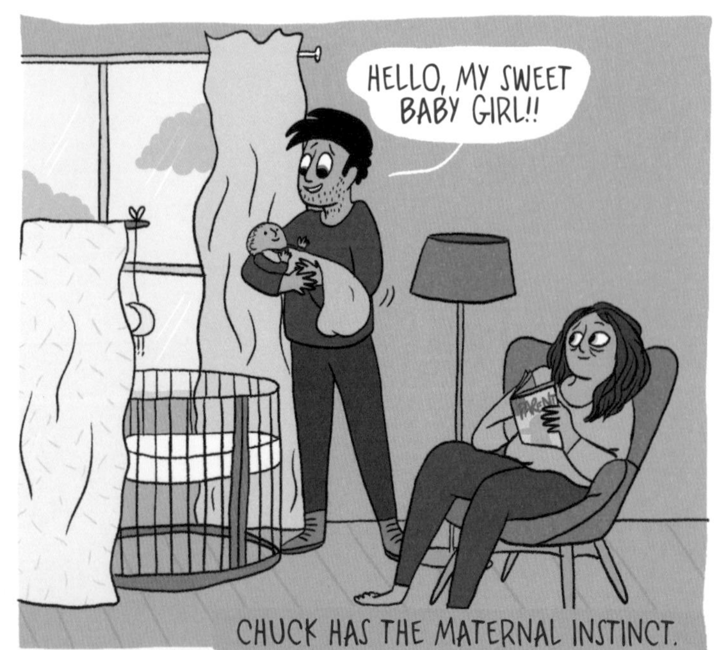
HELLO, MY SWEET BABY GIRL!!
CHUCK HAS THE MATERNAL INSTINCT.

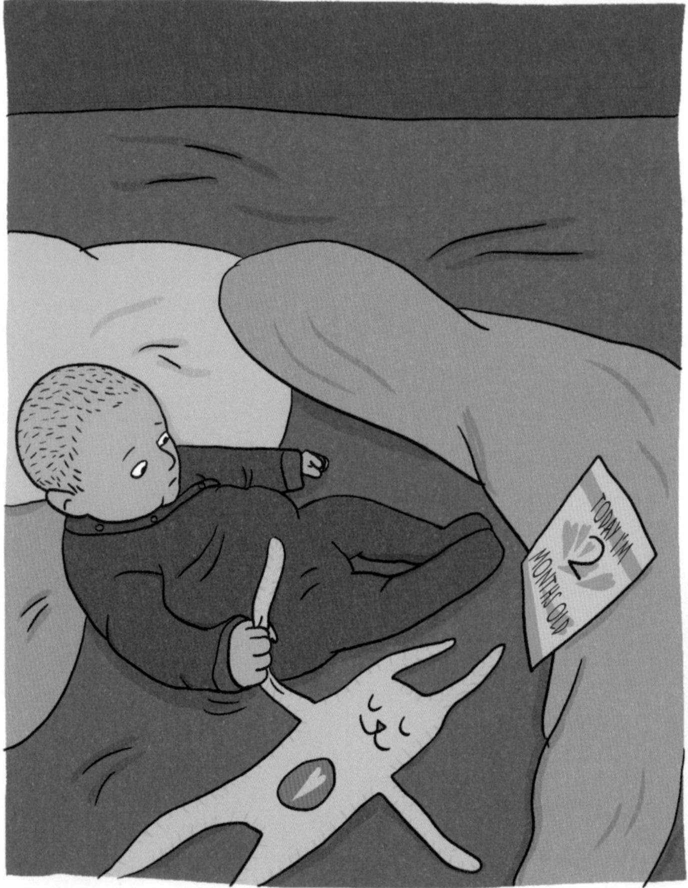
TODAY I'M
2
MONTHS OLD

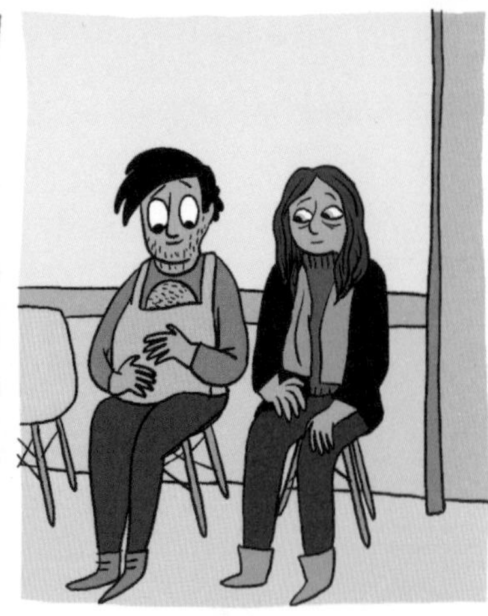

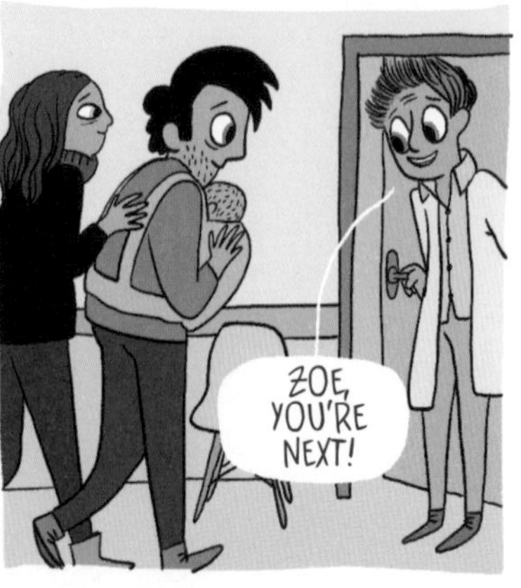
ZOE, YOU'RE NEXT!

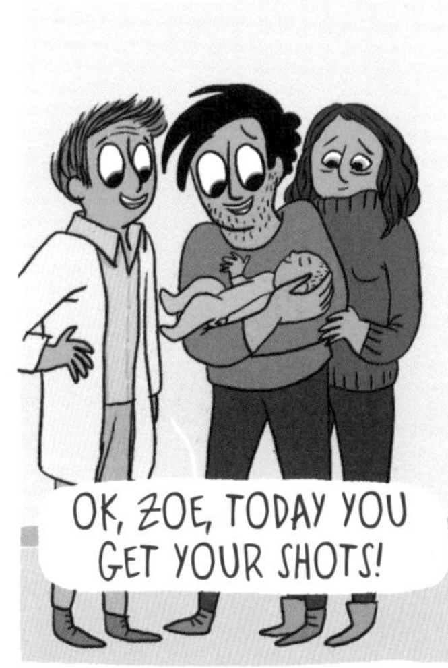
OK, ZOE, TODAY YOU GET YOUR SHOTS!

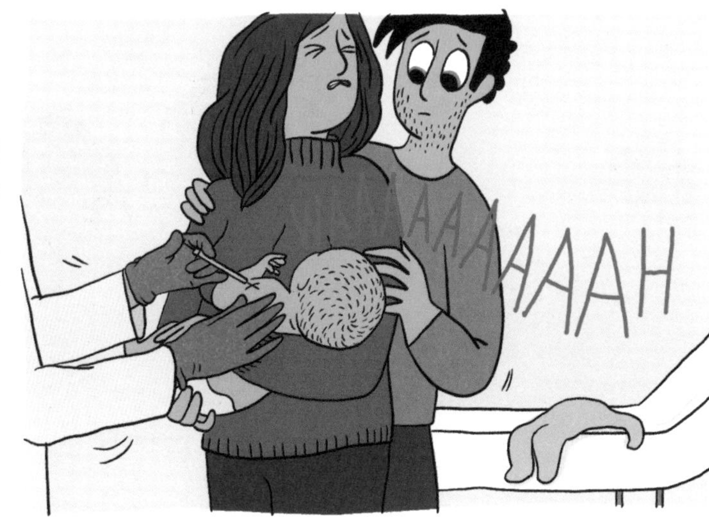
WAHAAAAAAAH

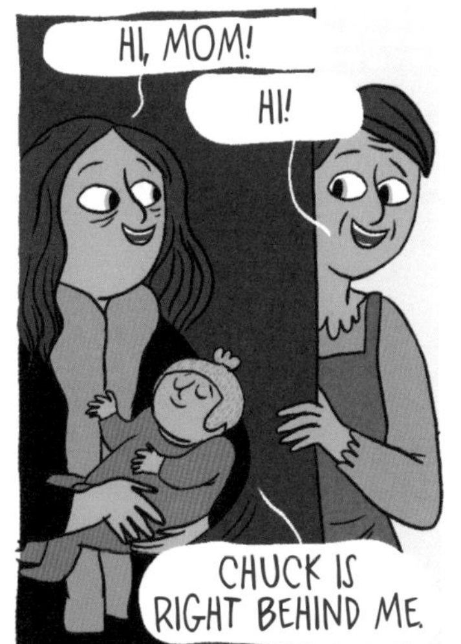
HI, MOM!
HI!
CHUCK IS RIGHT BEHIND ME.

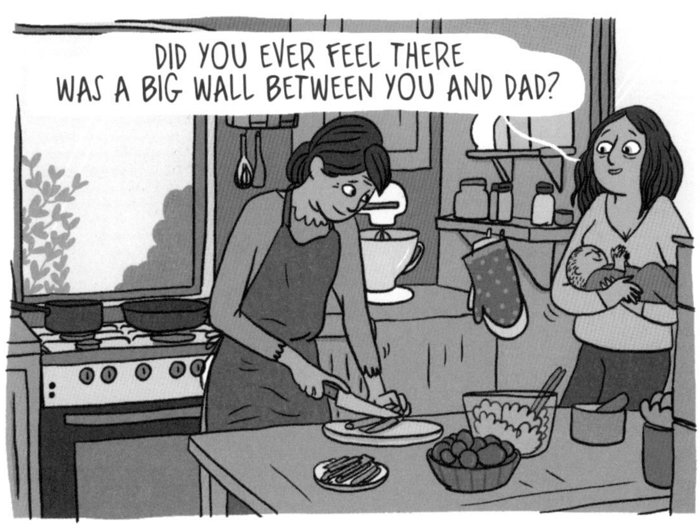
DID YOU EVER FEEL THERE WAS A BIG WALL BETWEEN YOU AND DAD?

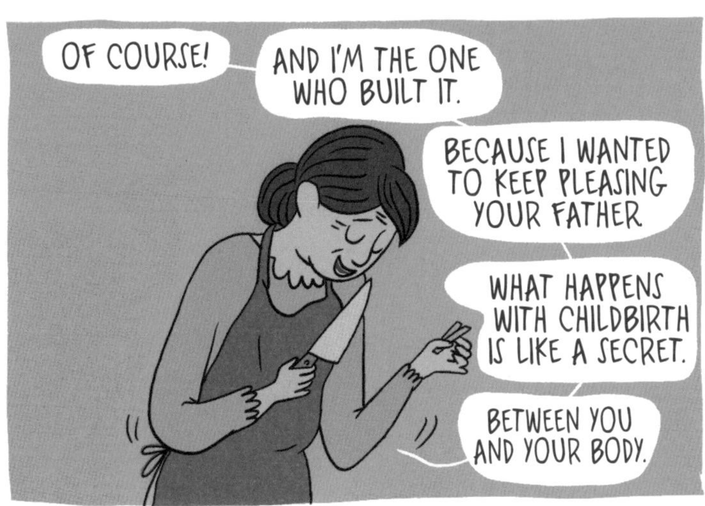
OF COURSE!
AND I'M THE ONE WHO BUILT IT.
BECAUSE I WANTED TO KEEP PLEASING YOUR FATHER.
WHAT HAPPENS WITH CHILDBIRTH IS LIKE A SECRET.
BETWEEN YOU AND YOUR BODY.

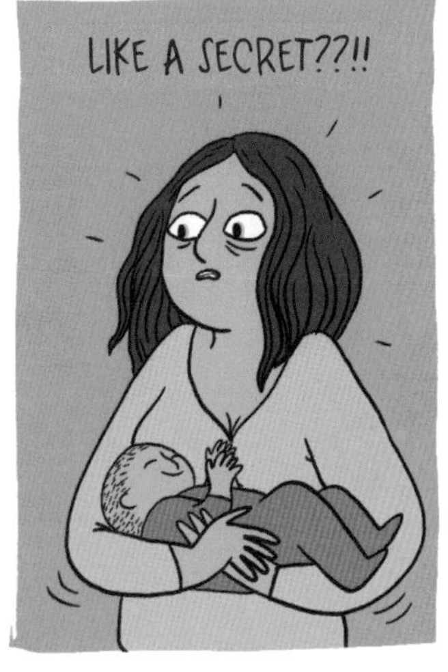
LIKE A SECRET??!!

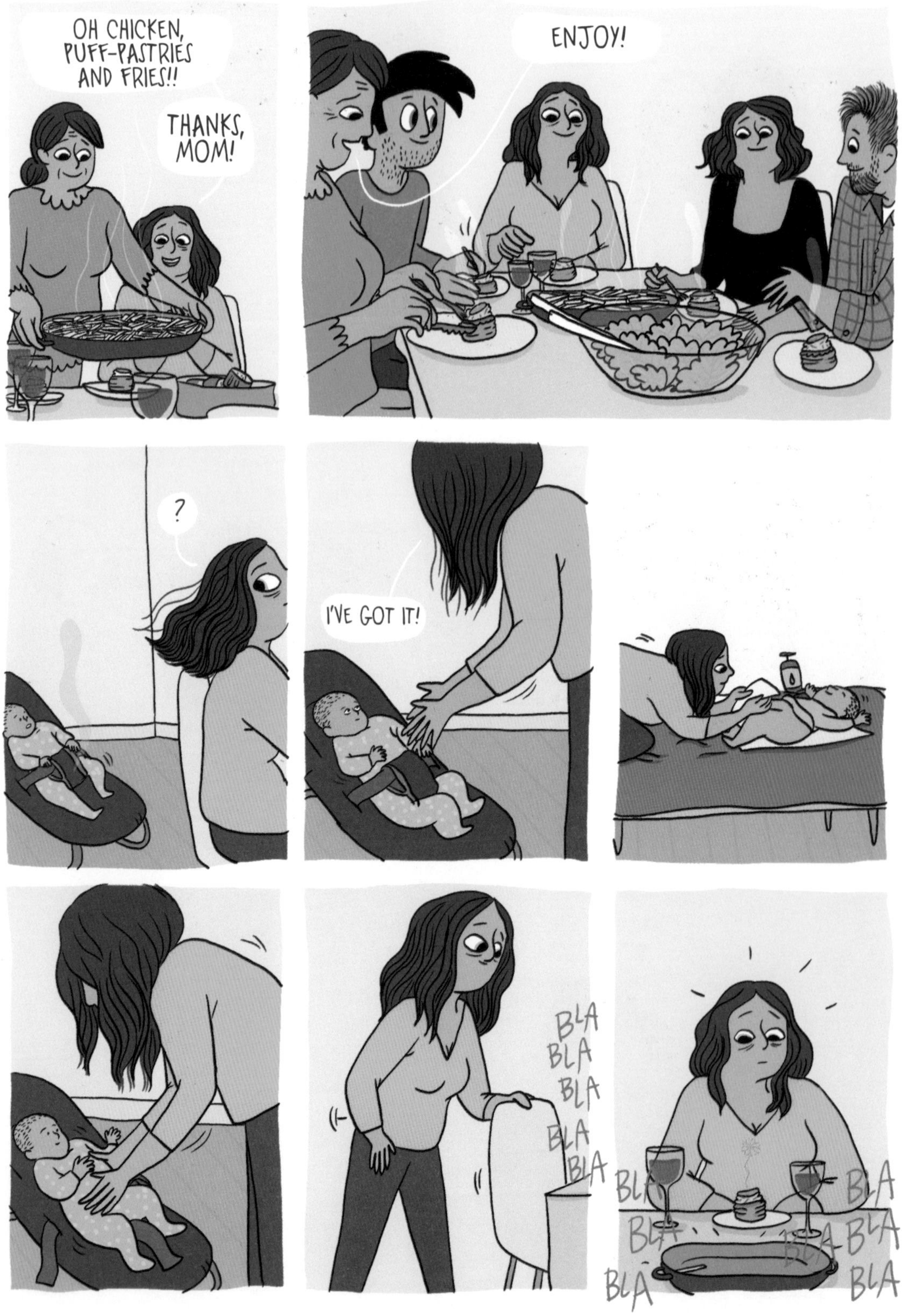

OH CHICKEN, PUFF-PASTRIES AND FRIES!!

THANKS, MOM!

ENJOY!

?

I'VE GOT IT!

BLA
BLA
BLA
BLA
BLA

BLA
BLA
BLA

BLA
BLA
BLA
BLA

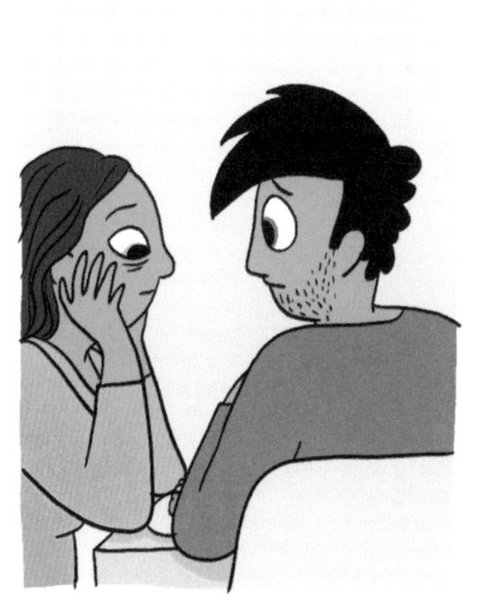

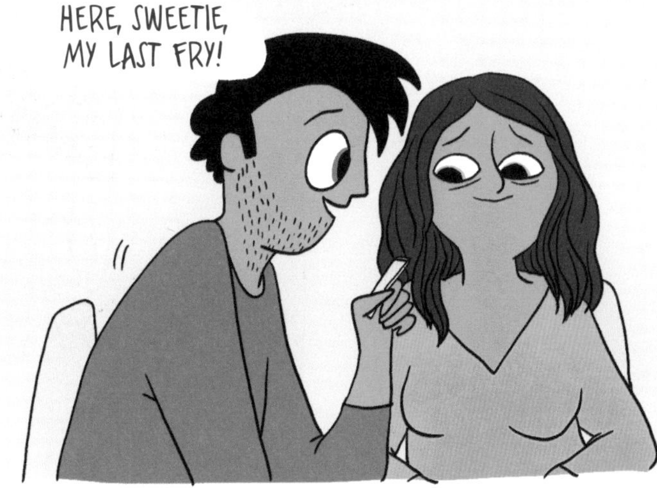
HERE, SWEETIE, MY LAST FRY!

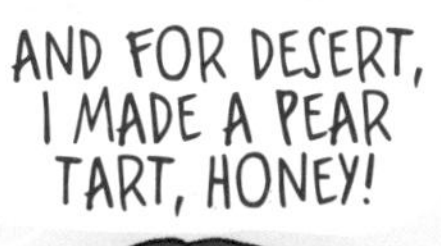
AND FOR DESERT, I MADE A PEAR TART, HONEY!

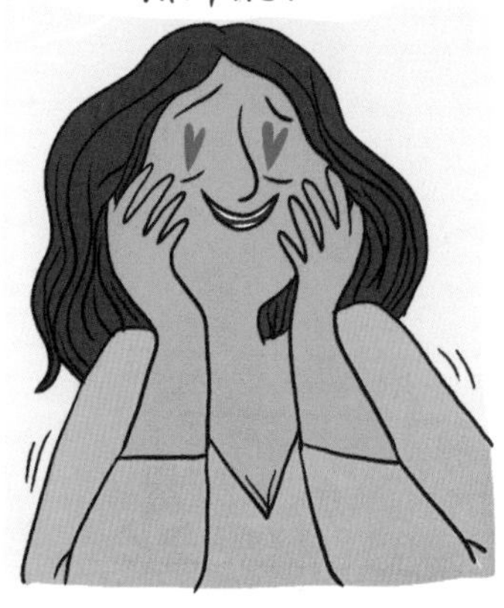

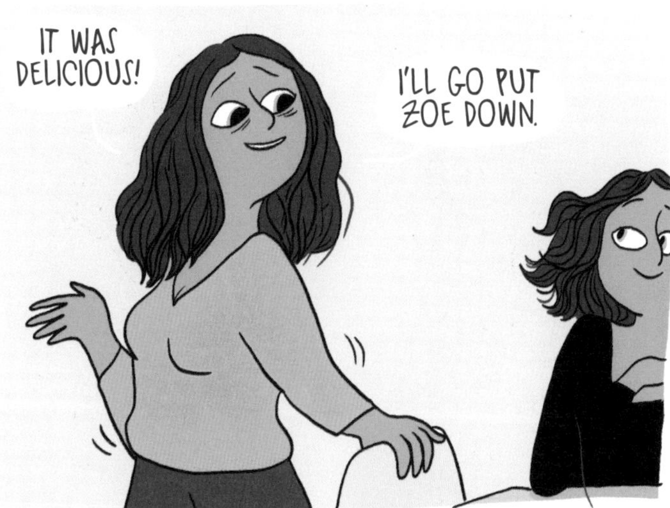
IT WAS DELICIOUS!
I'LL GO PUT ZOE DOWN.

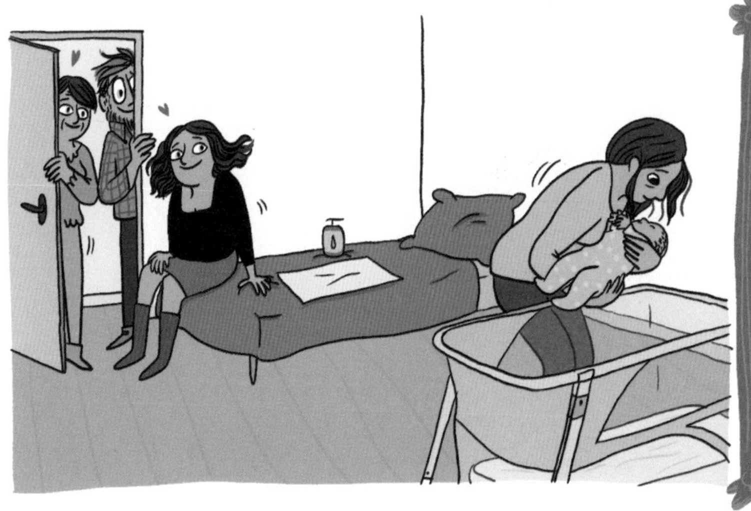

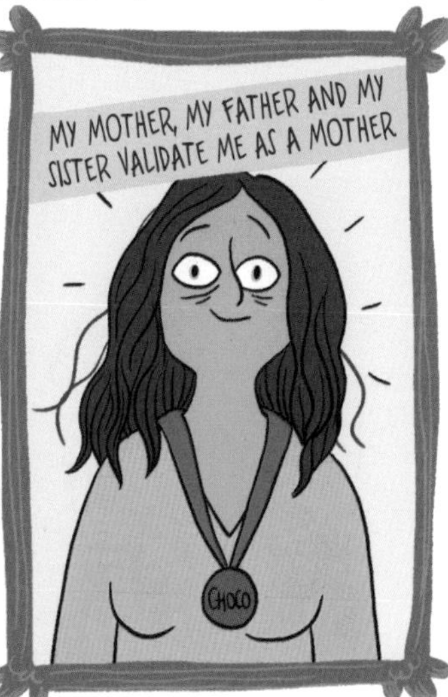
MY MOTHER, MY FATHER AND MY SISTER VALIDATE ME AS A MOTHER
CHOCO

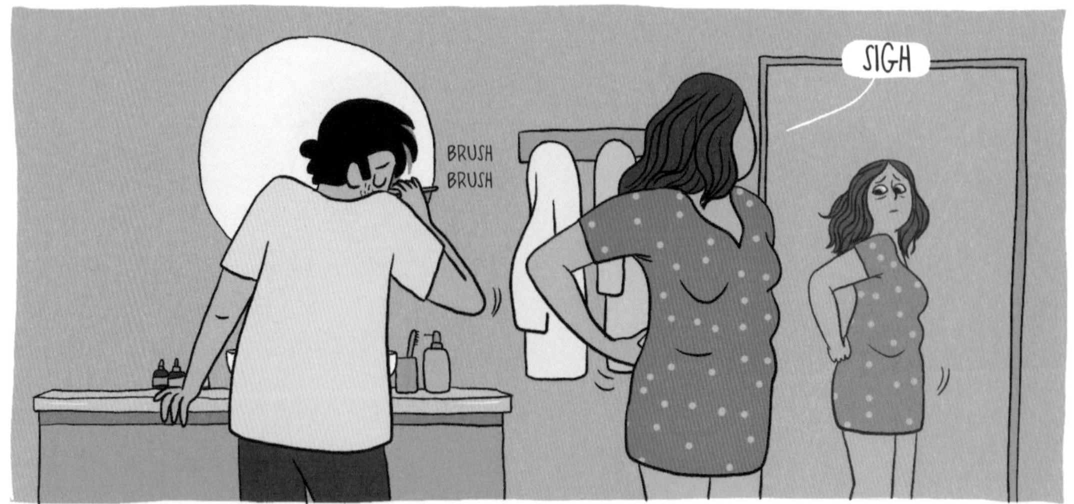
BRUSH
BRUSH
SIGH

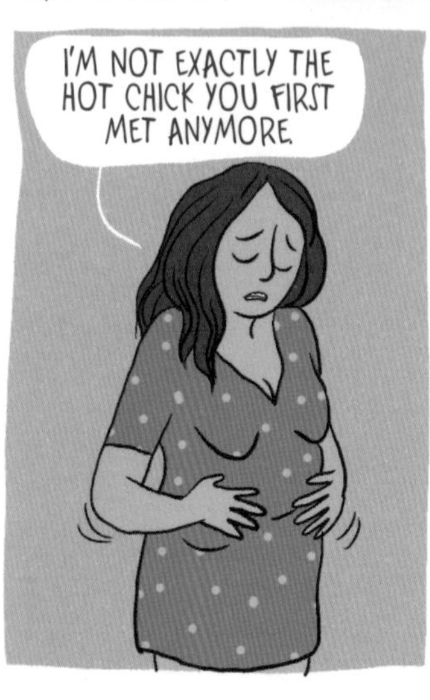
I'M NOT EXACTLY THE HOT CHICK YOU FIRST MET ANYMORE.

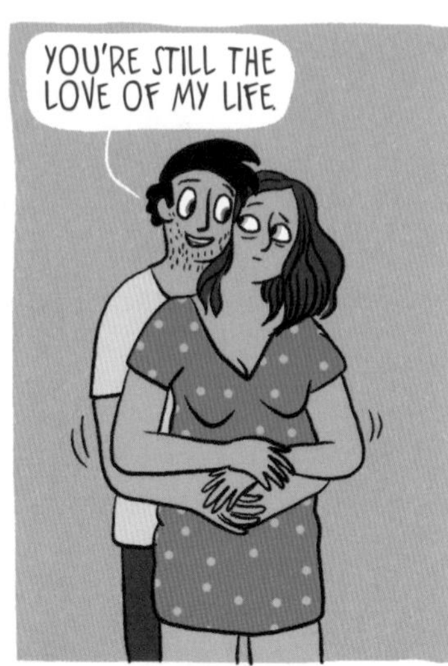
YOU'RE STILL THE LOVE OF MY LIFE.

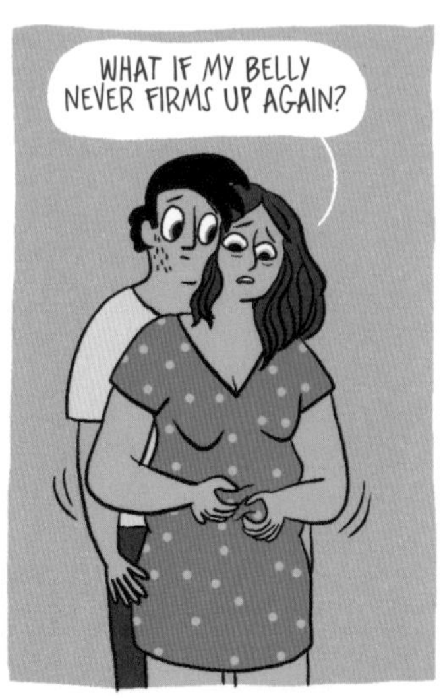
WHAT IF MY BELLY NEVER FIRMS UP AGAIN?

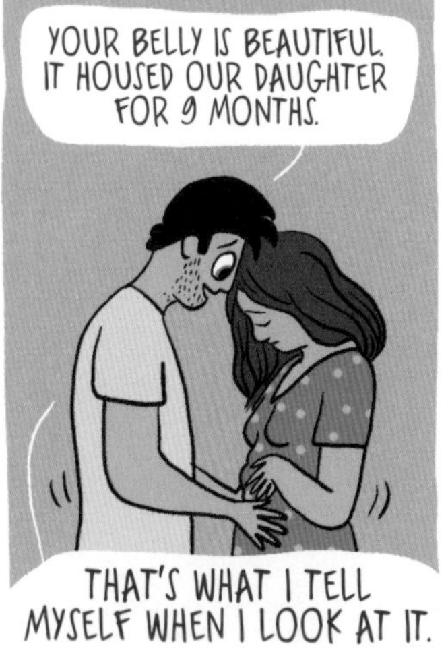
YOUR BELLY IS BEAUTIFUL. IT HOUSED OUR DAUGHTER FOR 9 MONTHS.
THAT'S WHAT I TELL MYSELF WHEN I LOOK AT IT.

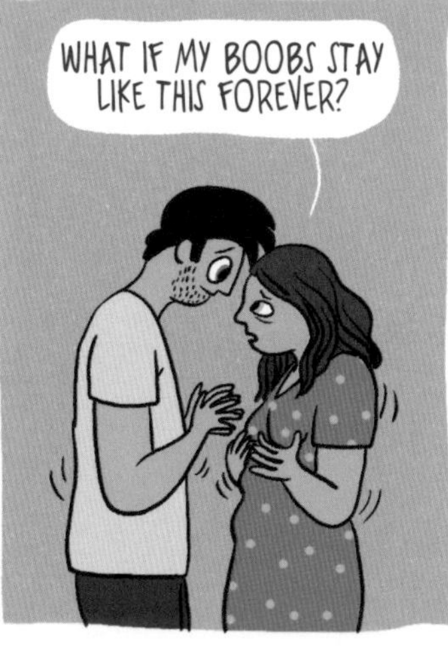
WHAT IF MY BOOBS STAY LIKE THIS FOREVER?

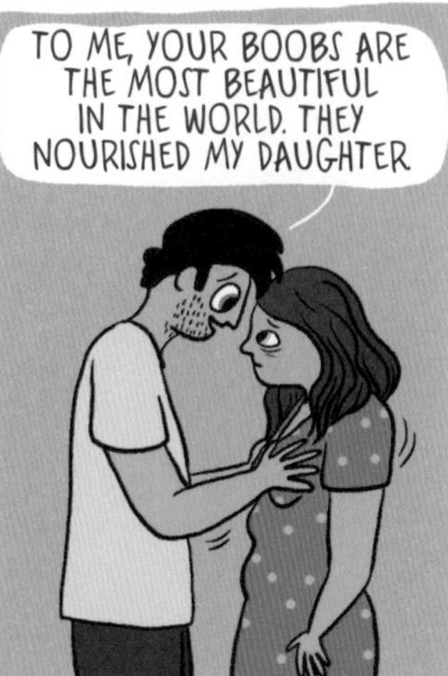
TO ME, YOUR BOOBS ARE THE MOST BEAUTIFUL IN THE WORLD. THEY NOURISHED MY DAUGHTER

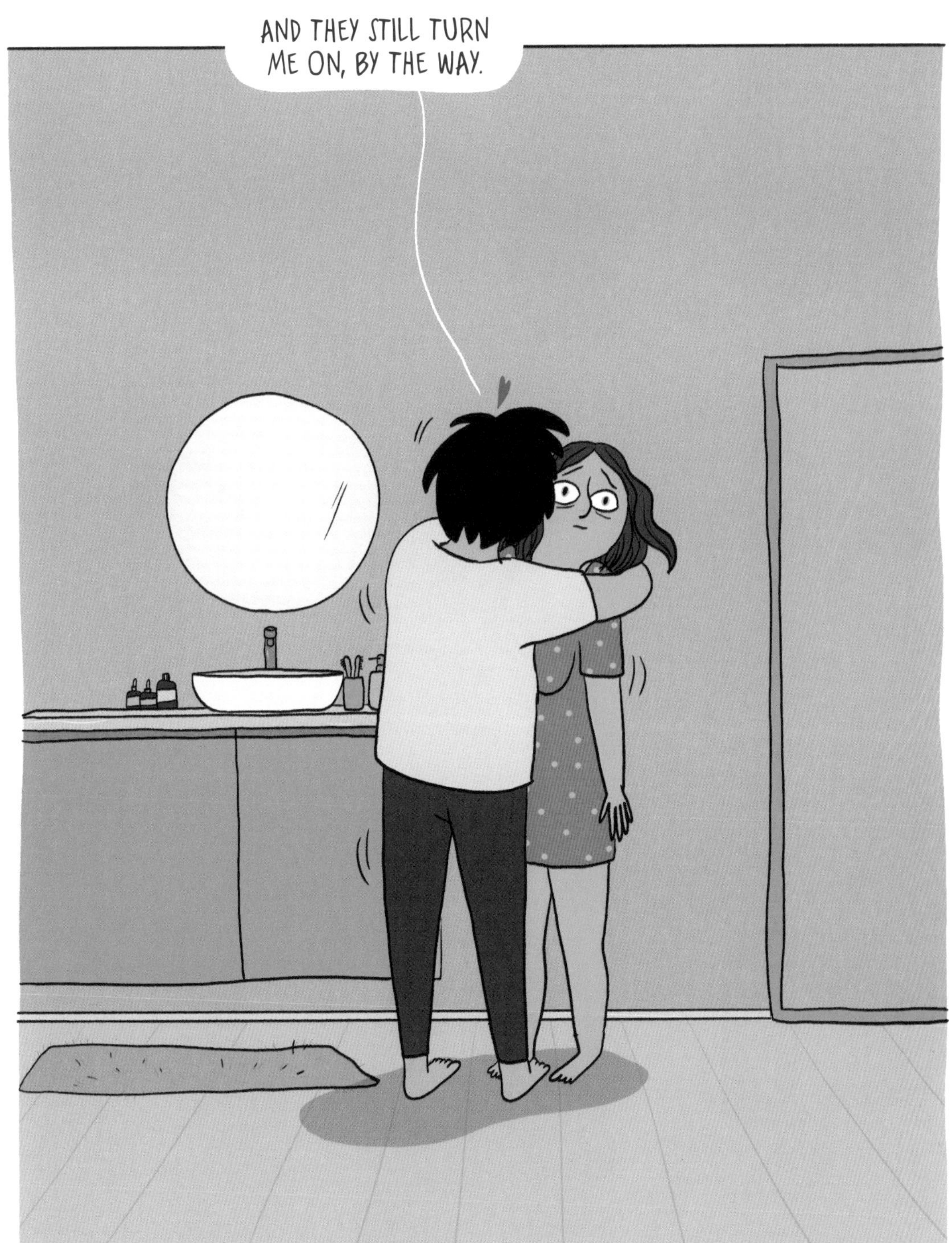
AND THEY STILL TURN ME ON, BY THE WAY.

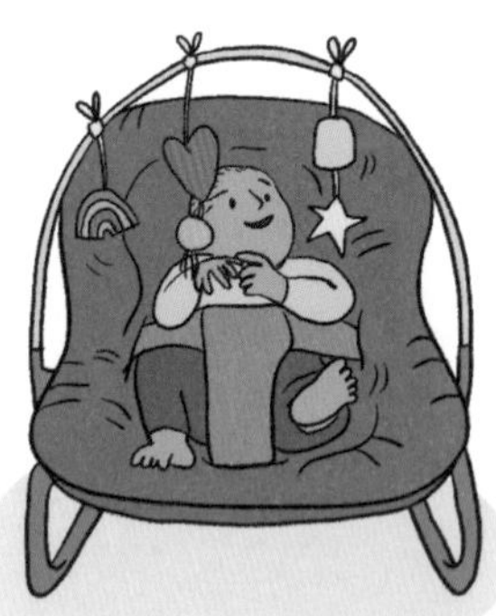
OH, LOOK, SHE'S SMILING!

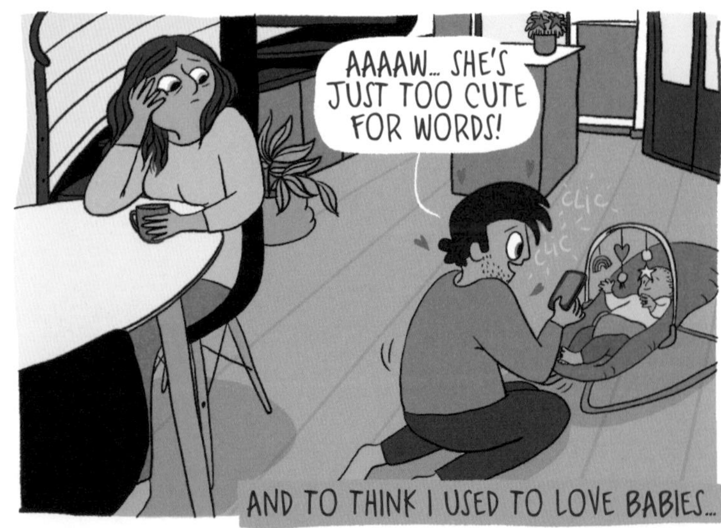
AAAAW... SHE'S JUST TOO CUTE FOR WORDS!
CLIC
CLIC
AND TO THINK I USED TO LOVE BABIES...

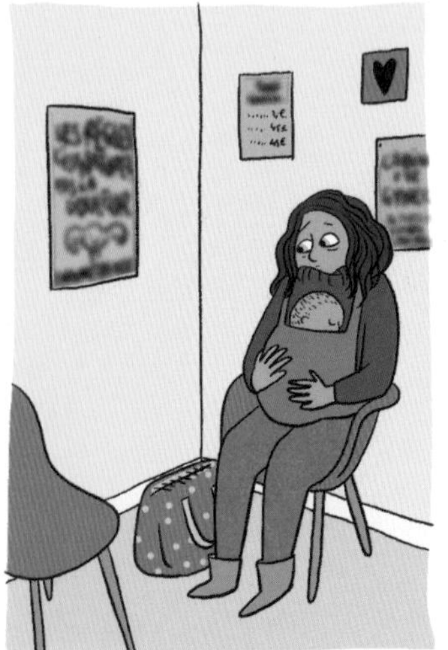

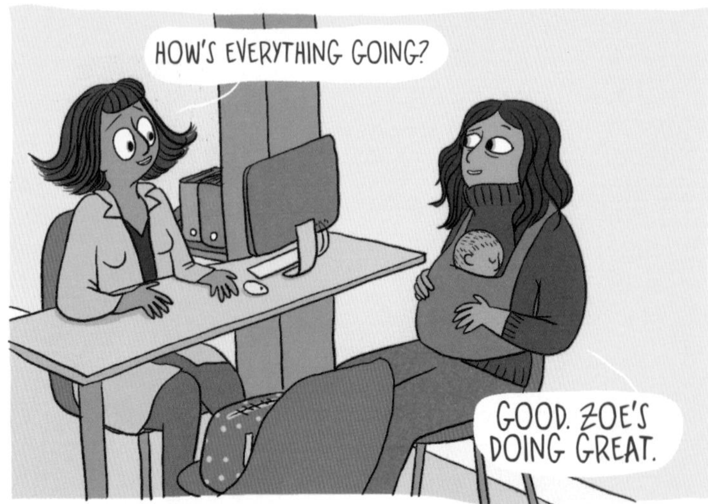
HOW'S EVERYTHING GOING?
GOOD. ZOE'S DOING GREAT.

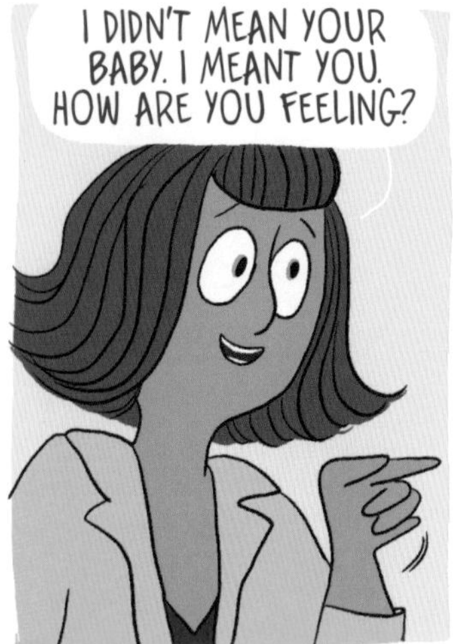
I DIDN'T MEAN YOUR BABY. I MEANT YOU. HOW ARE YOU FEELING?

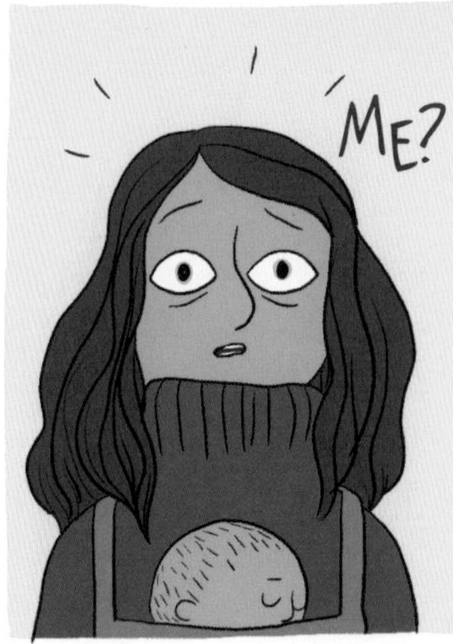
ME?

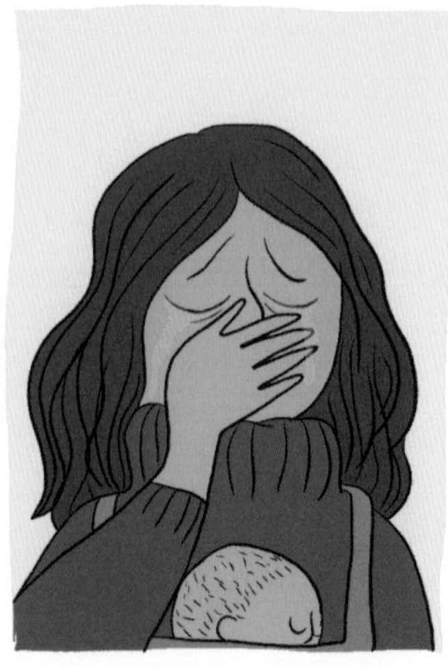

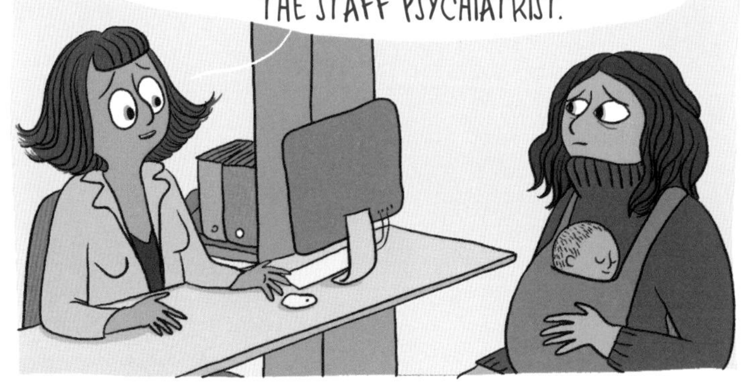

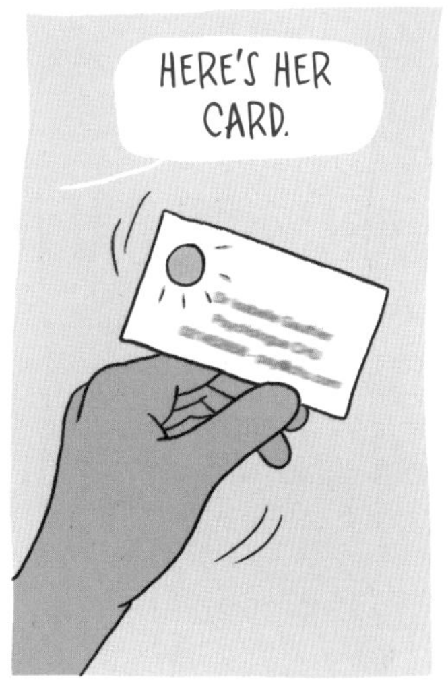

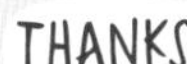

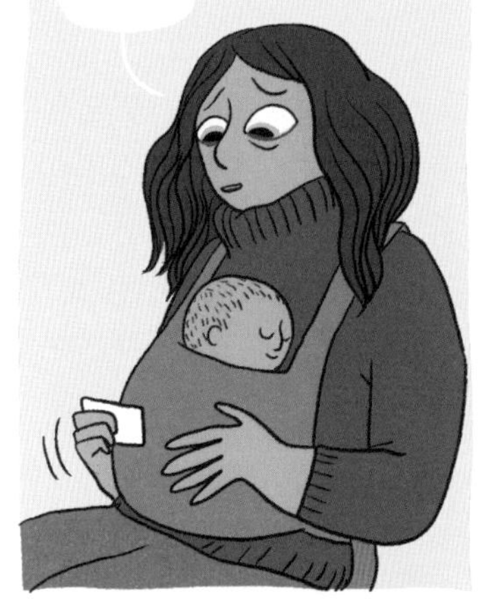

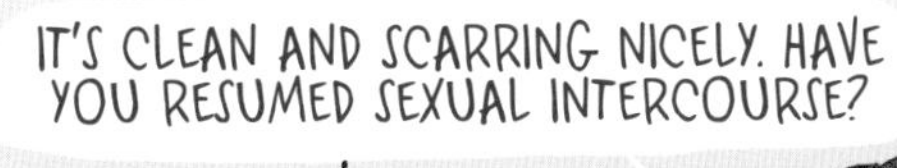

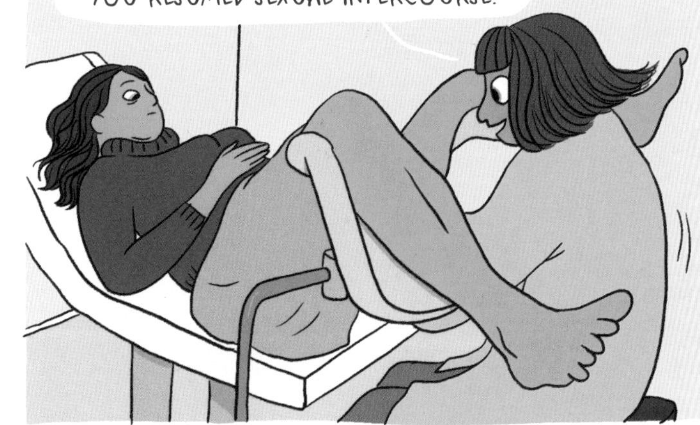

I'M HAUNTED BY THE IMAGE OF MY DAUGHTER COMING OUT OF MY VAGINA WITH A VENTOUSE, AND THE ONE OF THE MIDWIFE STITCHING ME UP DOWN THERE. WHERE IT STILL HURTS AT TIMES. HOW ON EARTH CAN I THINK ABOUT SEX?

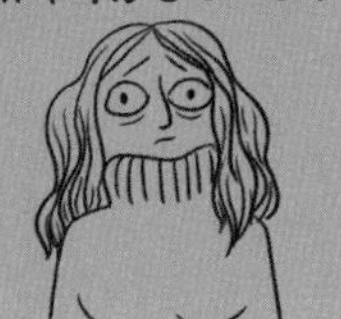

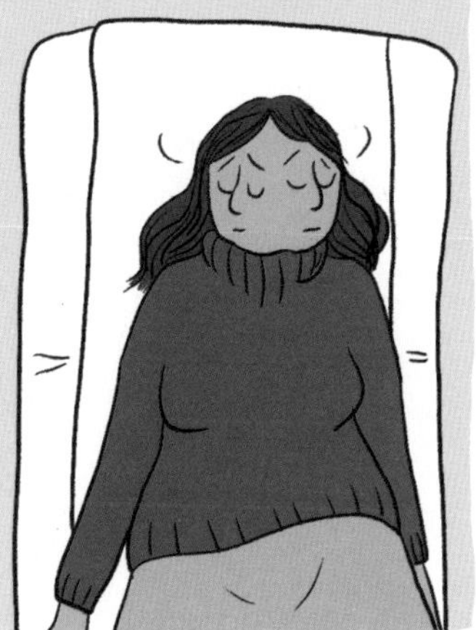

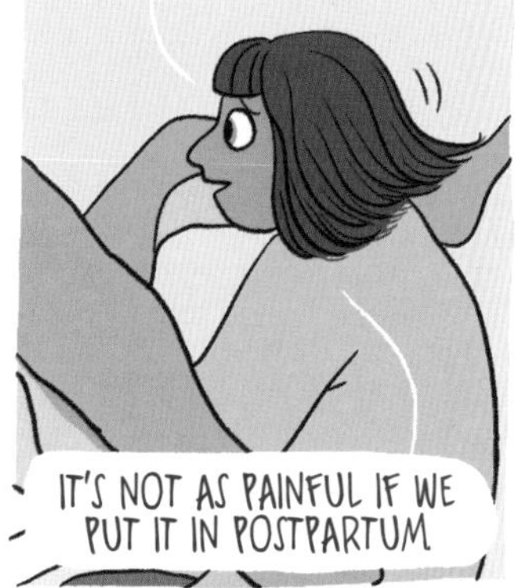

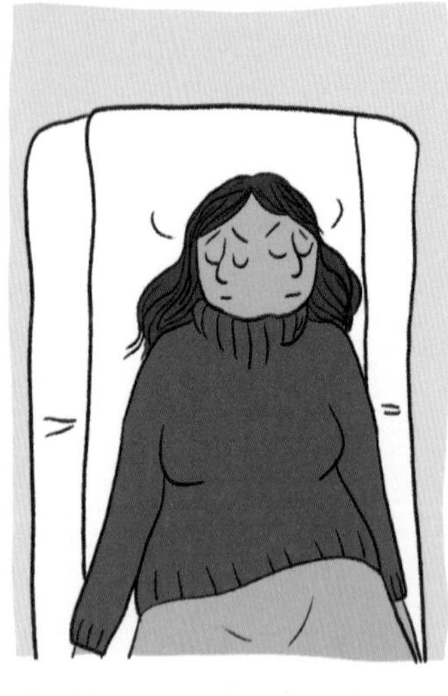

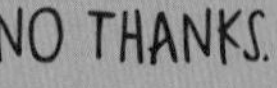

I'M NOT READY FOR SOMEONE TO GO RUMMAGING AROUND IN THERE AGAIN.

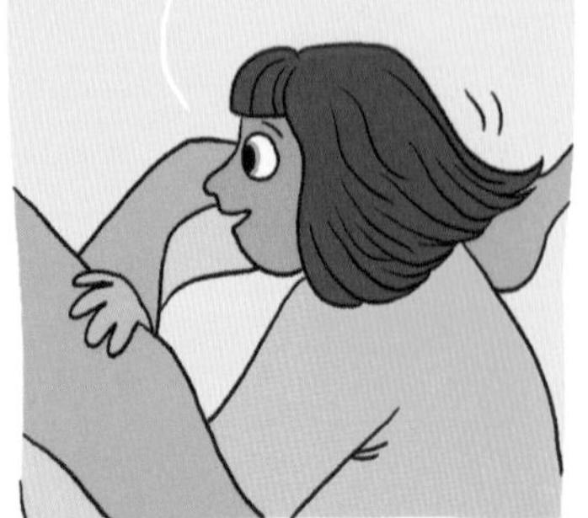

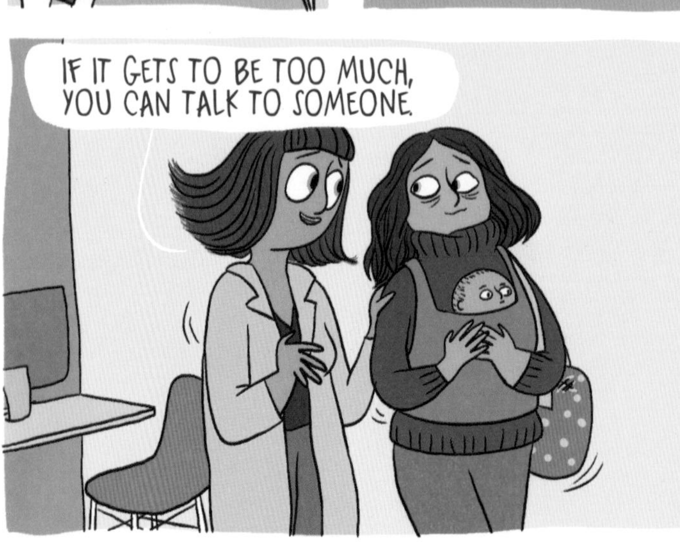

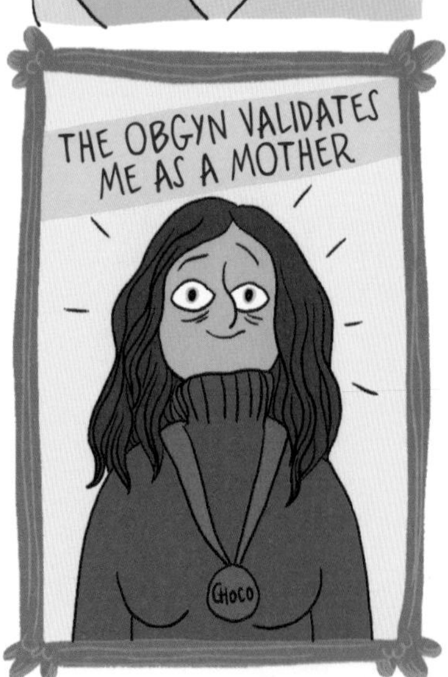

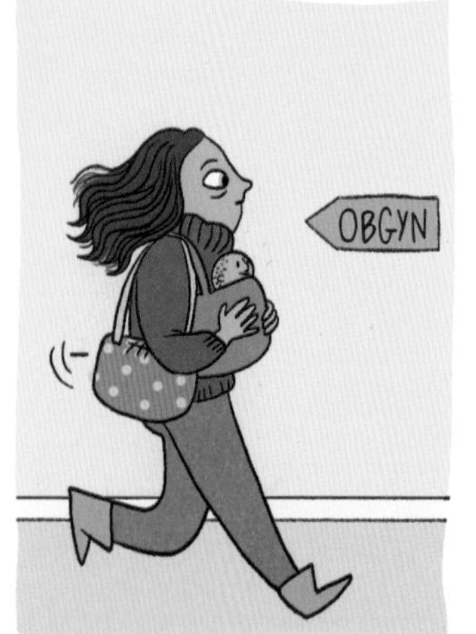

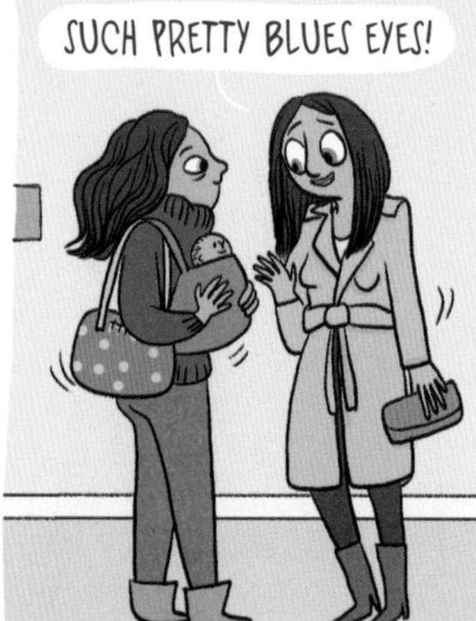

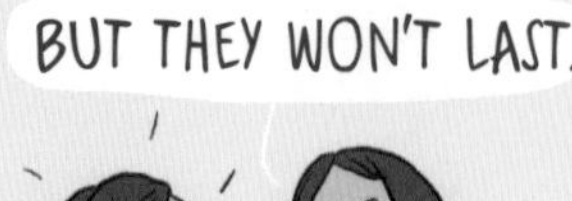

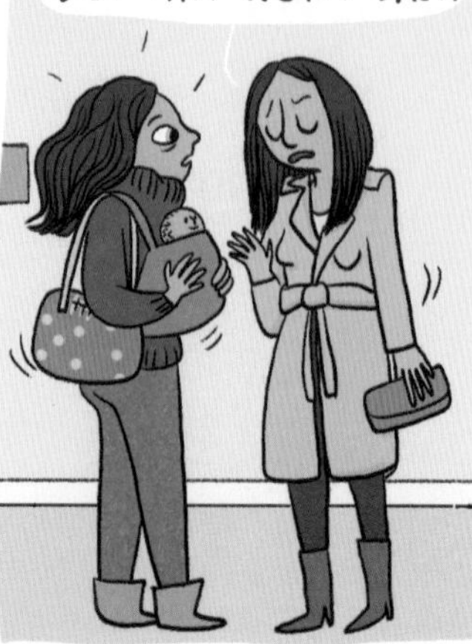

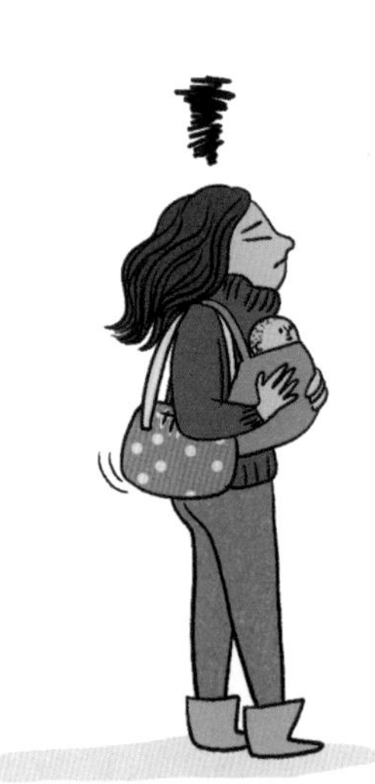

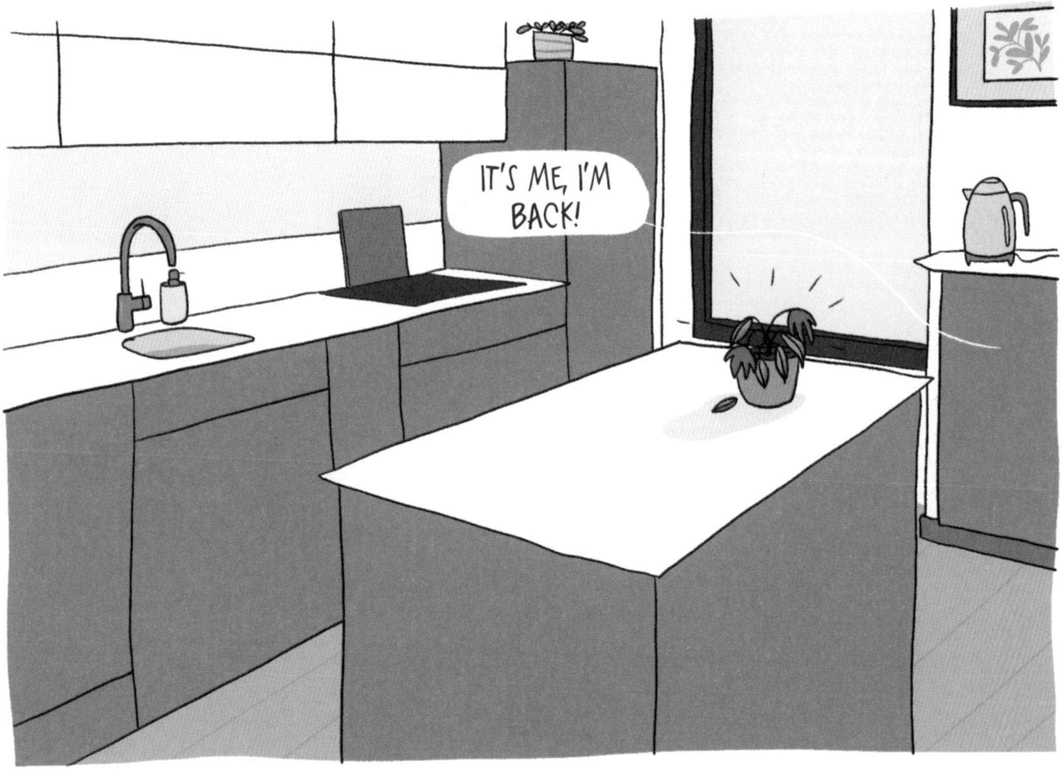

IT'S ME, I'M BACK!

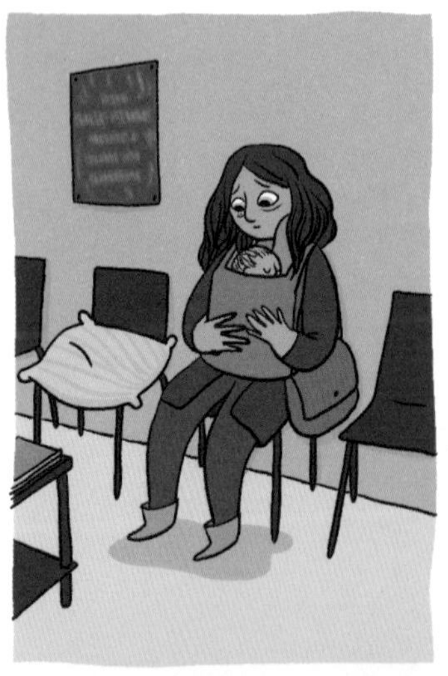

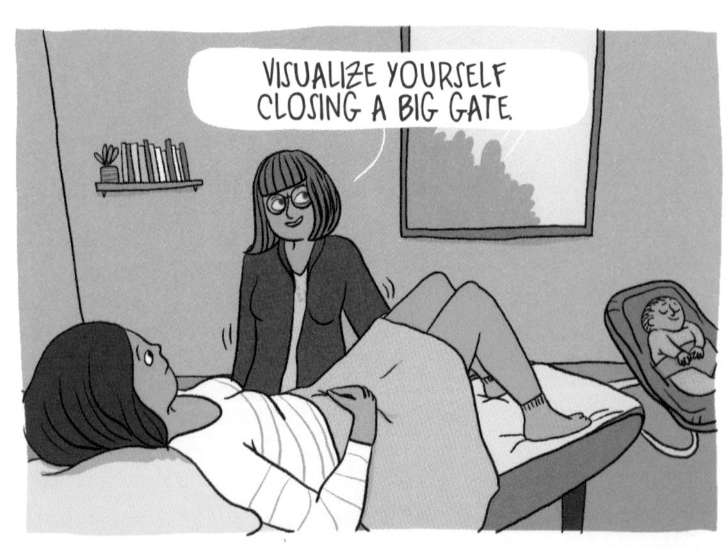
VISUALIZE YOURSELF CLOSING A BIG GATE.

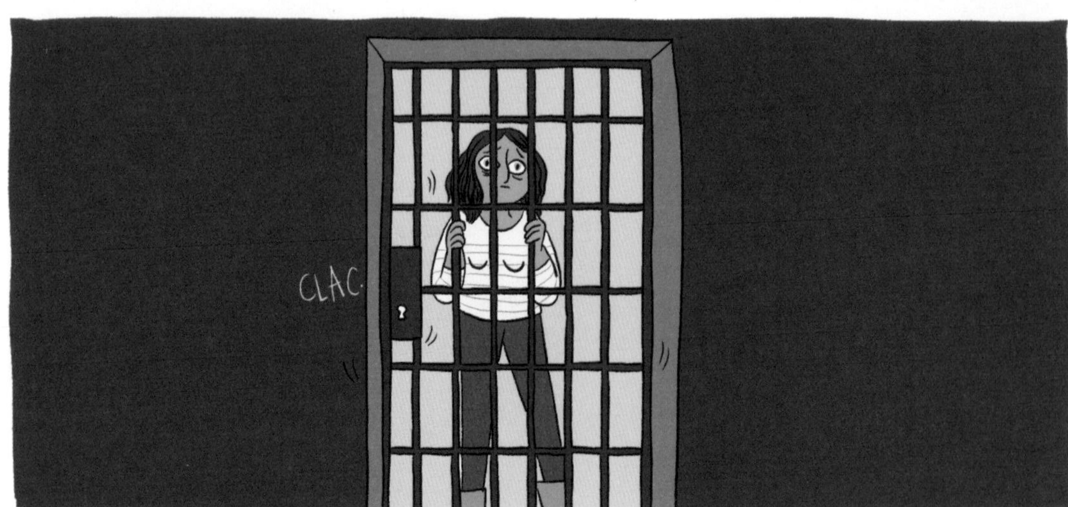
CLAC.

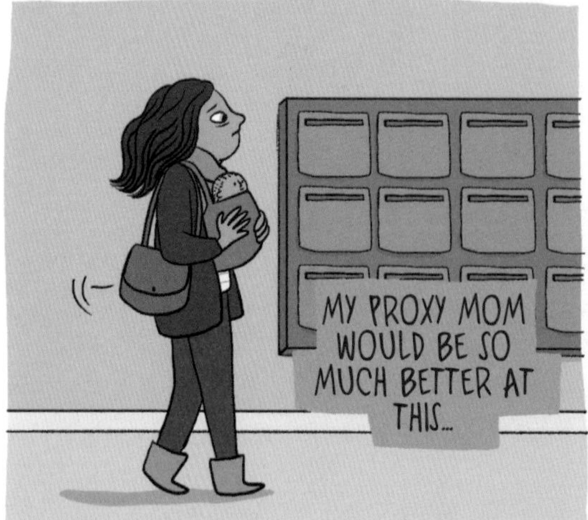
MY PROXY MOM WOULD BE SO MUCH BETTER AT THIS...

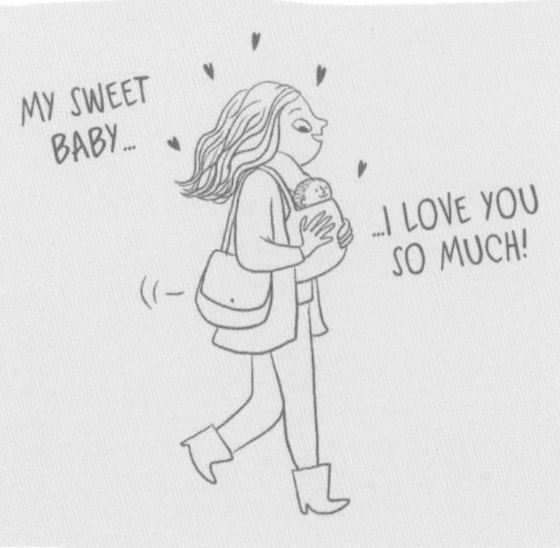
MY SWEET BABY...
...I LOVE YOU SO MUCH!

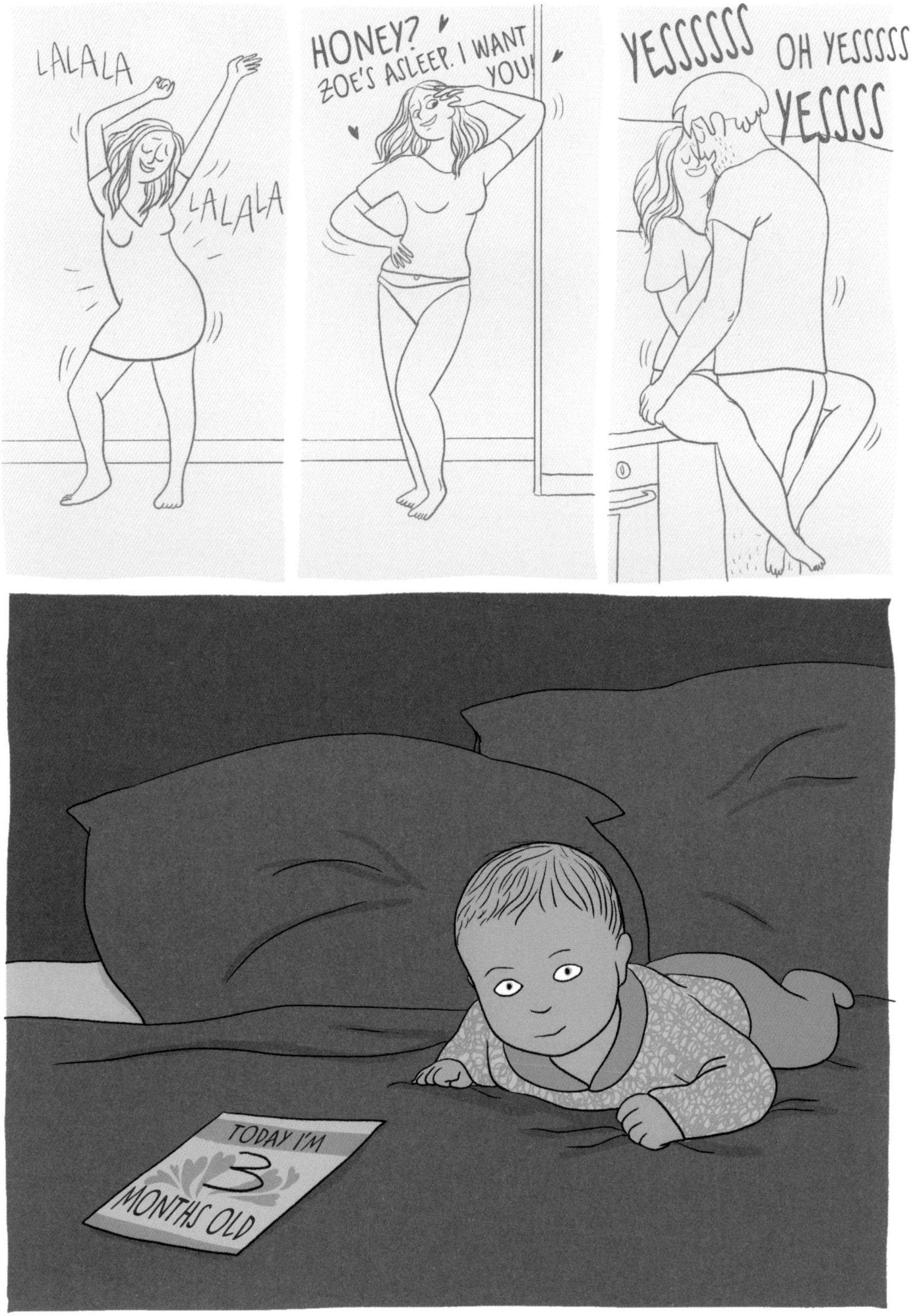

LALALA
LALALA
HONEY? ZOE'S ASLEEP. I WANT YOU!
YESSSSSS
OH YESSSSS
YESSSS

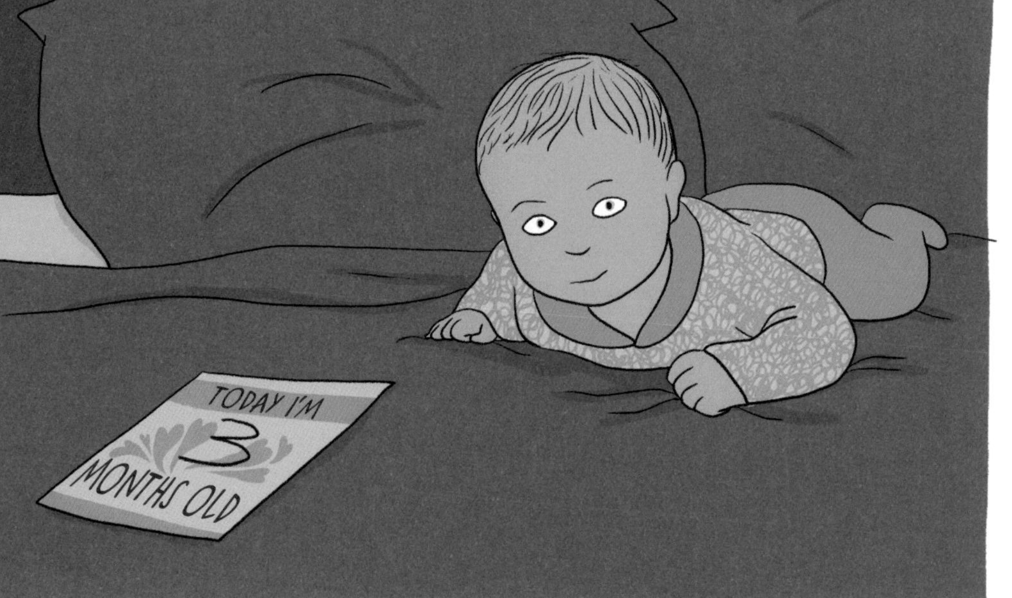
TODAY I'M
3
MONTHS OLD

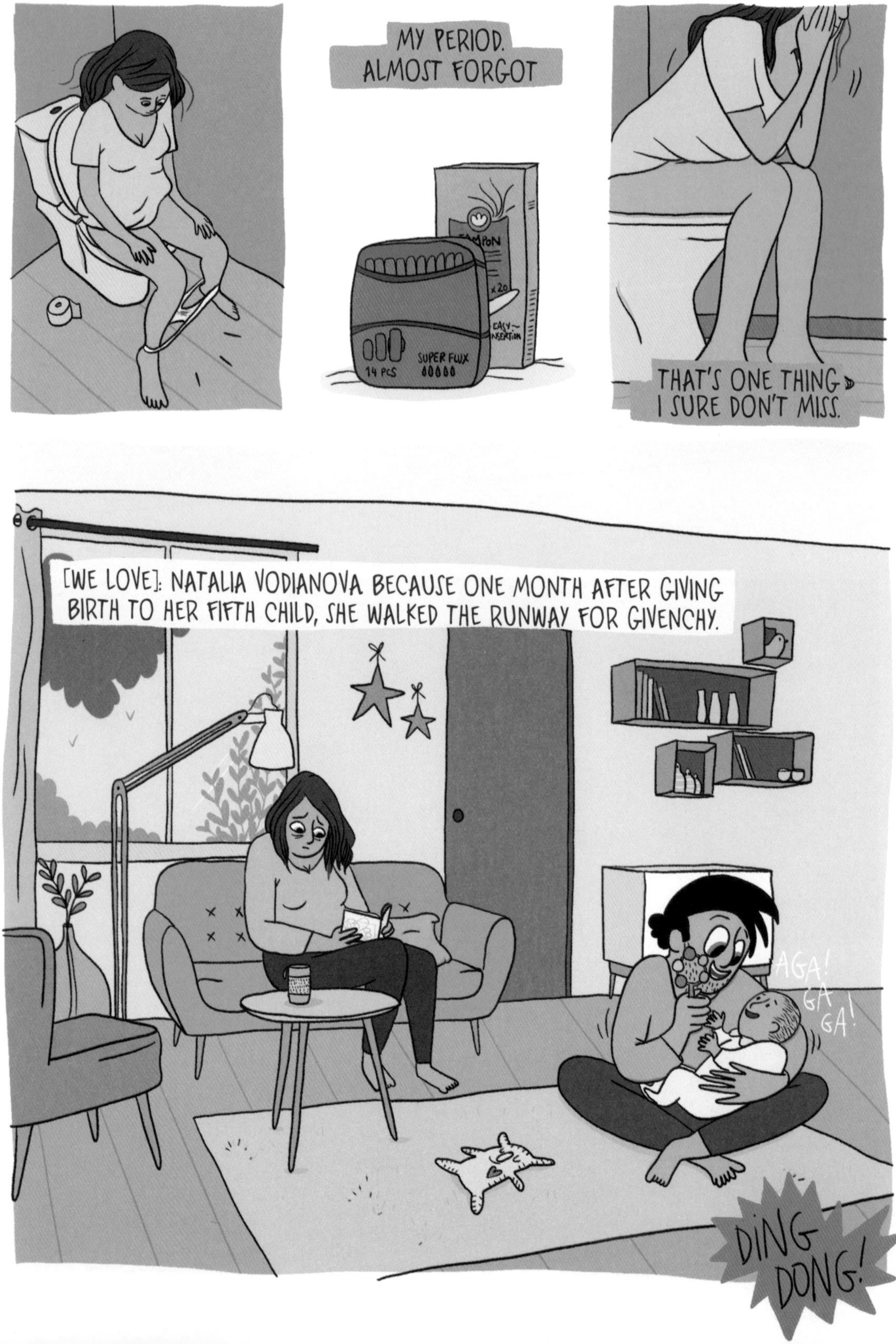

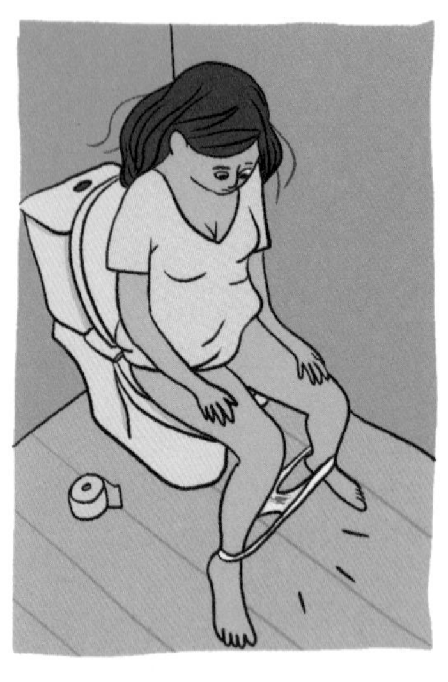

MY PERIOD.
ALMOST FORGOT

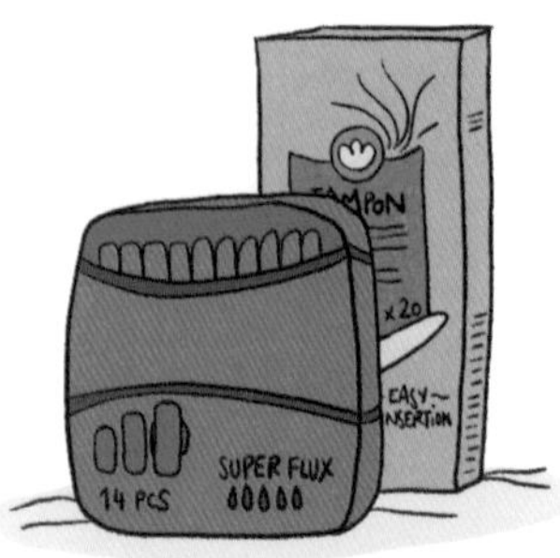

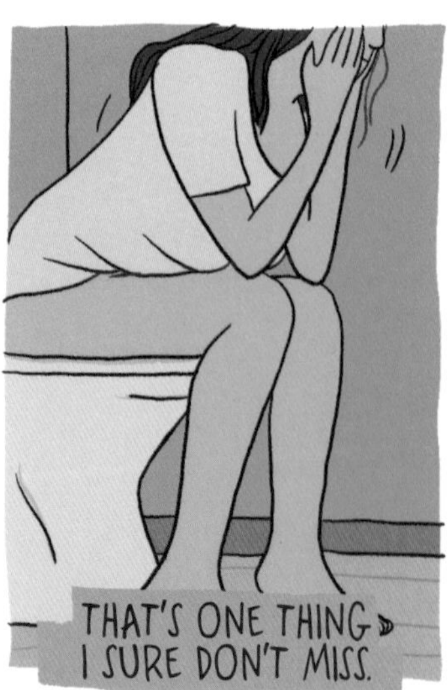

[WE LOVE]: NATALIA VODIANOVA BECAUSE ONE MONTH AFTER GIVING BIRTH TO HER FIFTH CHILD, SHE WALKED THE RUNWAY FOR GIVENCHY.

AGA! GA GA!

DING DONG!

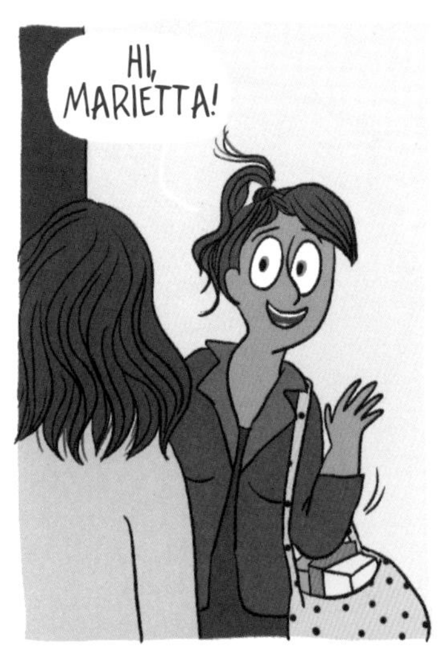
HI, MARIETTA!

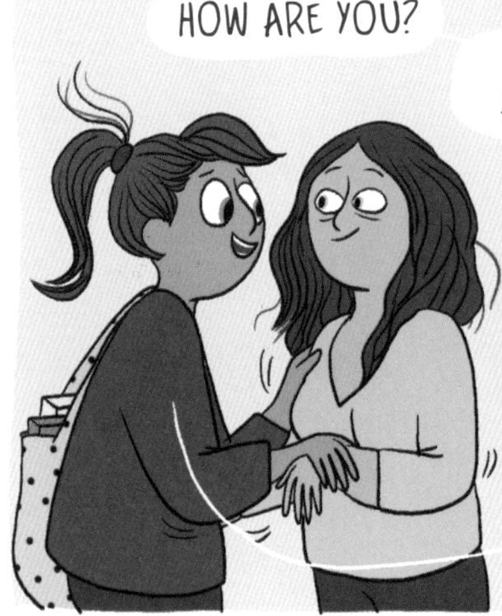
HOW ARE YOU?
WHAT DID YOU FEEL, AFTER GIVING BIRTH?
DO YOU REALIZE THERE ARE THREE OF YOU FROM NOW ON?
YOU MUST BE SO HAPPY TO HAVE HER!

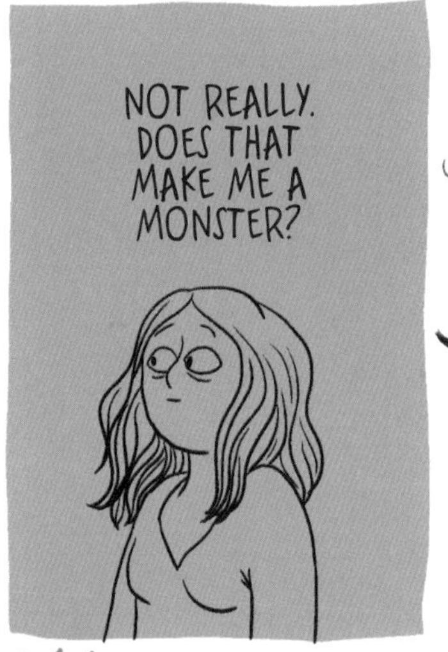
NOT REALLY. DOES THAT MAKE ME A MONSTER?

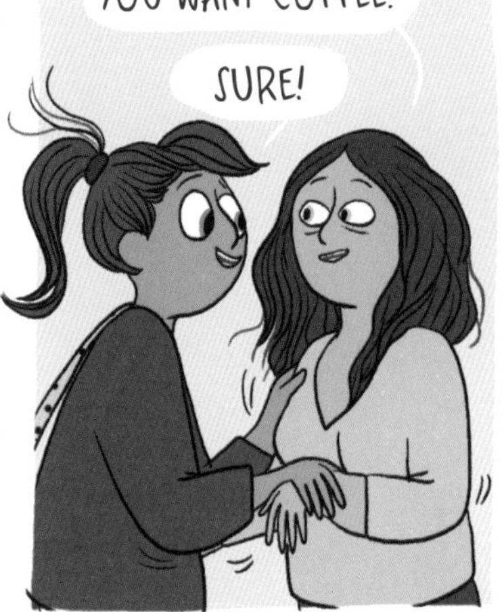
YOU WANT COFFEE?
SURE!

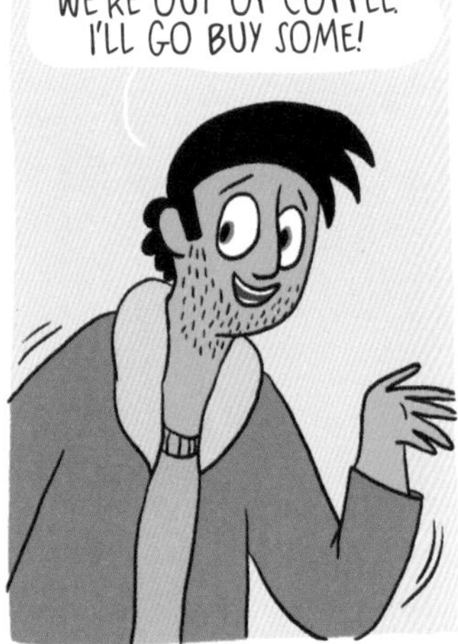
WE'RE OUT OF COFFEE. I'LL GO BUY SOME!

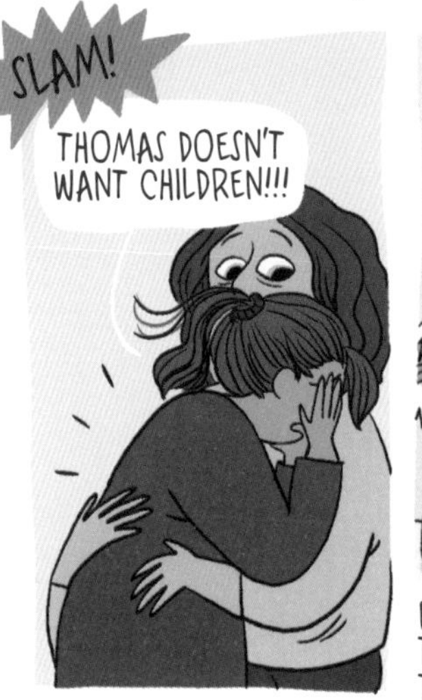
SLAM!
THOMAS DOESN'T WANT CHILDREN!!!

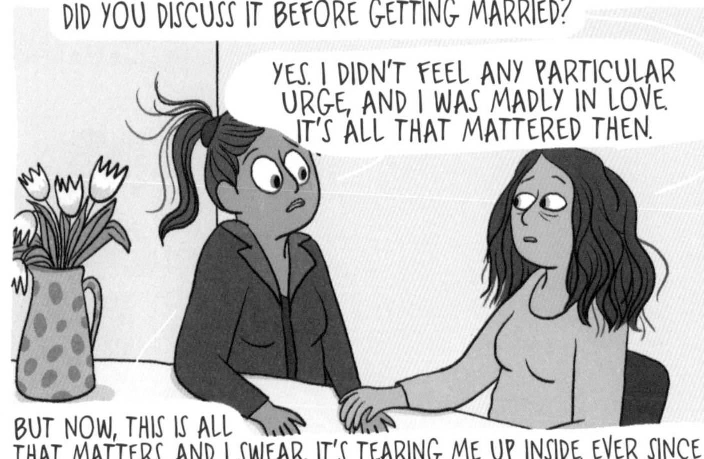
DID YOU DISCUSS IT BEFORE GETTING MARRIED?
YES. I DIDN'T FEEL ANY PARTICULAR URGE, AND I WAS MADLY IN LOVE. IT'S ALL THAT MATTERED THEN.
BUT NOW, THIS IS ALL THAT MATTERS, AND I SWEAR, IT'S TEARING ME UP INSIDE. EVER SINCE I TURNED 35, IT'S ALL I CAN THINK ABOUT. I KEEP THINKING MY EGGS ARE OLD AND IT'S NOW OR NEVER.

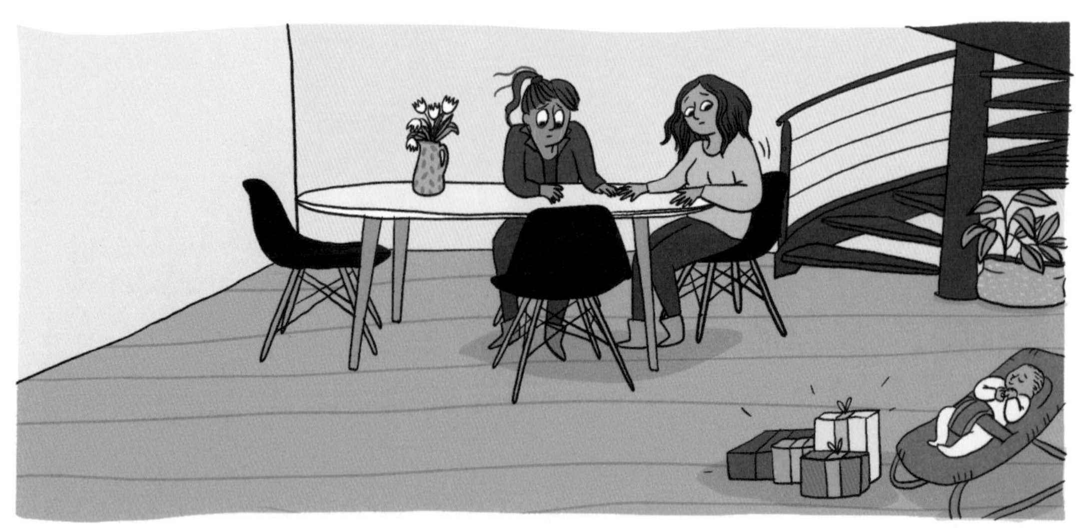

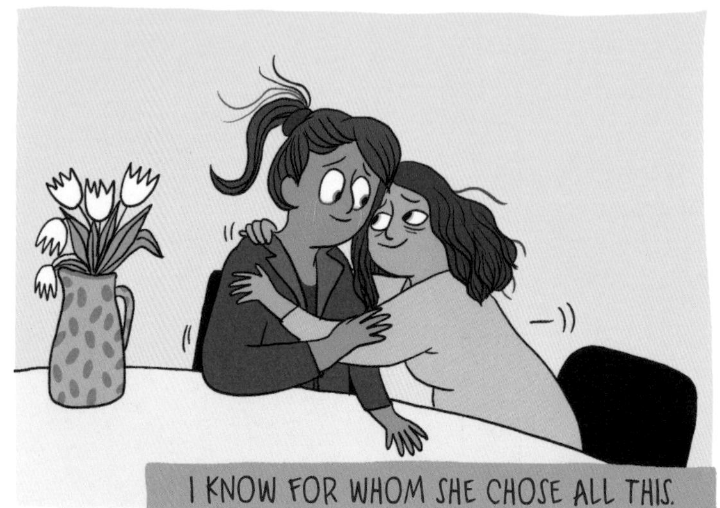
I KNOW FOR WHOM SHE CHOSE ALL THIS.

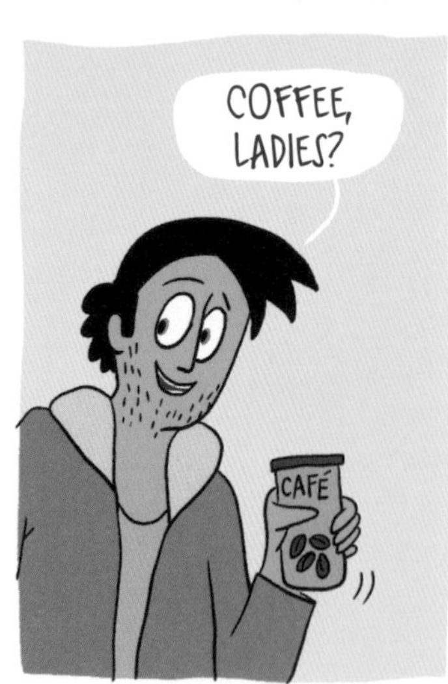
COFFEE, LADIES?
CAFÉ

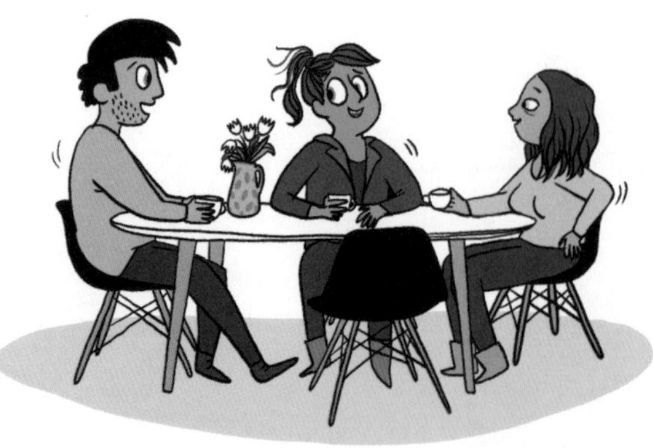
blablablablabla...

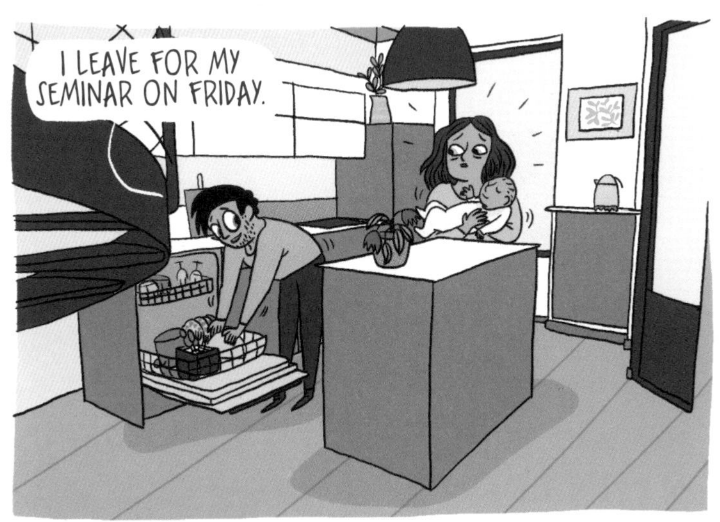
I LEAVE FOR MY SEMINAR ON FRIDAY.

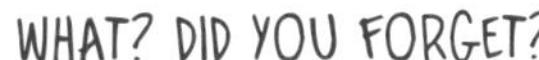
WHAT? DID YOU FORGET?

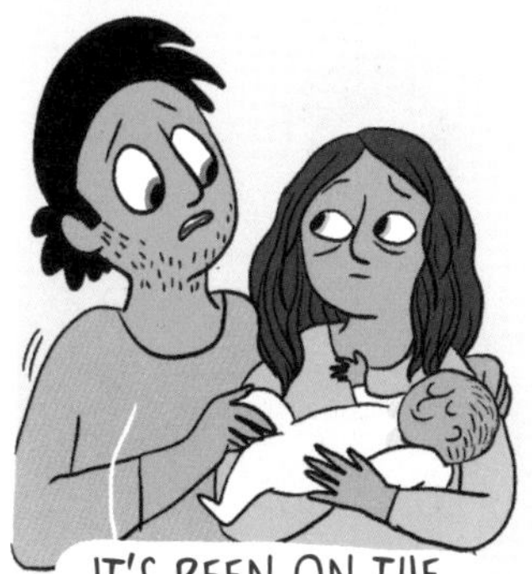
IT'S BEEN ON THE CALENDAR FOR MONTHS.

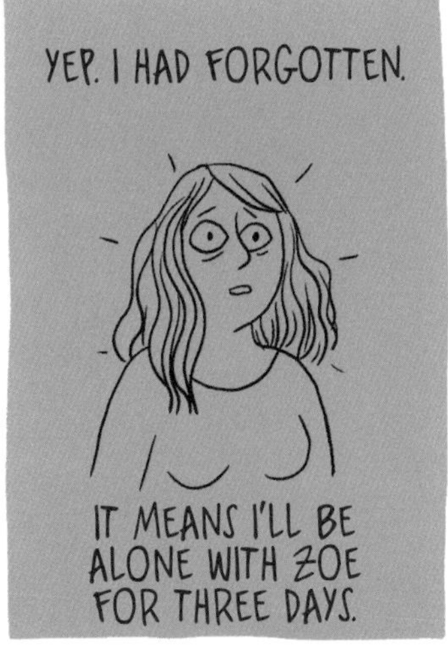
YEP. I HAD FORGOTTEN.
IT MEANS I'LL BE ALONE WITH ZOE FOR THREE DAYS.

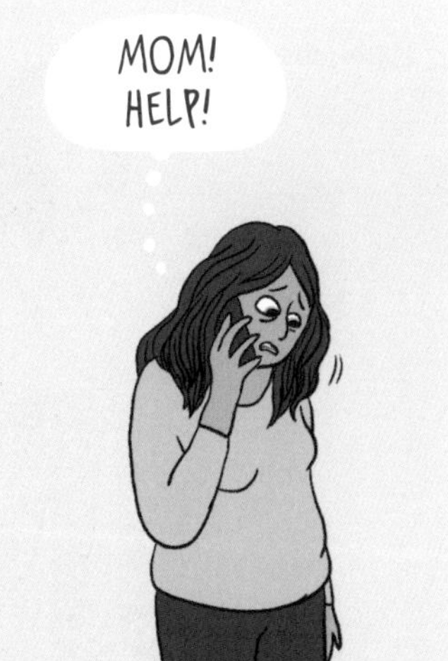
MOM! HELP!

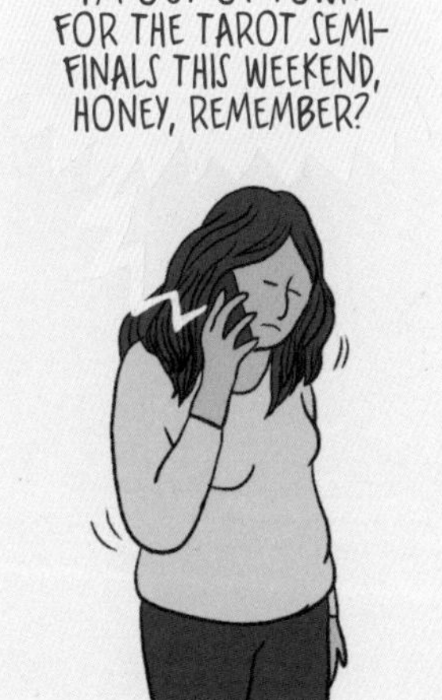
I'M OUT OF TOWN FOR THE TAROT SEMI-FINALS THIS WEEKEND, HONEY, REMEMBER?

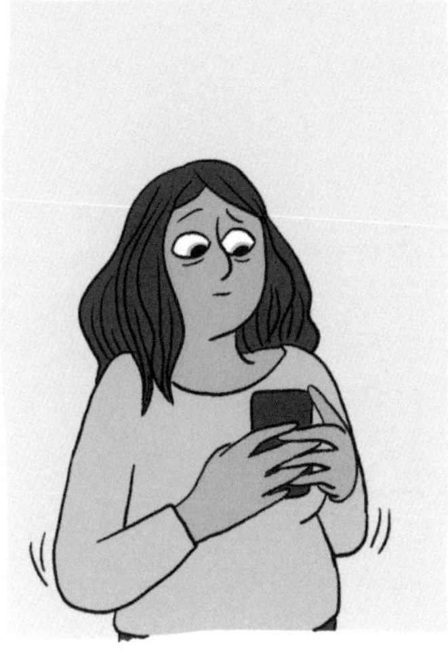

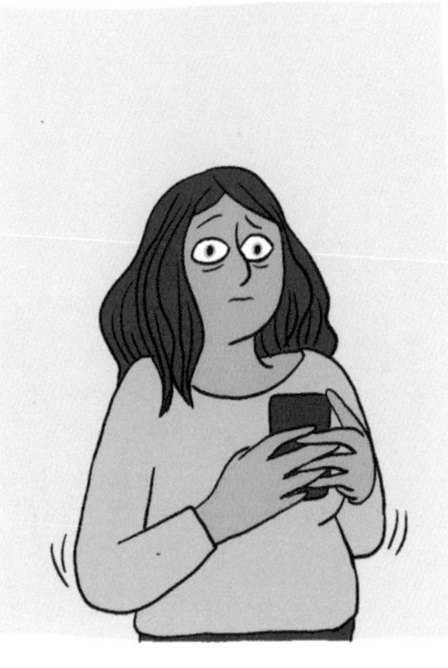

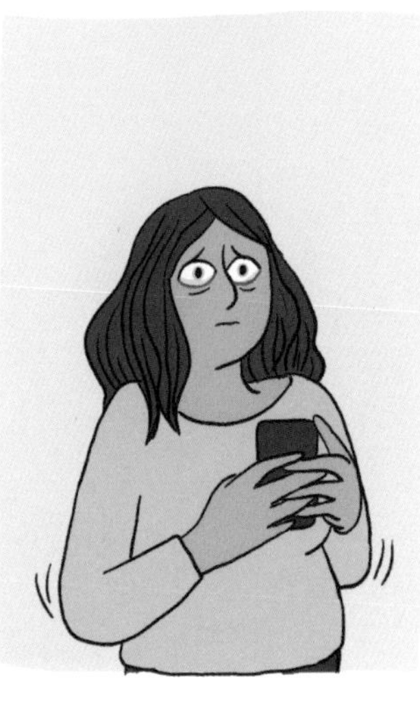

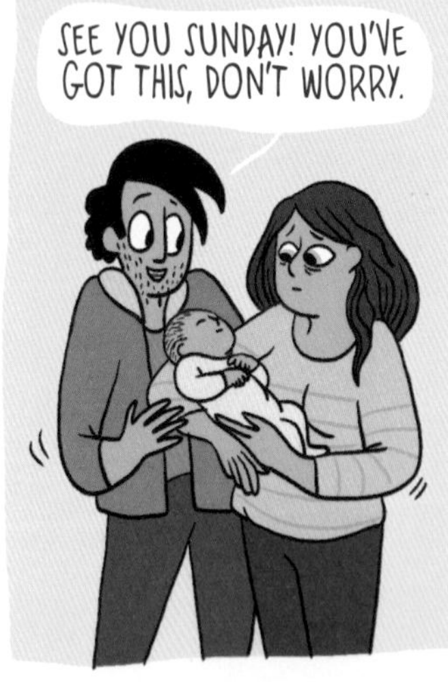
SEE YOU SUNDAY! YOU'VE GOT THIS, DON'T WORRY.
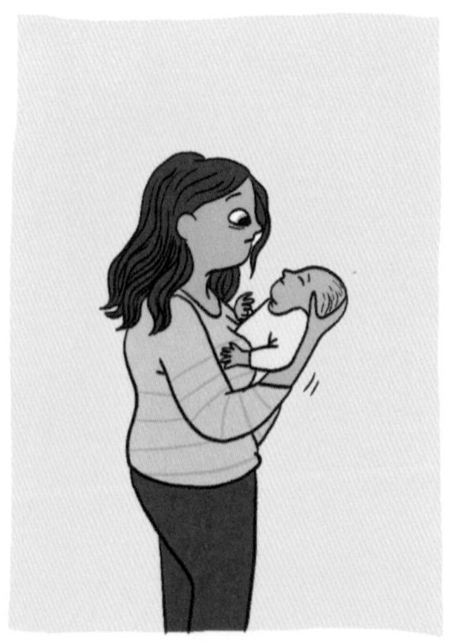
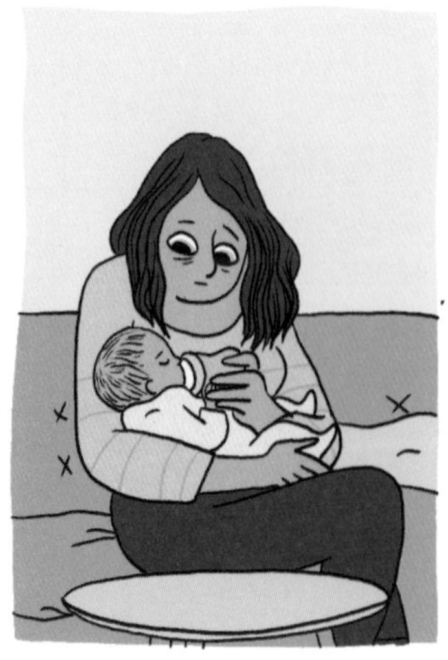
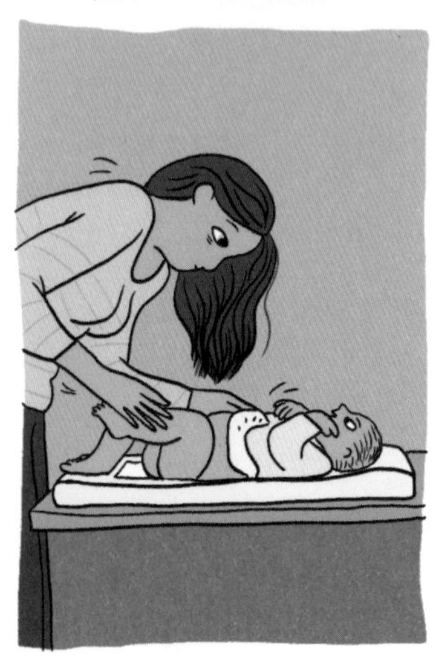
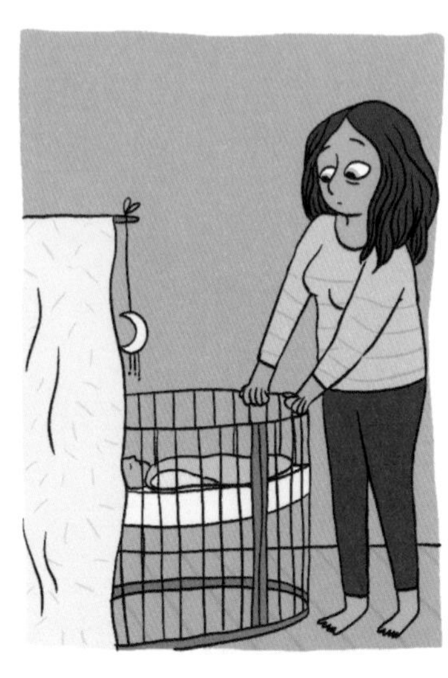
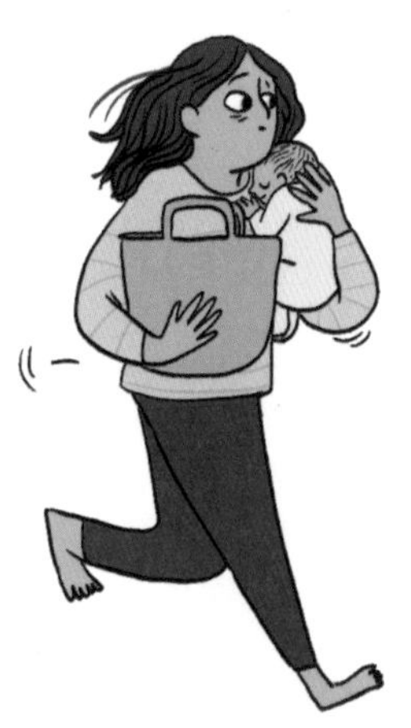
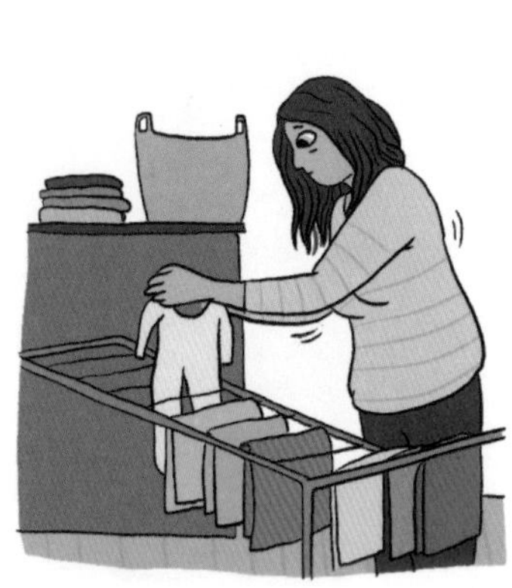
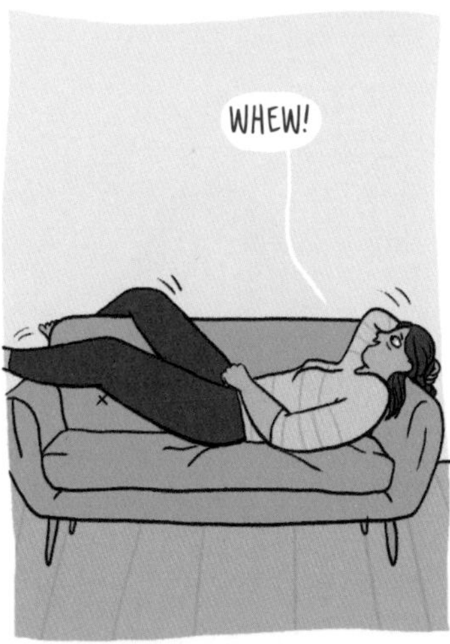
WHEW!
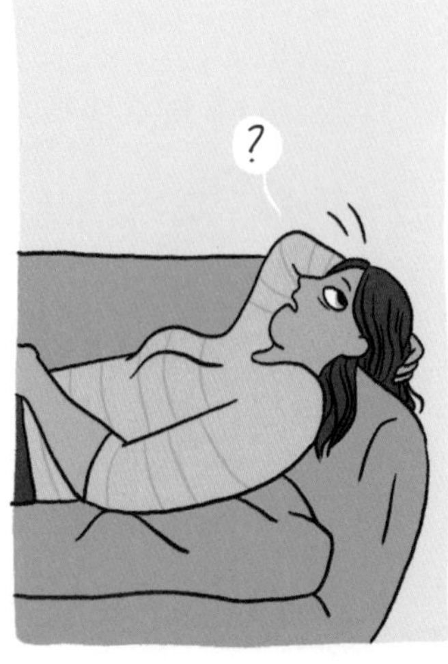
?

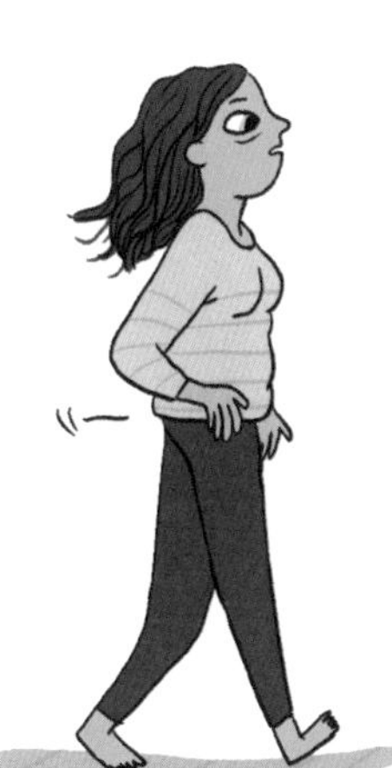

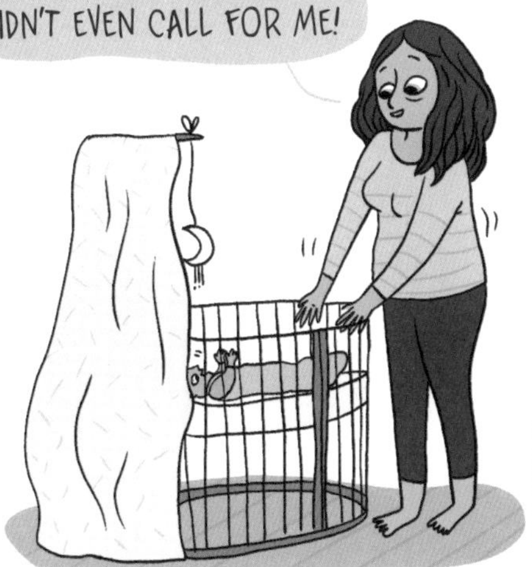
OH! SHE WAS AWAKE AND DIDN'T EVEN CALL FOR ME!

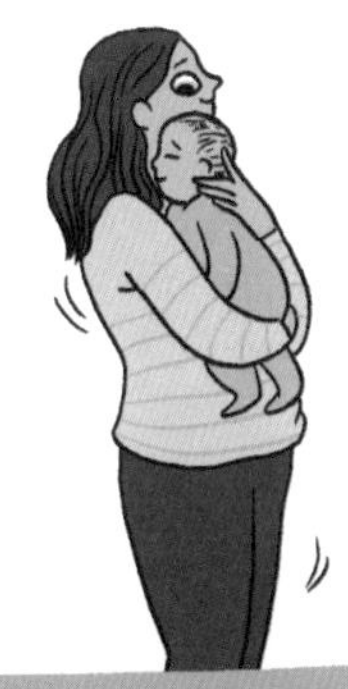
COULD SHE BE TRYING TO MAKE IT EASIER FOR ME FOR THE NEXT THREE DAYS?

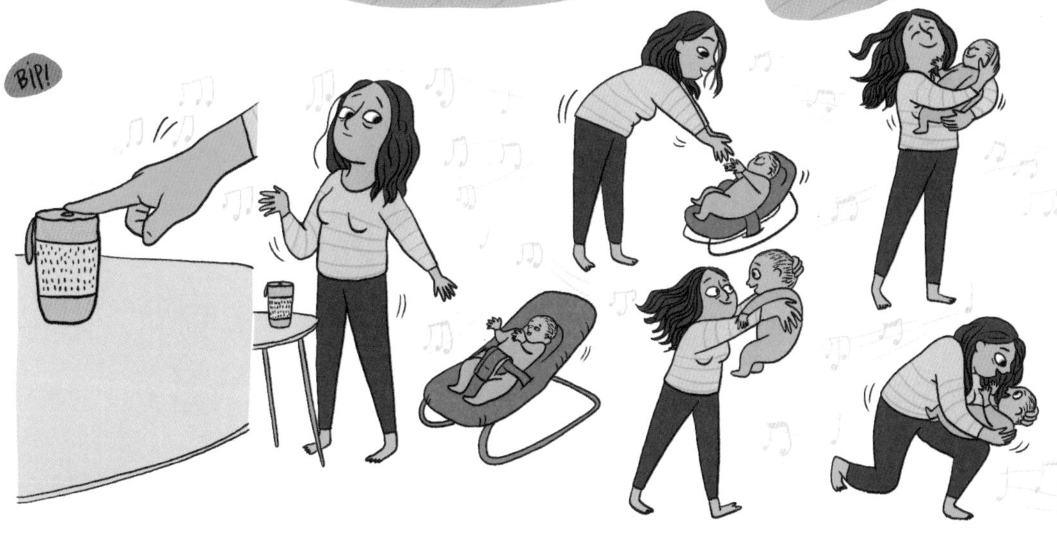
BIP!

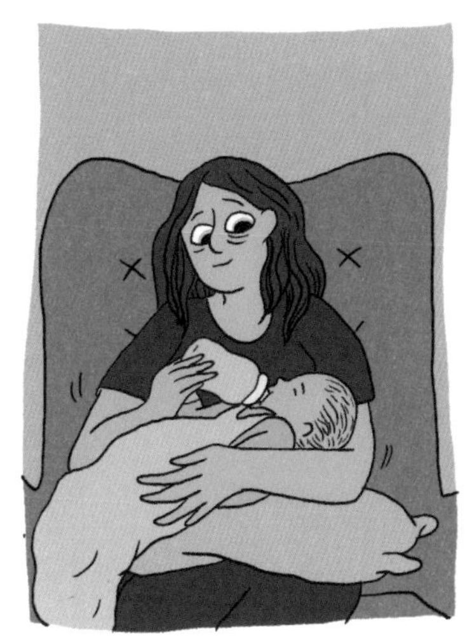

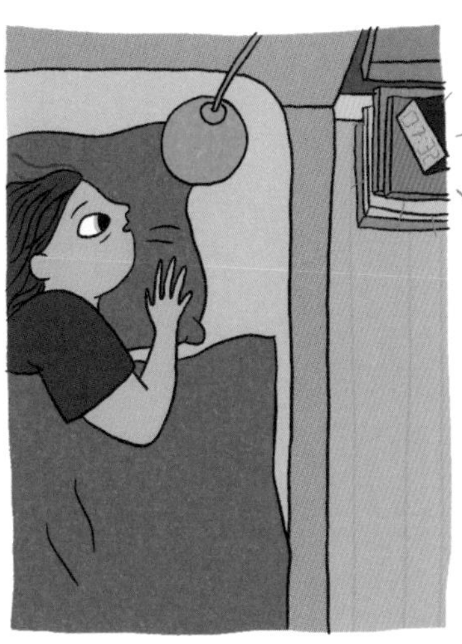

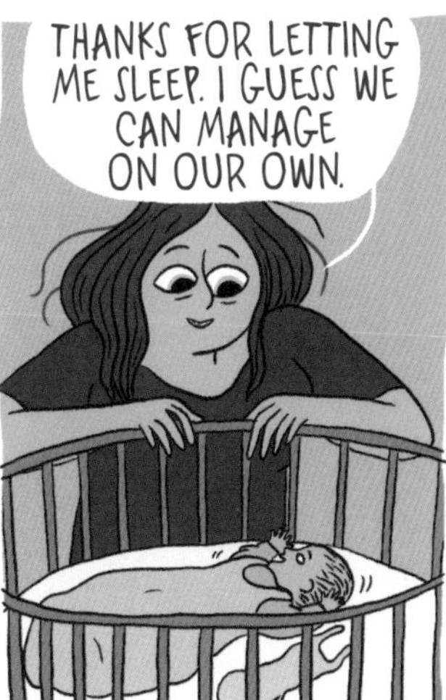
THANKS FOR LETTING ME SLEEP. I GUESS WE CAN MANAGE ON OUR OWN.

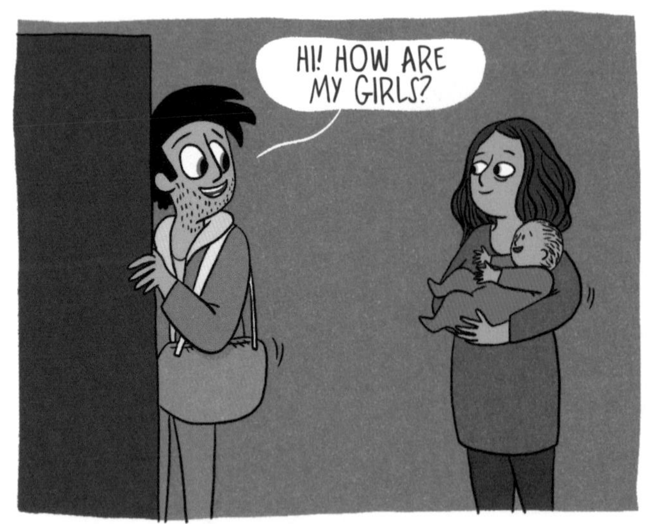

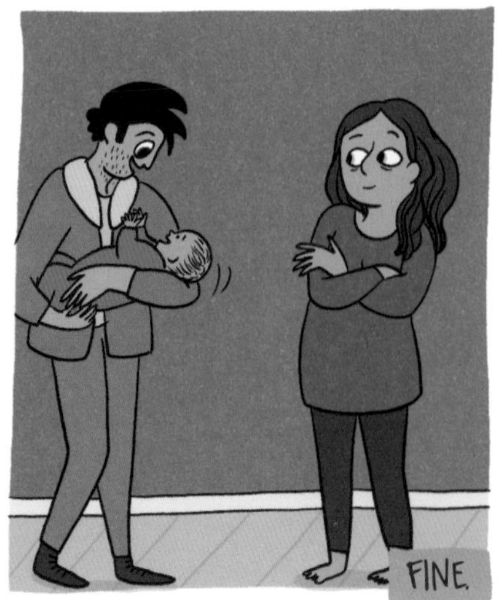

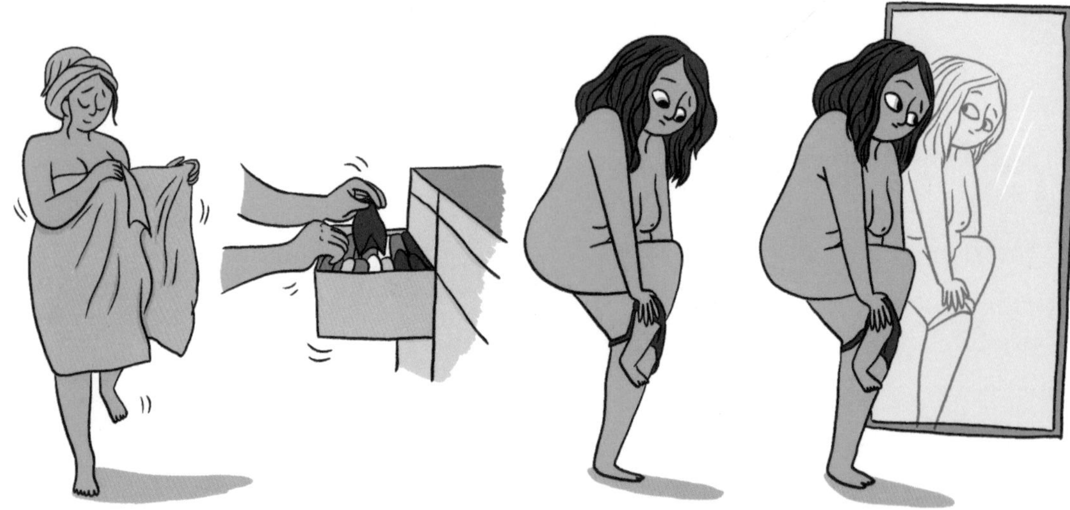

I'M AT WAR AGAINST MY BODY. BUT IT'S A LETHARGIC WAR I'M TOO TIRED TO FIGHT, AND I HAVE NO ENERGY. I'M THIS CLOSE TO SURRENDERING. I LIVE IN A STATE BEYOND EXHAUSTION, A STATE FOR WHICH NO WORD HAS BEEN INVENTED.

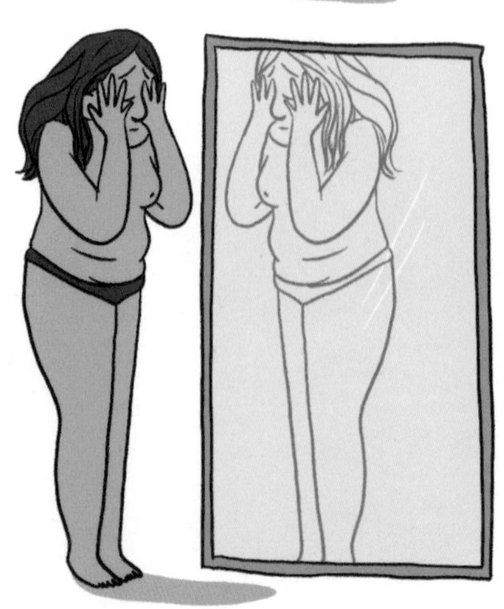

I WISH I DIDN'T EVEN HAVE A BODY.

JUST ARMS,
FOR HOLDING ZOE.
I'D LIKE TO FORGET ABOUT MY BODY, BUT IT WON'T LE ME.
I'M IN THE SAME SORRY STATE AS MY POINSETTIA
IS IT TRUE IT TAKES OUR BODY 9 MONTHS TO MAKE A BABY AND 9 MONTHS TO GET OVER IT?
MY FOURTH TRIMESTER WILL LAST AS LONG AS IT TAKES.

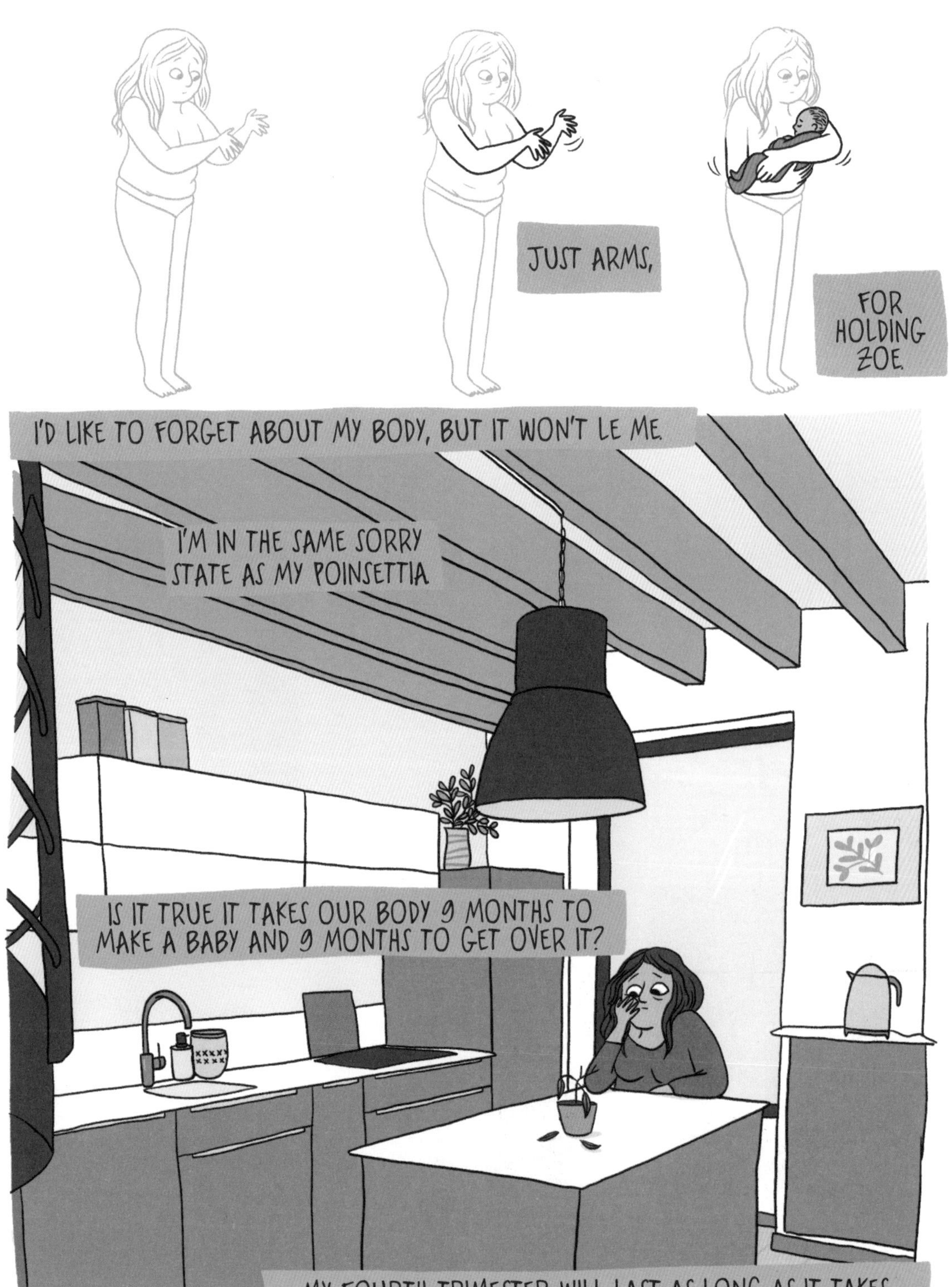

MYRTLE BERTIN

CERTIFIED
CHILD CARE
PROFESSIONAL

DING DONG

HELLO!

AND THIS IS THE NURSERY!
DIAPERS

PERFECTLY NORMAL, DON'T WORRY. SEE YOU LATER!
WAAAAAH

DING DONG

SHE STOPPED CRYING AS SOON AS YOU LEFT.

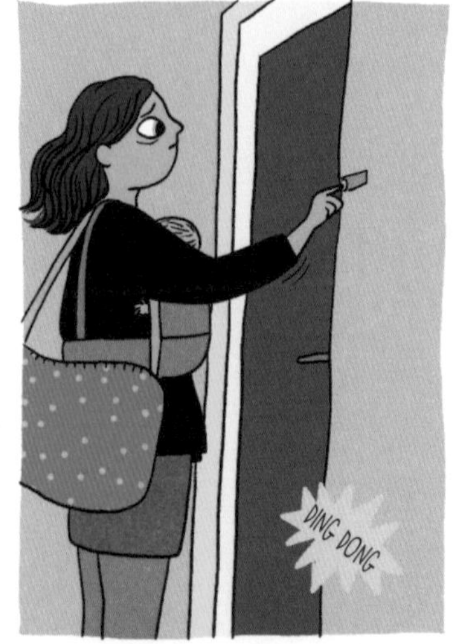

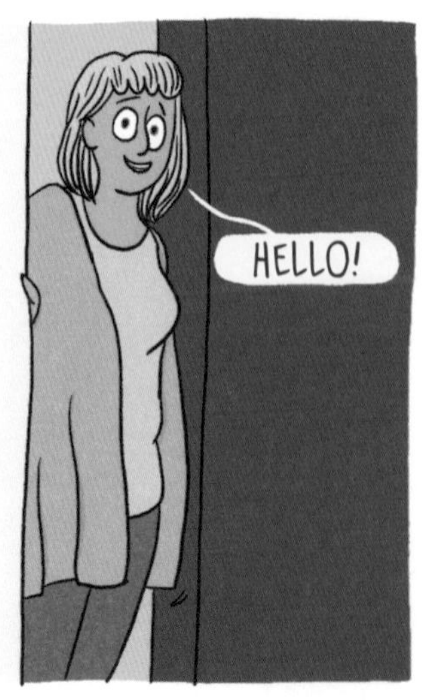

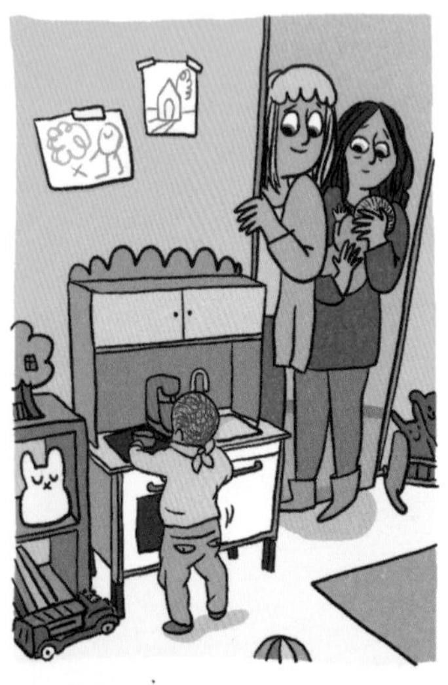

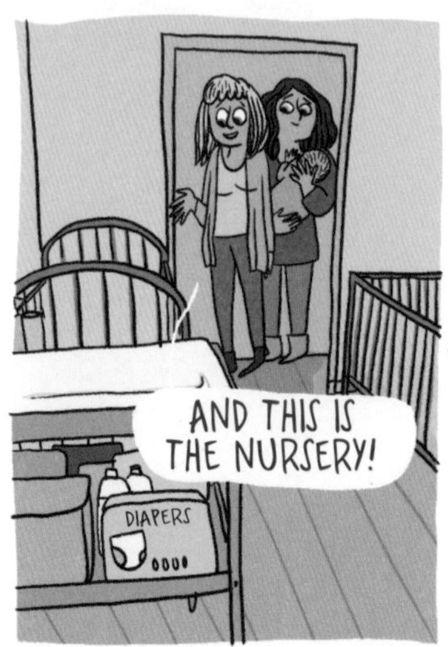

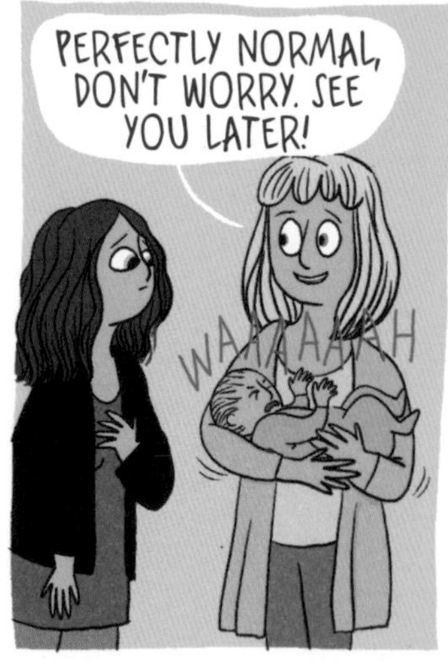

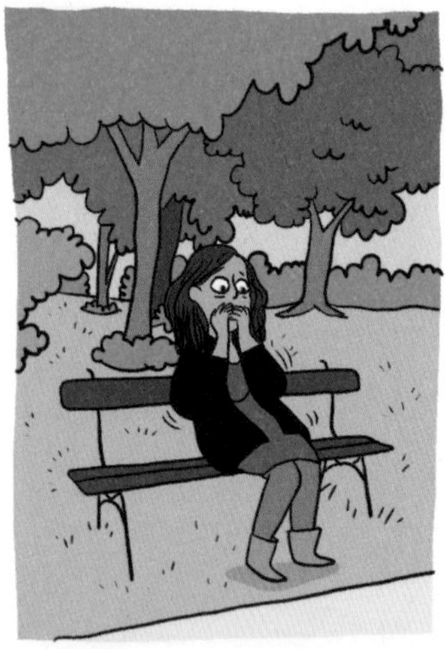

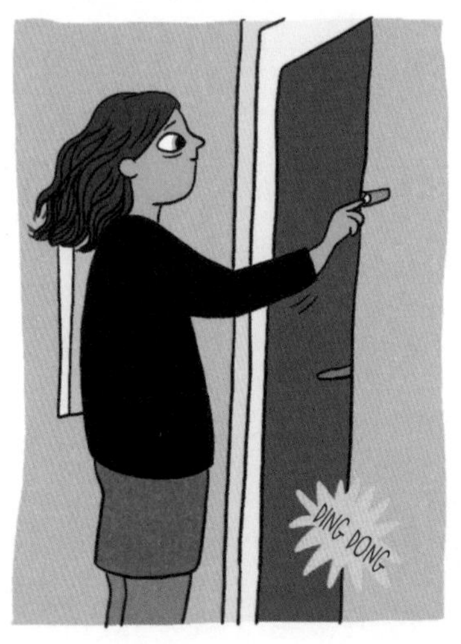

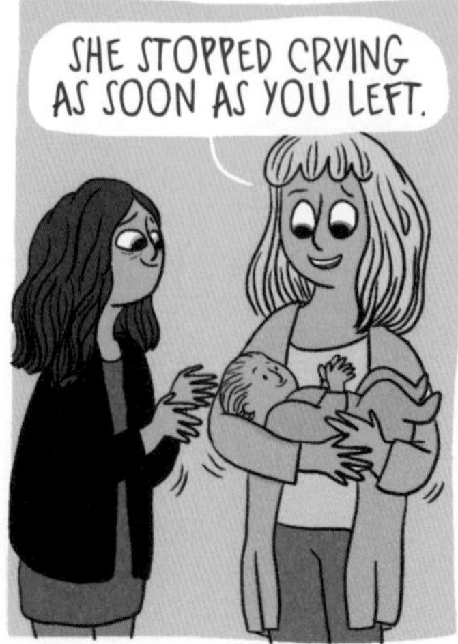

Zoe Child Care
Trial Period
Day 1

Separation hard
on Mommy.
Plan on a
longer trial
period.

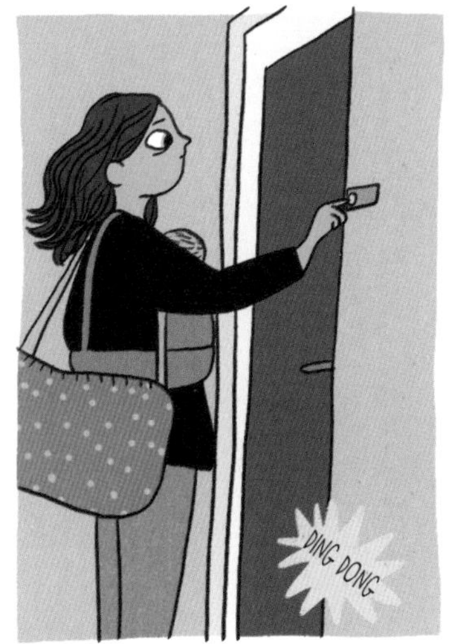

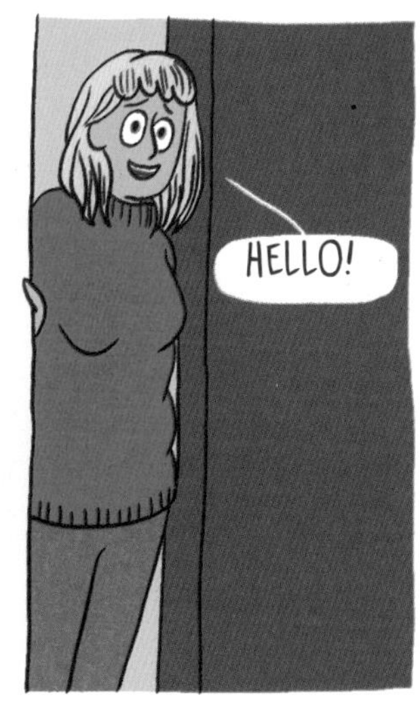

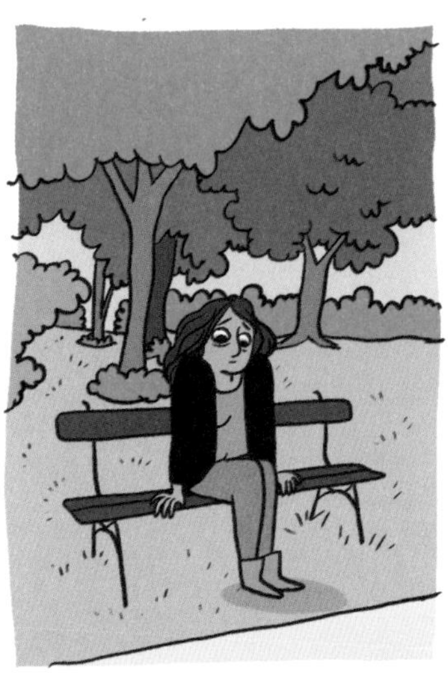

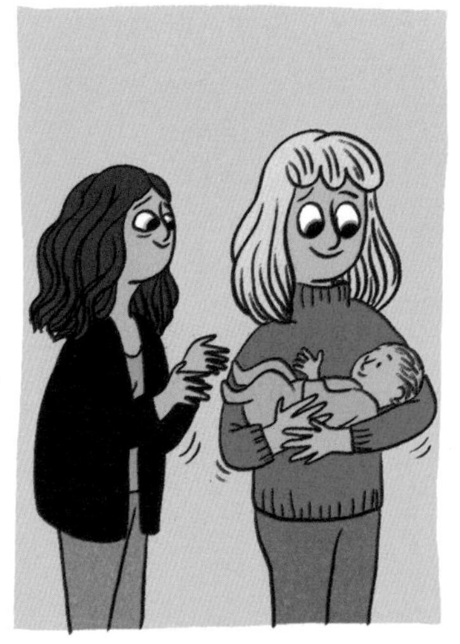

Zoe Child Care
Trial period

Day 3

Mommy: progress.
Zoe: N/A

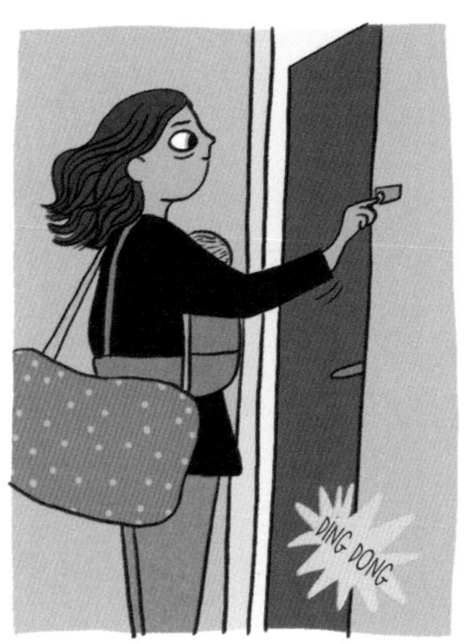

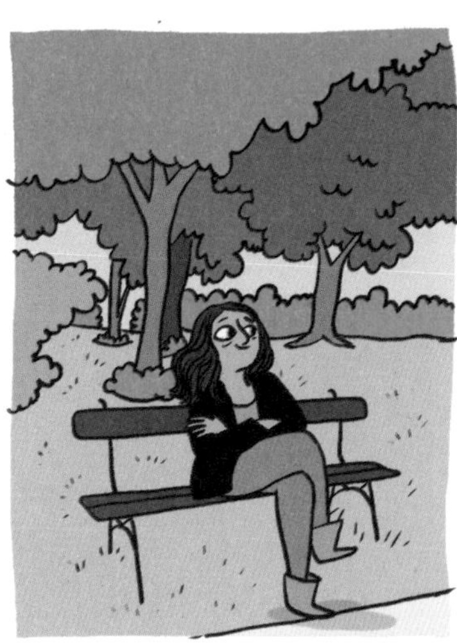

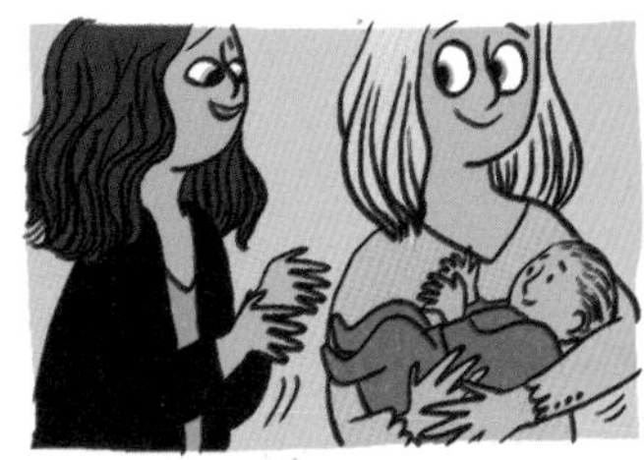

Zoe Child Care Trial period
Day 5
Mommy: peace of mind.
Zoe: getting used to it.
Successful trial period.
New schedule
starts Monday.

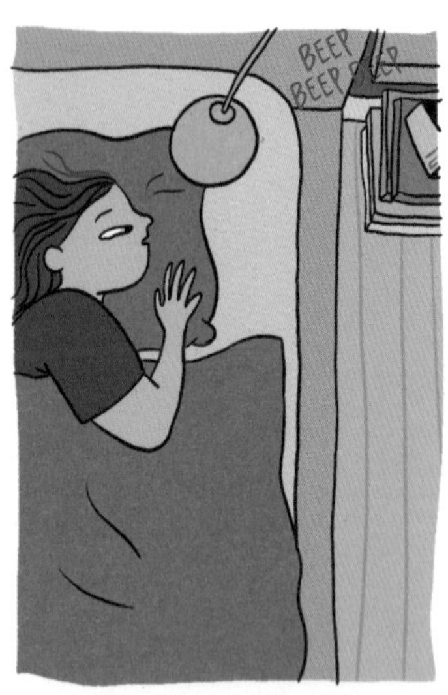
BEEP
BEEP

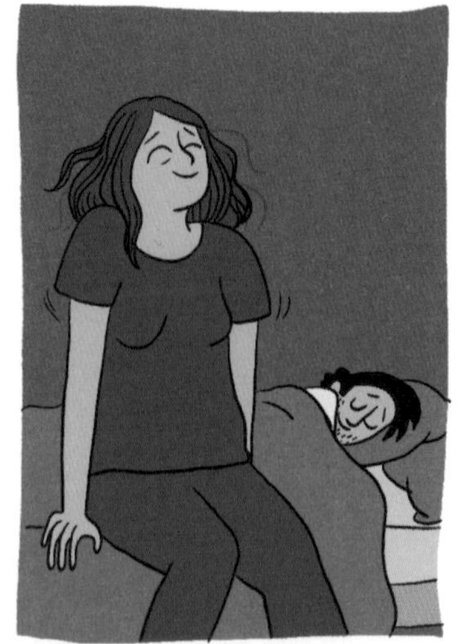

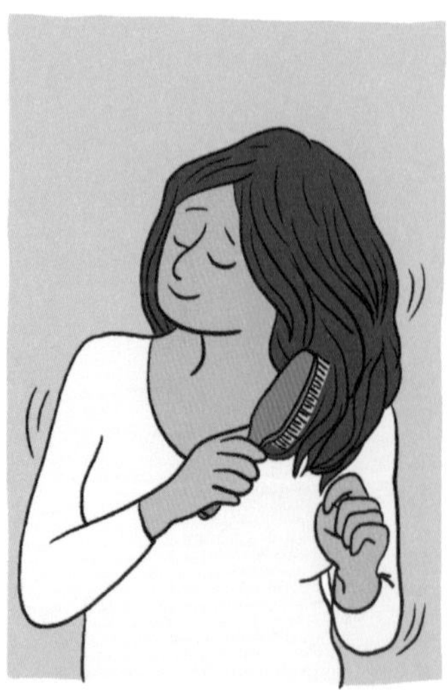

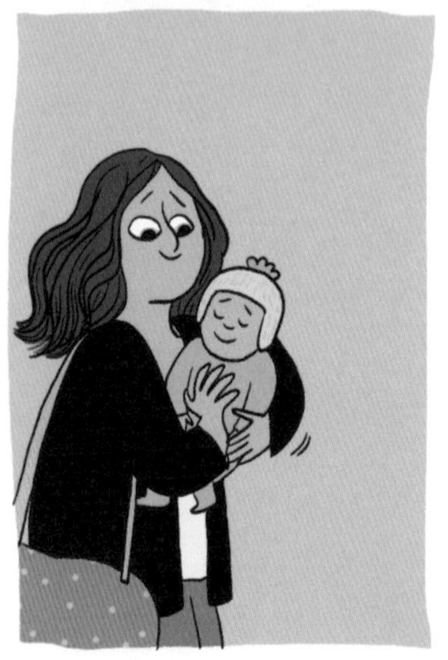

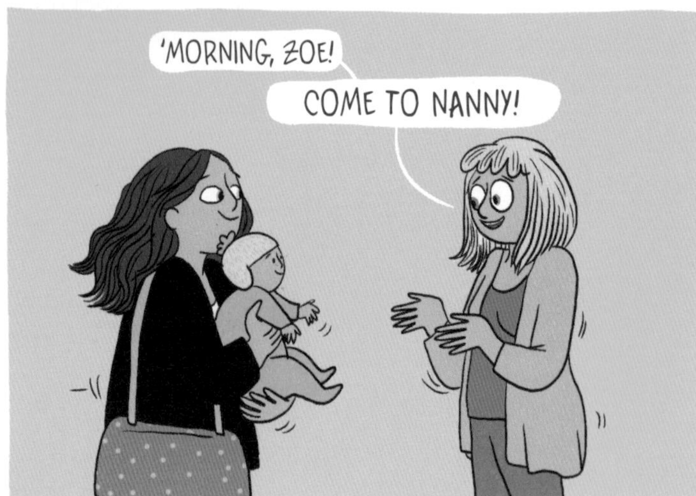
'MORNING, ZOE!
COME TO NANNY!

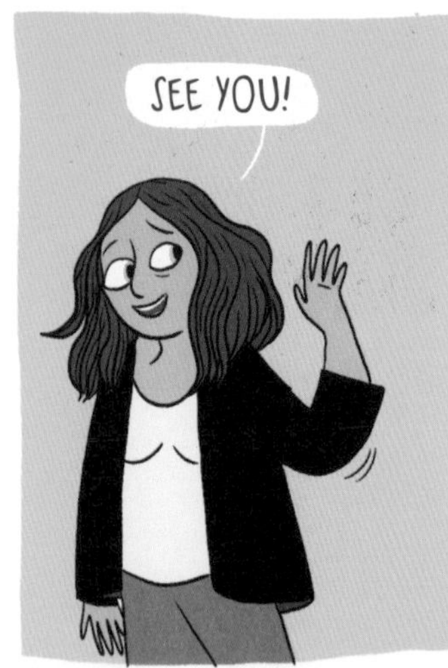
SEE YOU!

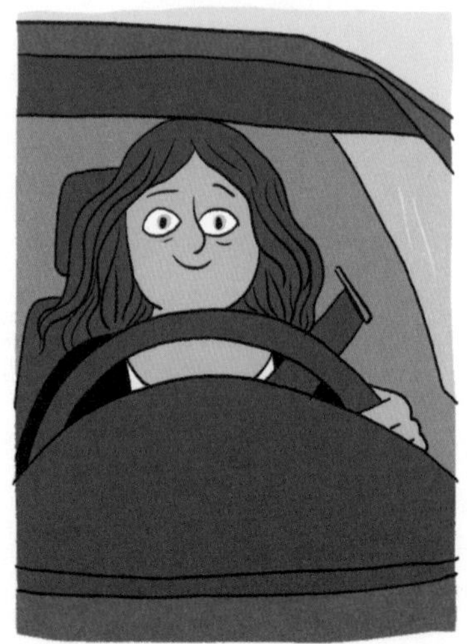

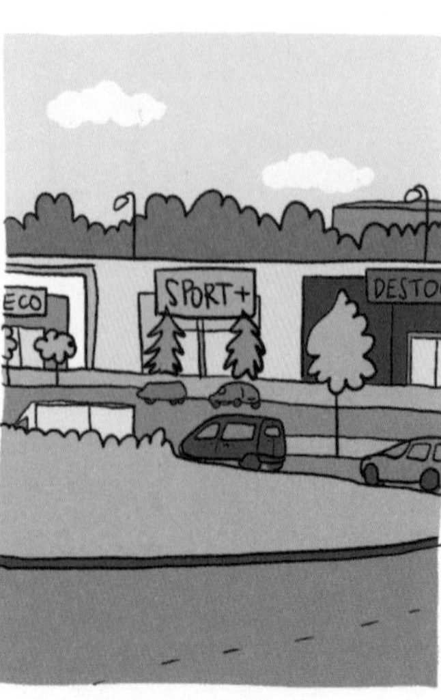
ECO
SPORT+
DESTOC

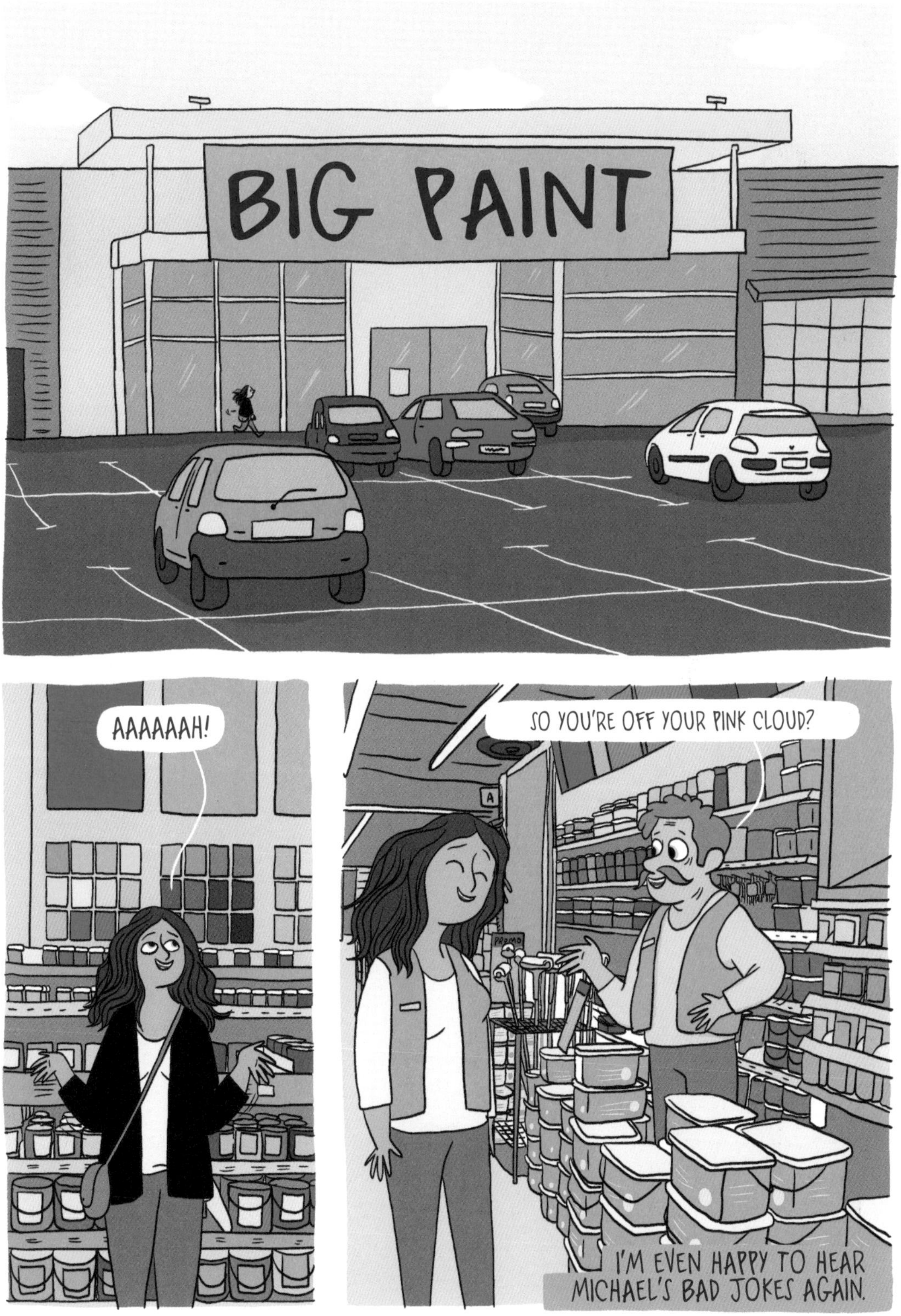

BIG PAINT

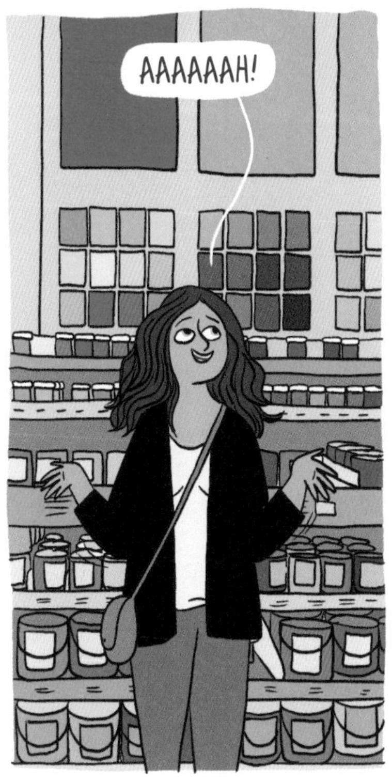
AAAAAAH!

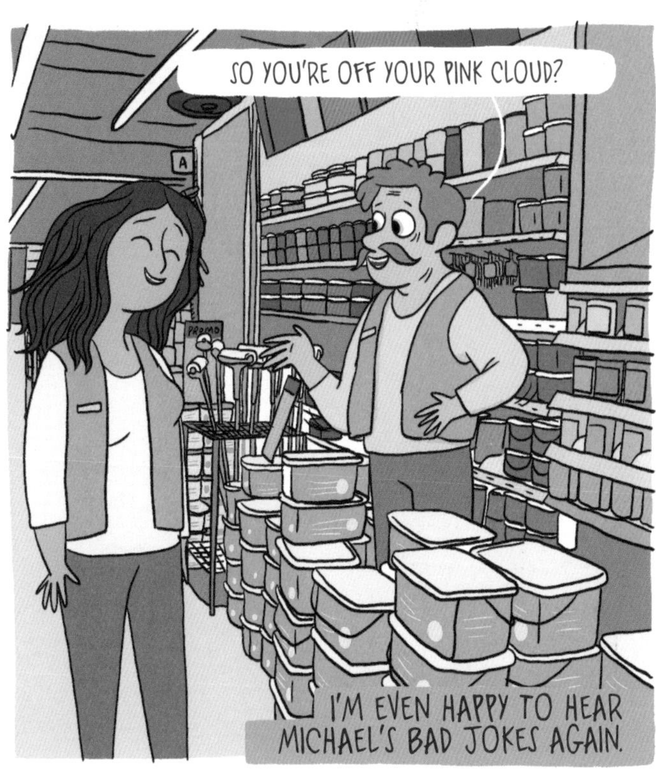
SO YOU'RE OFF YOUR PINK CLOUD?
I'M EVEN HAPPY TO HEAR MICHAEL'S BAD JOKES AGAIN.

IT'S FOR ZOE! FROM ALL OF US!

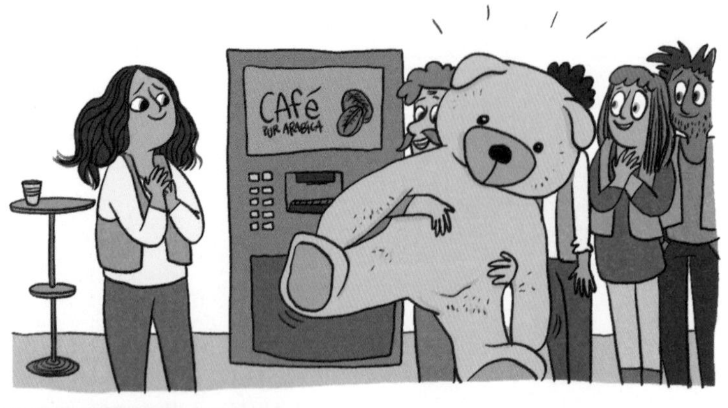

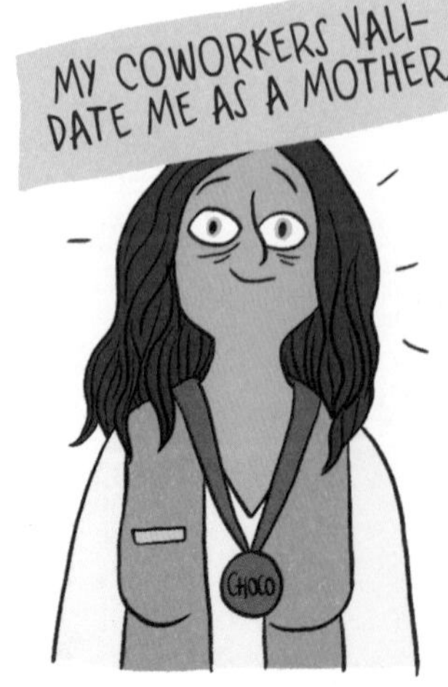

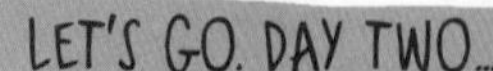

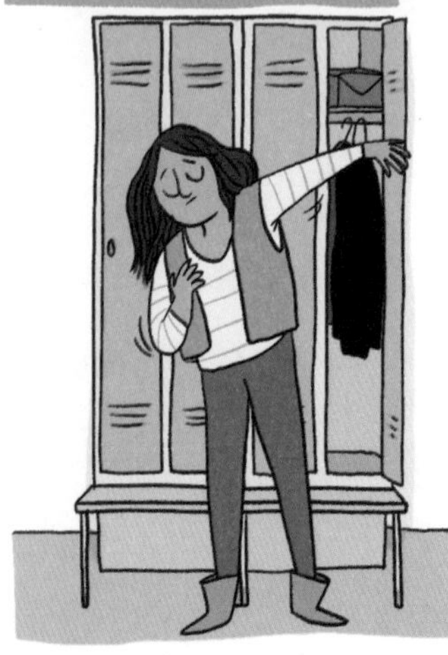

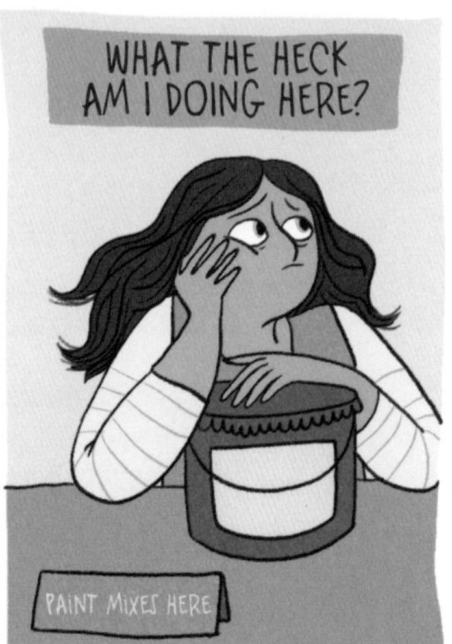

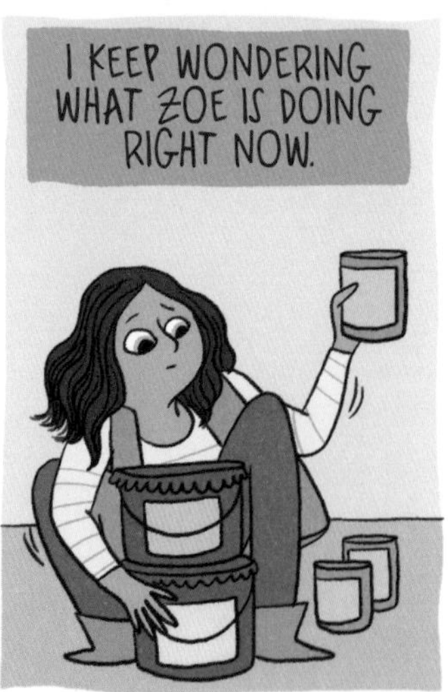

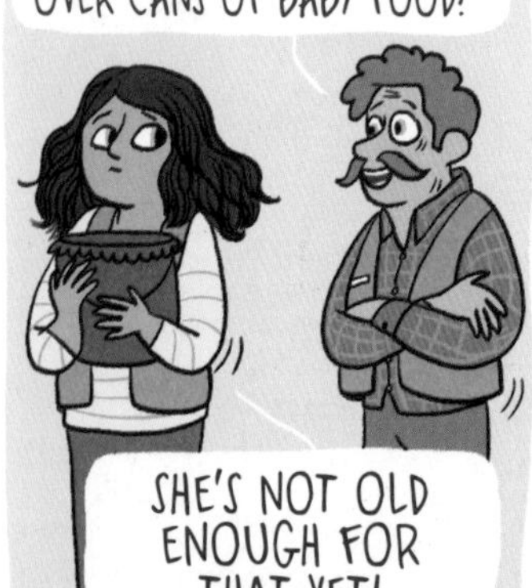

MICHAEL'S
JOKES
DON'T MAKE
ME LAUGH
ANYMORE.

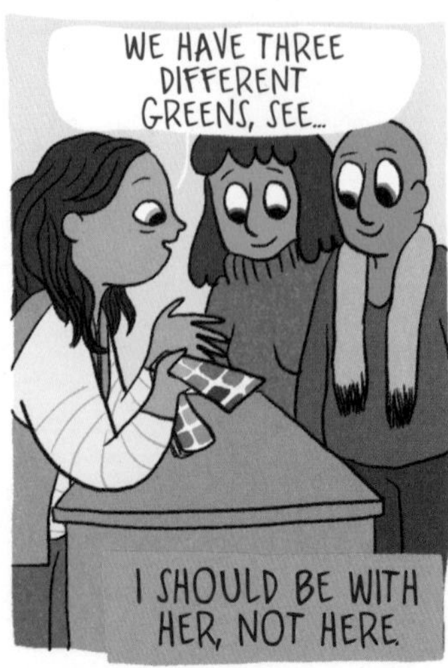

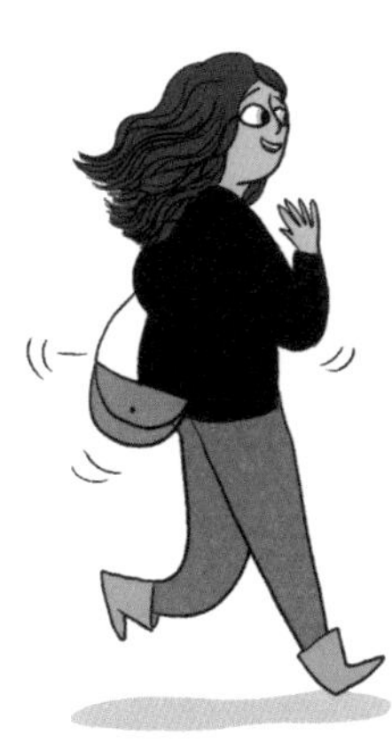

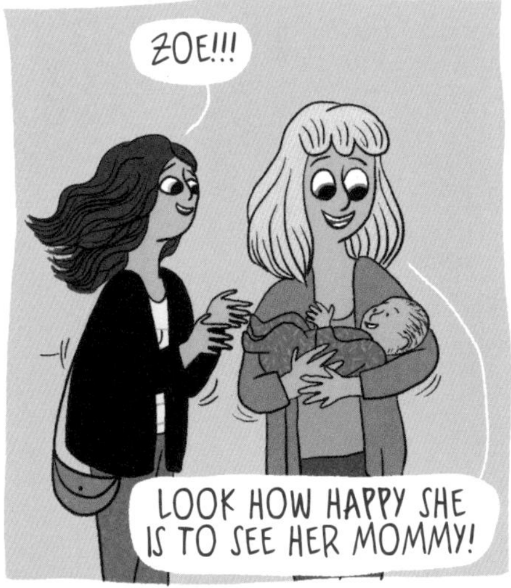
ZOE!!!
LOOK HOW HAPPY SHE IS TO SEE HER MOMMY!

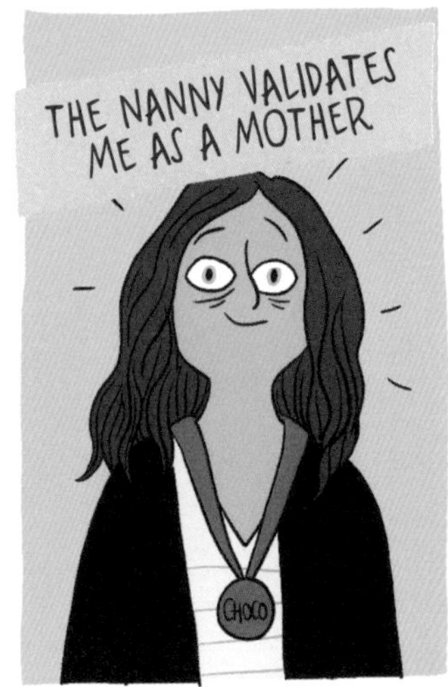
THE NANNY VALIDATES ME AS A MOTHER
CHOCO

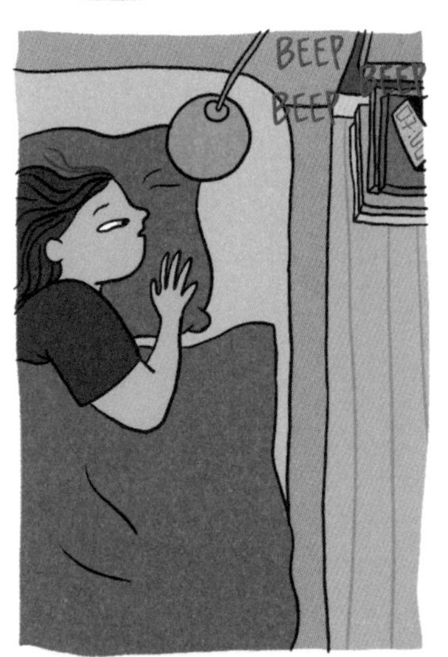
BEEP
BEEP

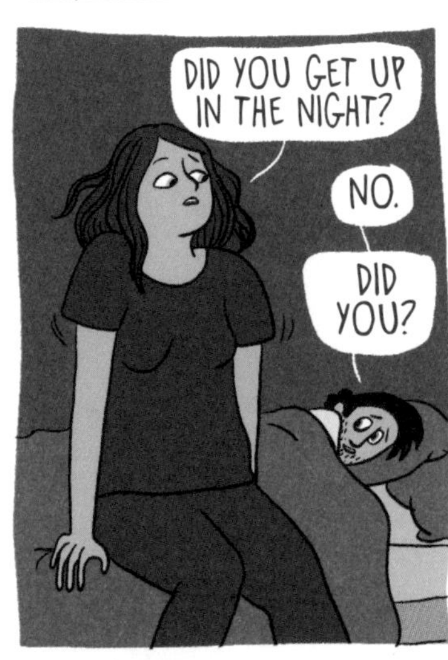
DID YOU GET UP IN THE NIGHT?
NO.
DID YOU?

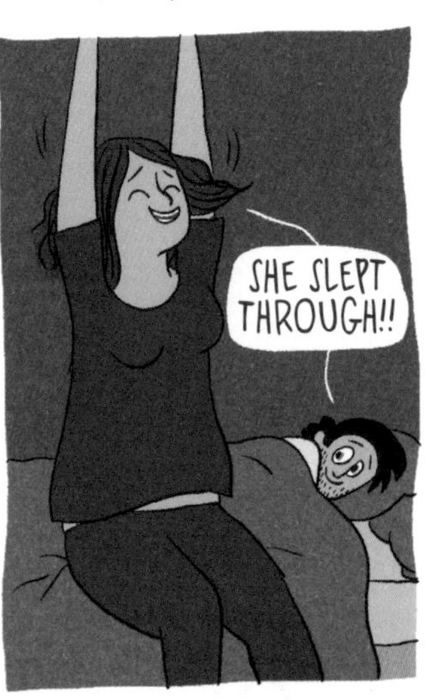
SHE SLEPT THROUGH!!

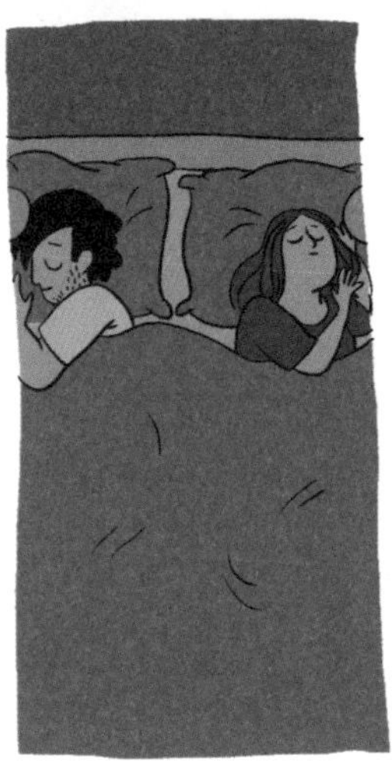

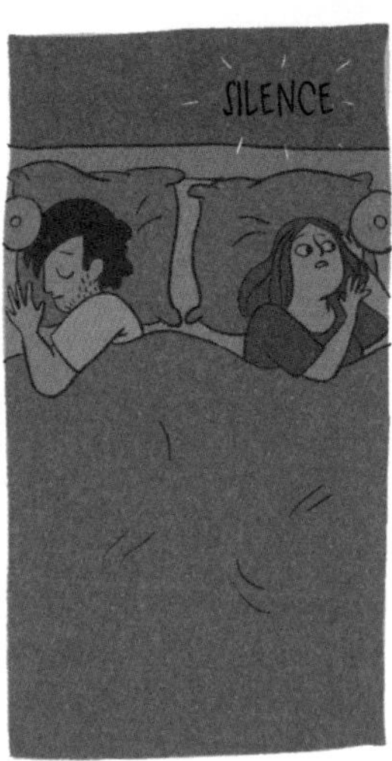
SILENCE

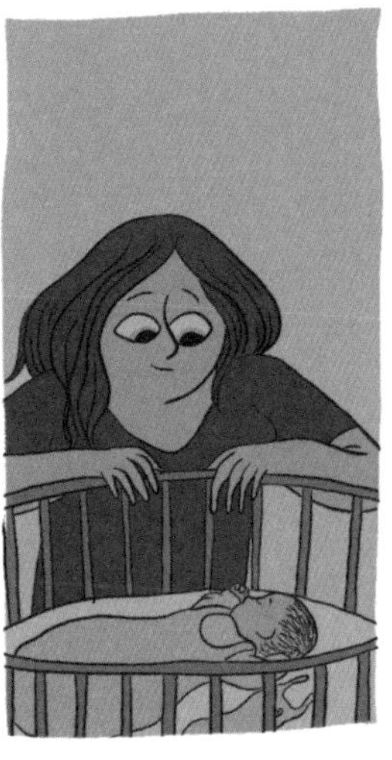

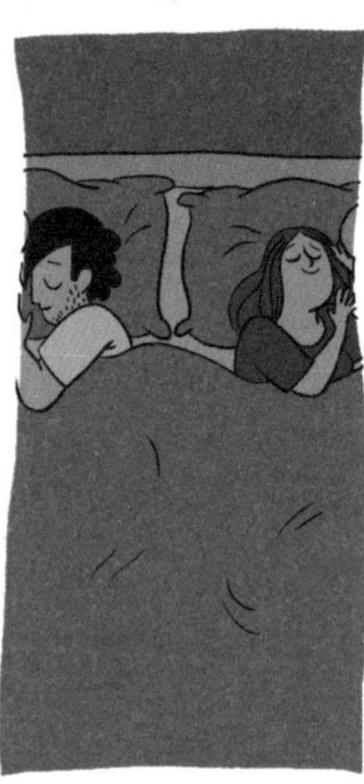

ZOE FINALLY MADE IT THROUGH THE NIGHT!
CAFé PUR ARABICA
SHE DID? THAT CAN CHANGE. BABIES GO THROUGH PHASES.

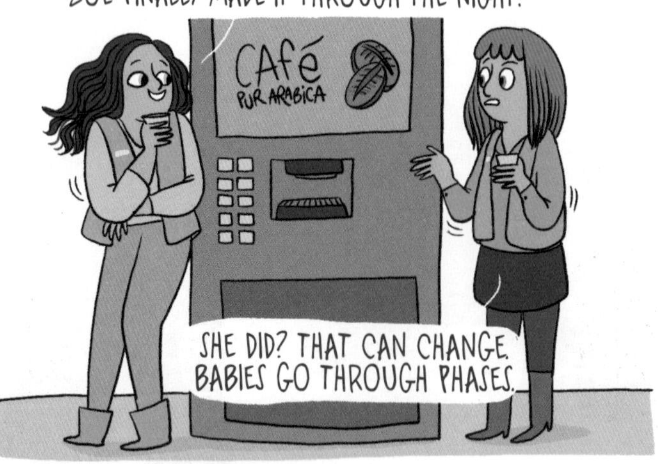

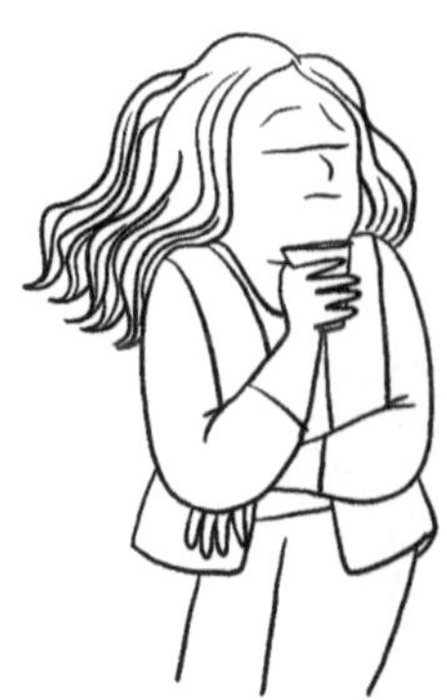

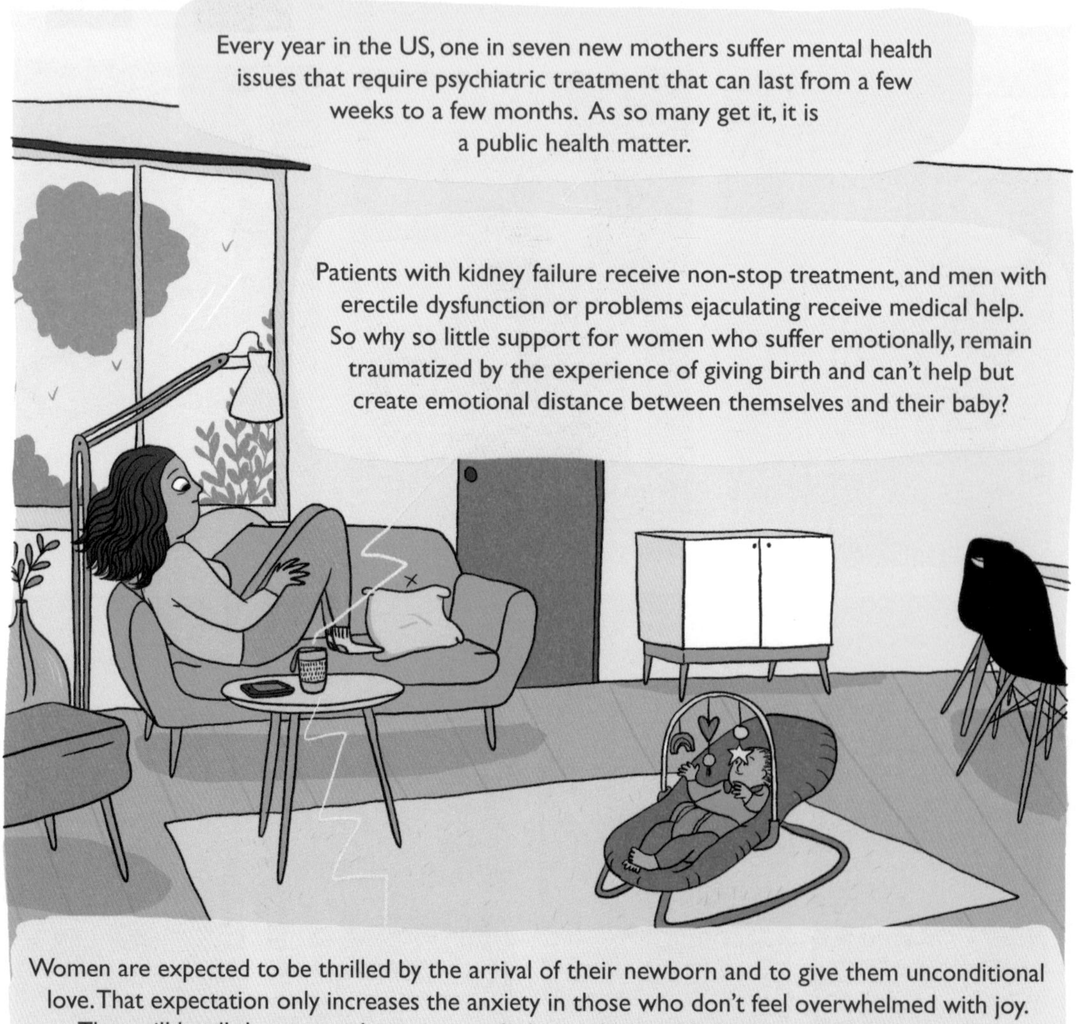

Every year in the US, one in seven new mothers suffer mental health issues that require psychiatric treatment that can last from a few weeks to a few months. As so many get it, it is a public health matter.

Patients with kidney failure receive non-stop treatment, and men with erectile dysfunction or problems ejaculating receive medical help. So why so little support for women who suffer emotionally, remain traumatized by the experience of giving birth and can't help but create emotional distance between themselves and their baby?

Women are expected to be thrilled by the arrival of their newborn and to give them unconditional love. That expectation only increases the anxiety in those who don't feel overwhelmed with joy. They will be all the more reluctant to seek the professional help they need and will suffer, if not in silence, then at least from being misunderstood by those close to them.

HI, KIDS!
HI MOM,
HI DAD!

OK, ZOE'S
ASLEEP!

I ALWAYS FIND THIS
PICTURE OF MOM
REALLY MOVING.
BECAUSE SHE WAS A
YOUNG WOMAN WHO
HADN'T MET MY DAD YET.

SHE HAD NO IDEA SHE WOULD
BECOME THE MOTHER OF DINA
AND ME, AND LEARN TO SPEAK
NORWEGIAN FOR LOVE.

THIS ONE'S MY
FAVORITE.
WHEN I
WAS 17.

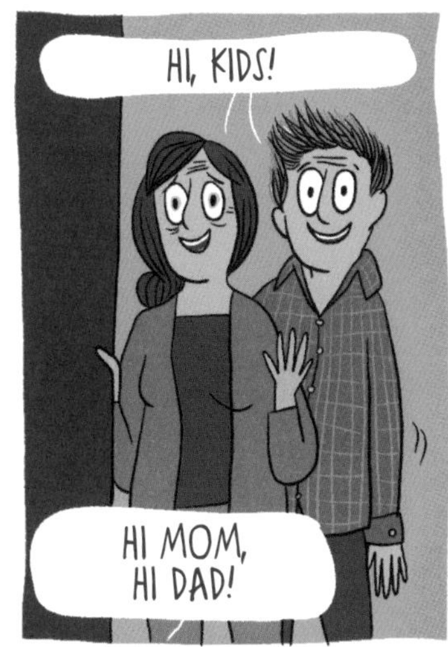

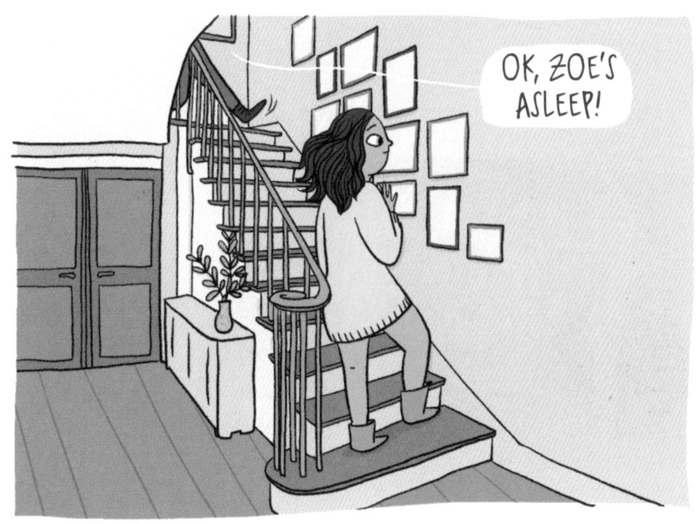

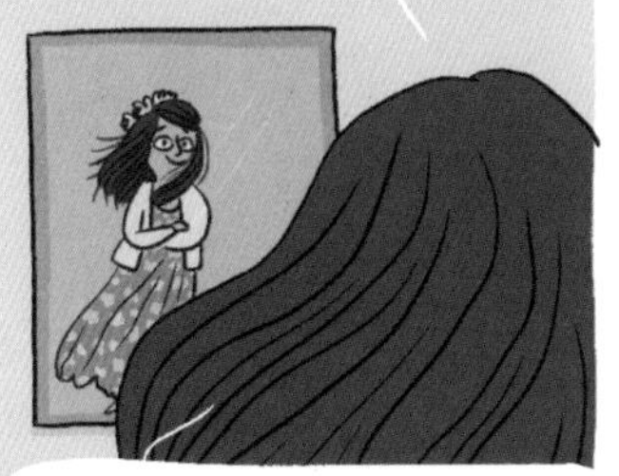

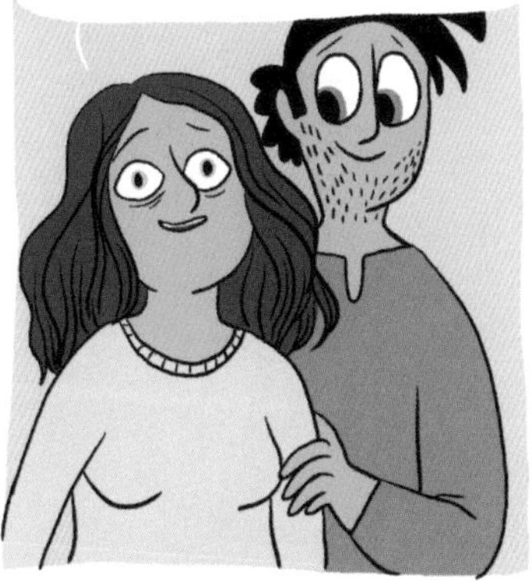

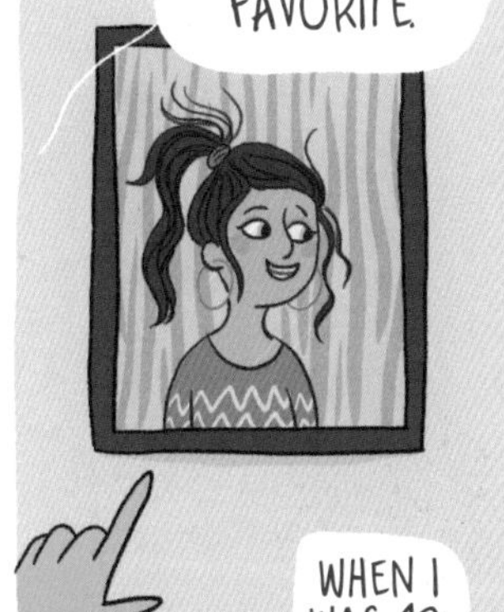

YOU HADN'T YET MET YOUR
AMAZING GUY AND DIDN'T
KNOW YOU WOULD BECOME
THE WONDERFUL MOTHER
OF OUR WONDERFUL ZOE.

CHUCK VALIDATES
ME AS A MOTHER
CHOCO

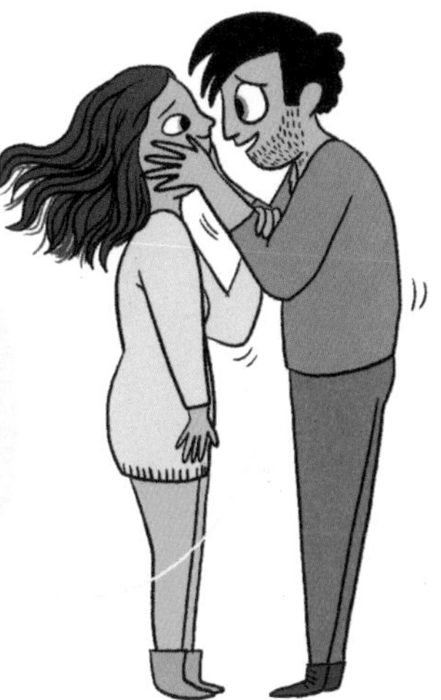

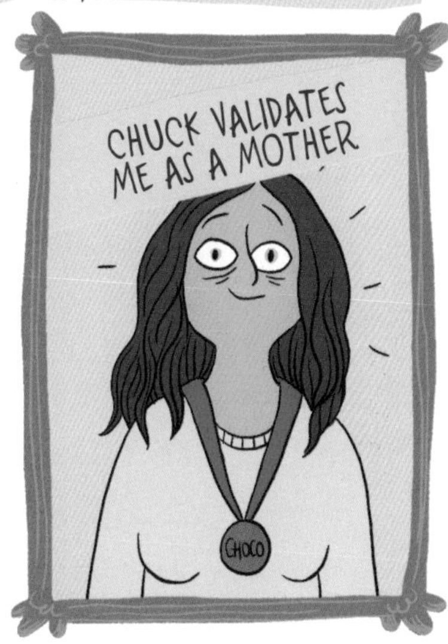

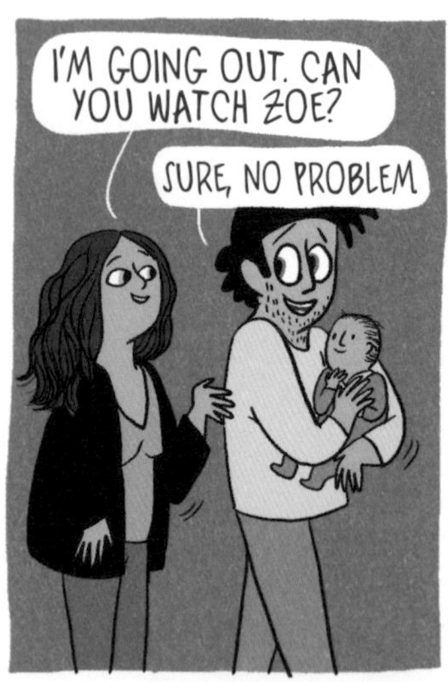
I'M GOING OUT. CAN YOU WATCH ZOE?
SURE, NO PROBLEM

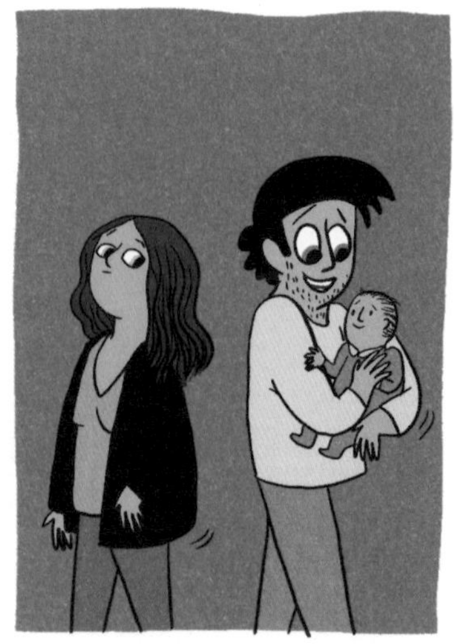

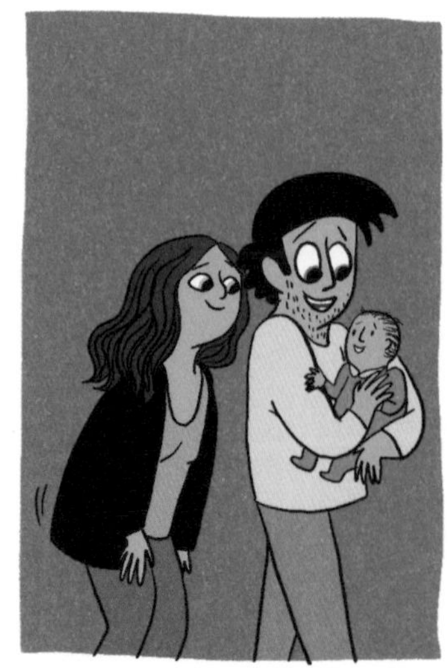

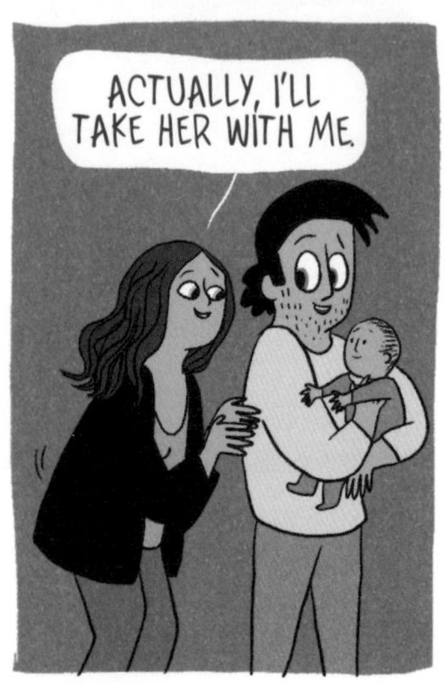
ACTUALLY, I'LL TAKE HER WITH ME.

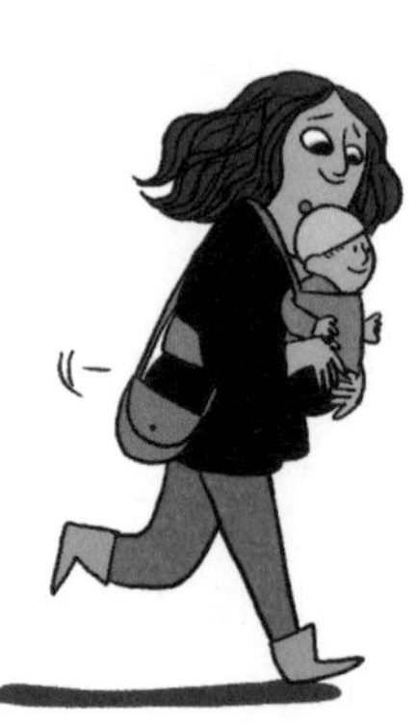

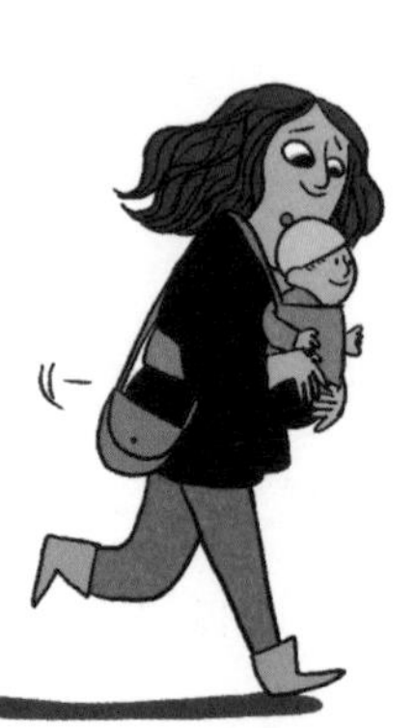

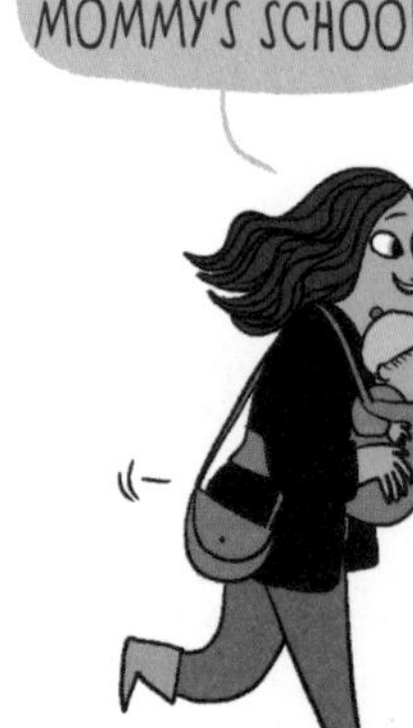
AND THAT WAS MOMMY'S SCHOOL.

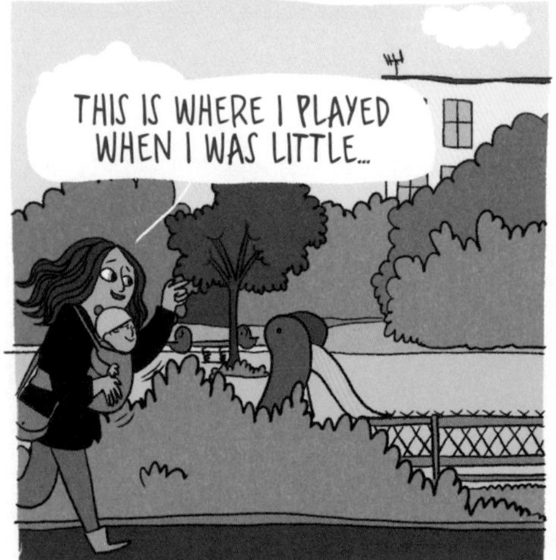
THIS IS WHERE I PLAYED WHEN I WAS LITTLE...

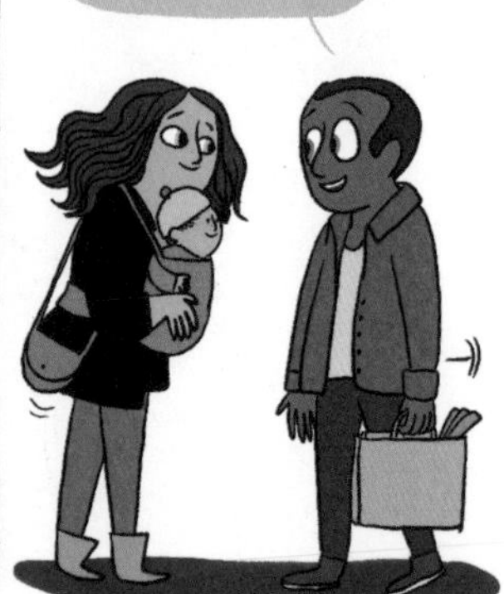
MARIETTA, HI! WHAT HAVE YOU BEEN UP TO?

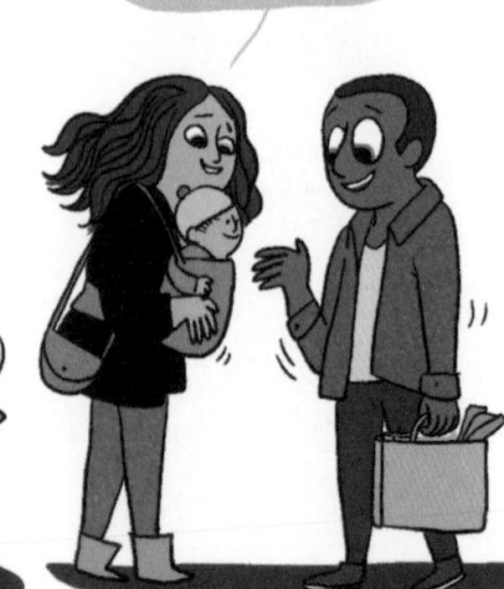
I'M ZOE'S MOTHER

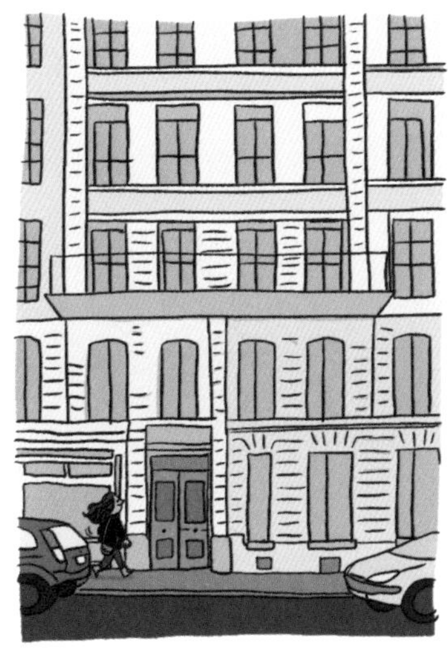

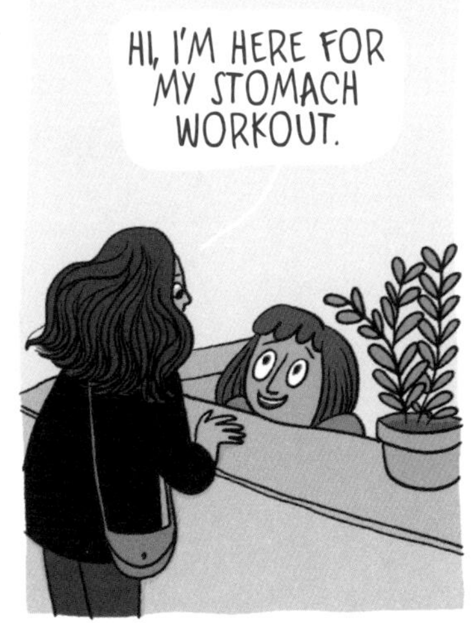
HI, I'M HERE FOR MY STOMACH WORKOUT.

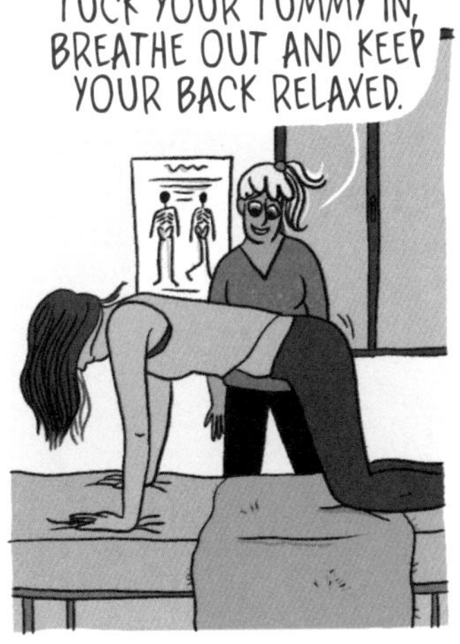
TUCK YOUR TUMMY IN, BREATHE OUT AND KEEP YOUR BACK RELAXED.

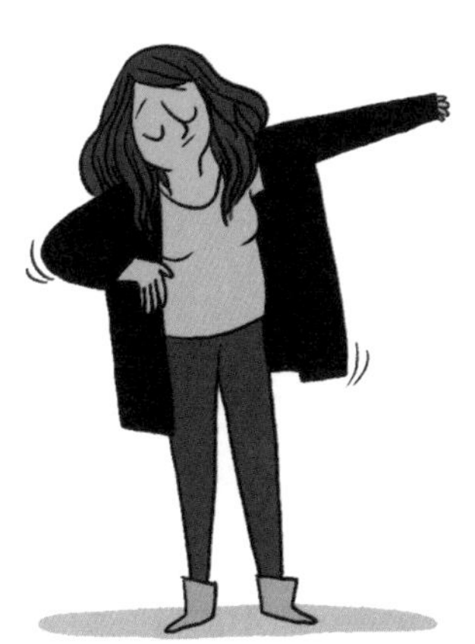

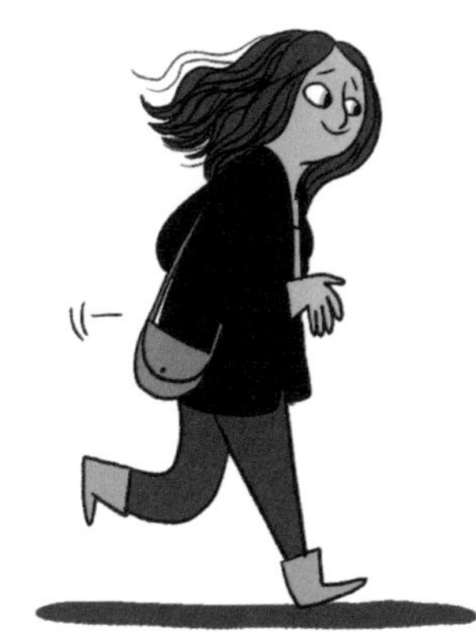

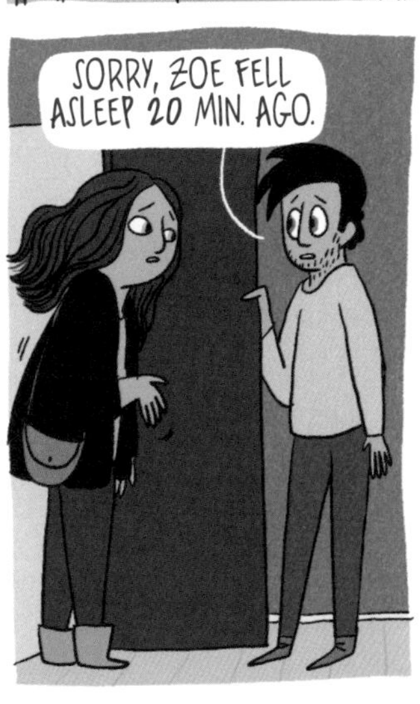
SORRY, ZOE FELL ASLEEP 20 MIN. AGO.

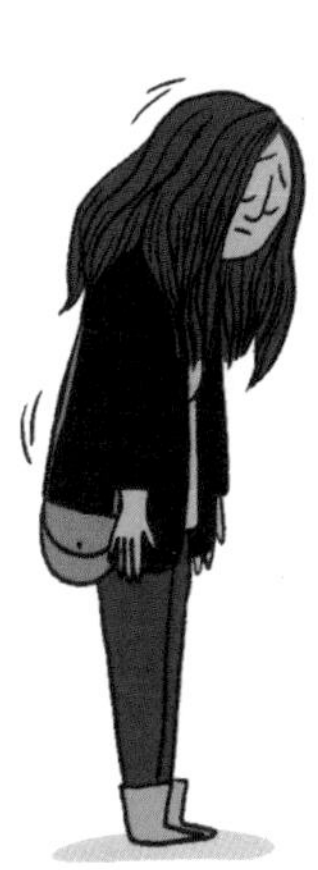

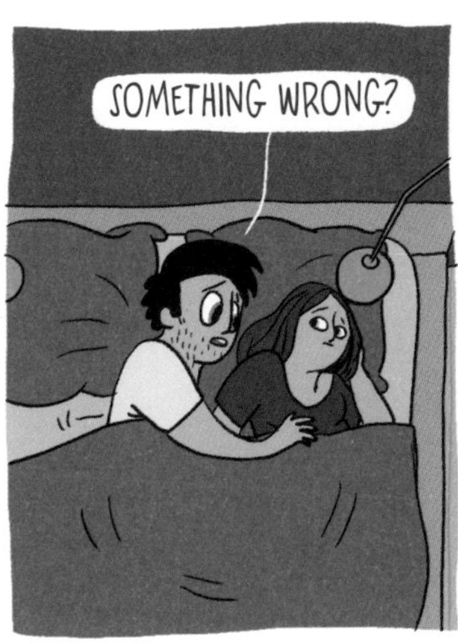
SOMETHING WRONG?

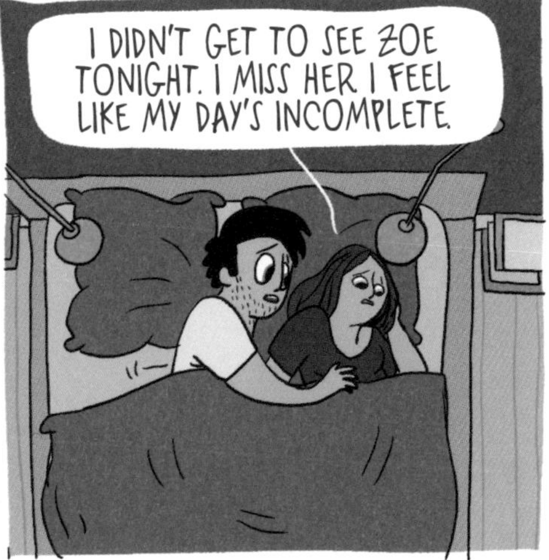
I DIDN'T GET TO SEE ZOE TONIGHT. I MISS HER I FEEL LIKE MY DAY'S INCOMPLETE.

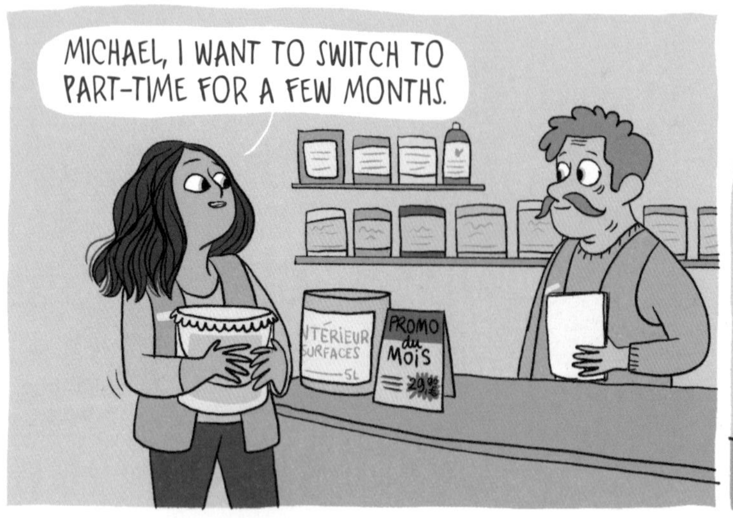
MICHAEL, I WANT TO SWITCH TO PART-TIME FOR A FEW MONTHS.
PROMO du MOIS

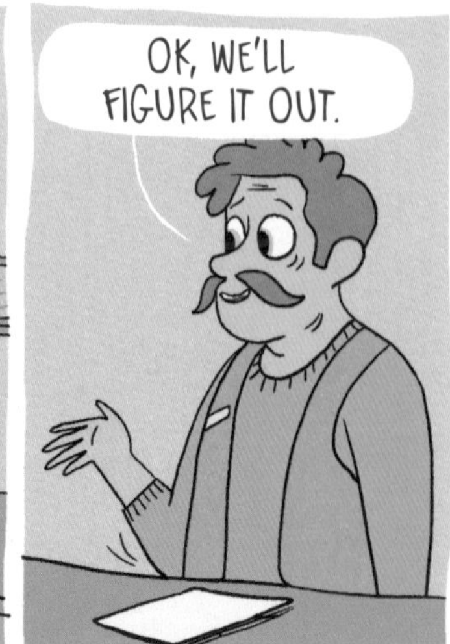
OK, WE'LL FIGURE IT OUT.

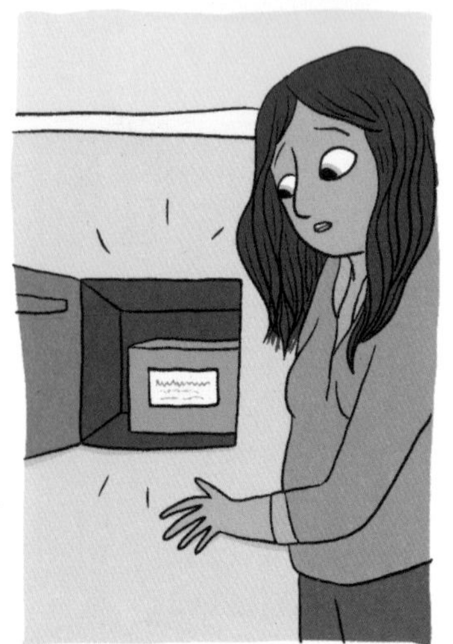

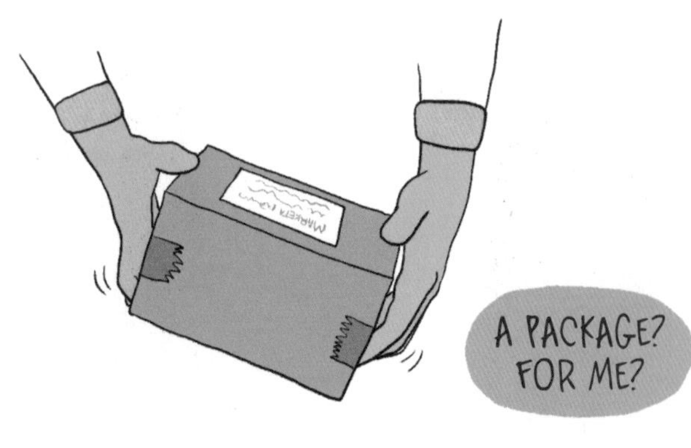
A PACKAGE? FOR ME?

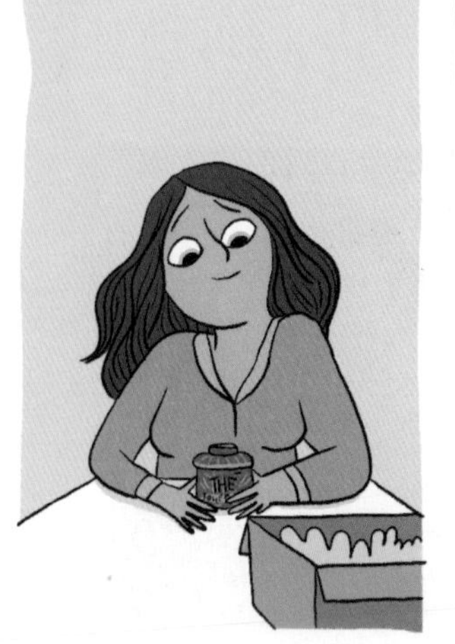

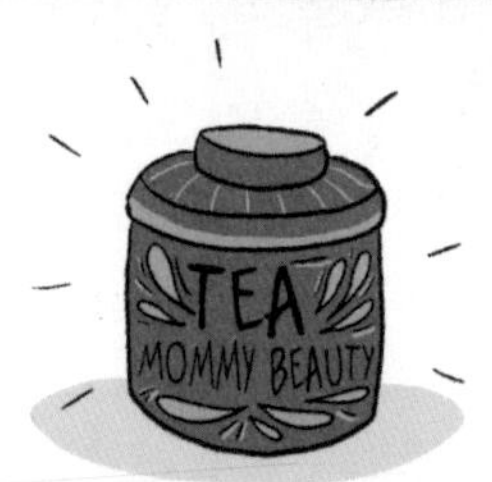
THIS TEA IS THE FIRST PRESENT FOR ME. AND JUST AS I THOUGHT, I NOW ONLY EXIST FOR WHAT I PRODUCED.
TEA
MOMMY BEAUTY

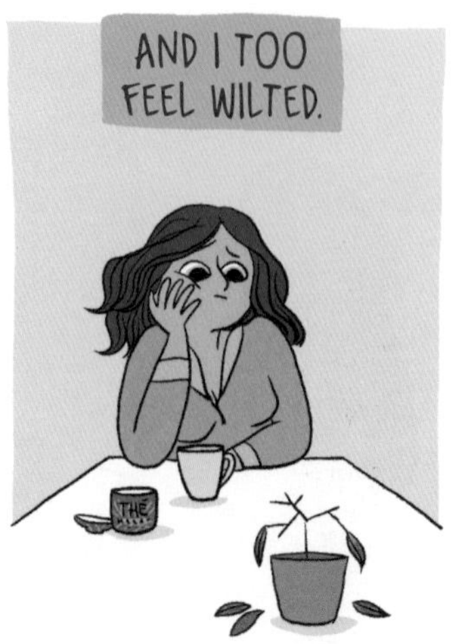
AND I TOO FEEL WILTED.

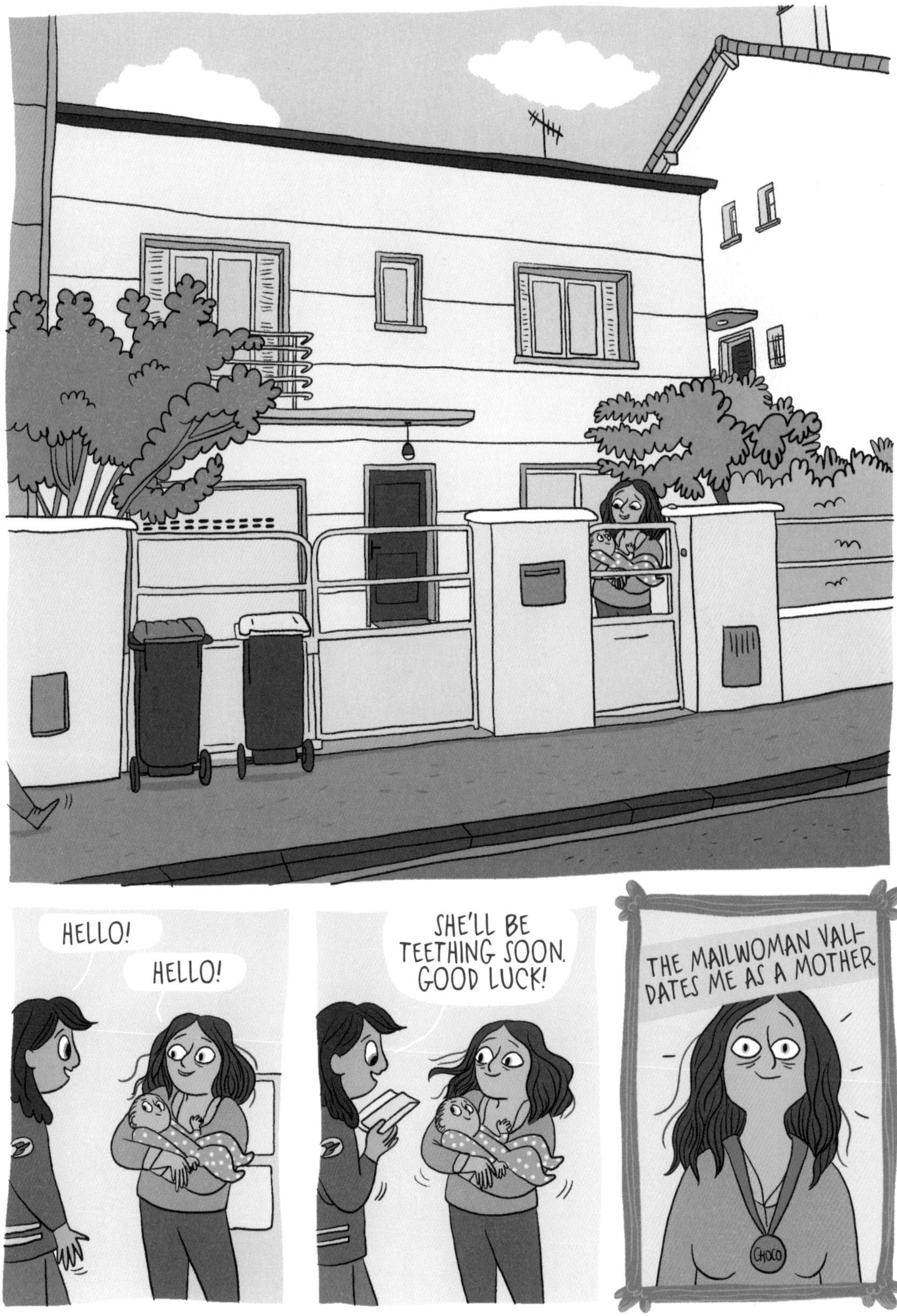

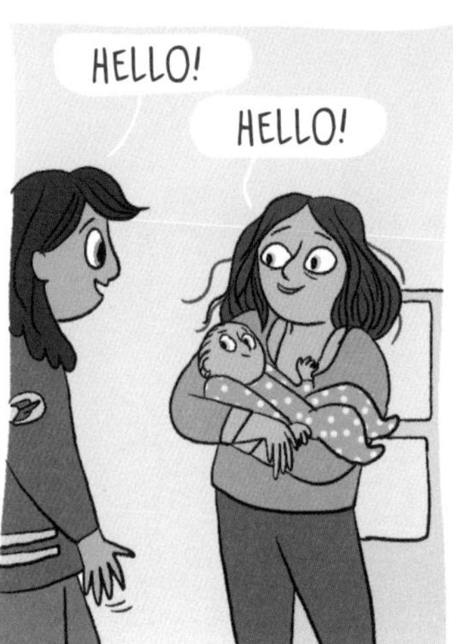
HELLO!
HELLO!

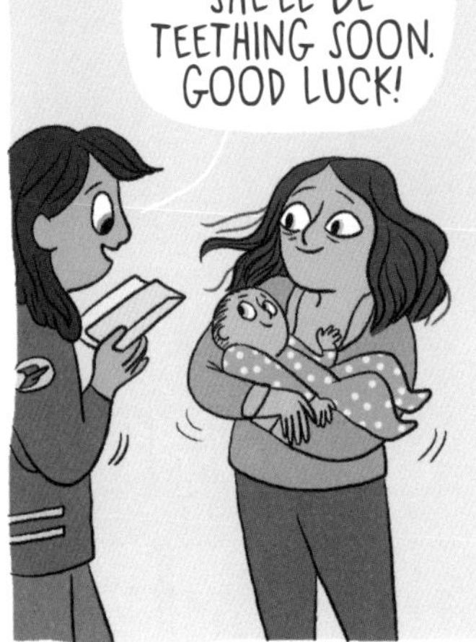
SHE'LL BE TEETHING SOON. GOOD LUCK!

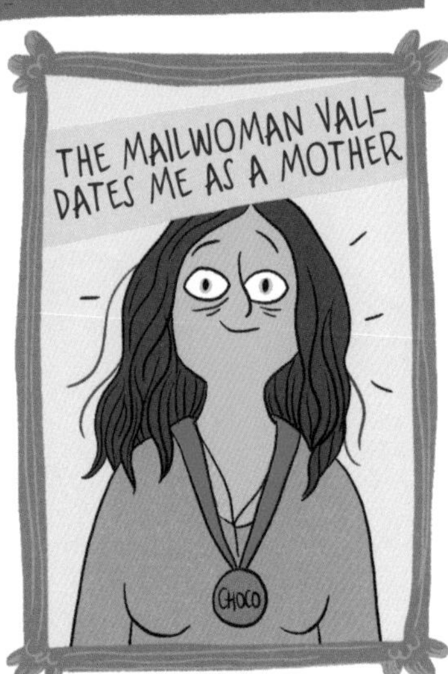
THE MAILWOMAN VALI-DATES ME AS A MOTHER
CHOCO

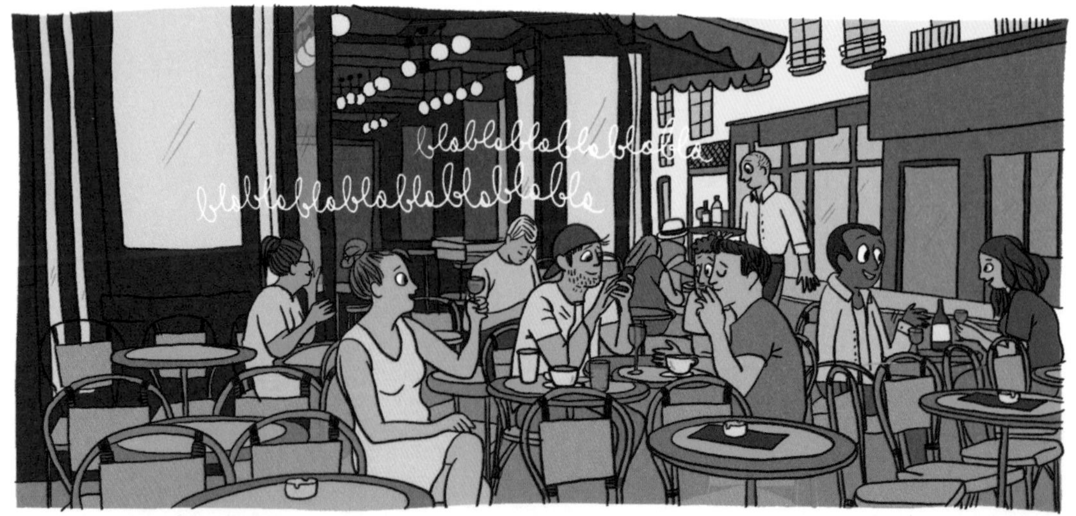

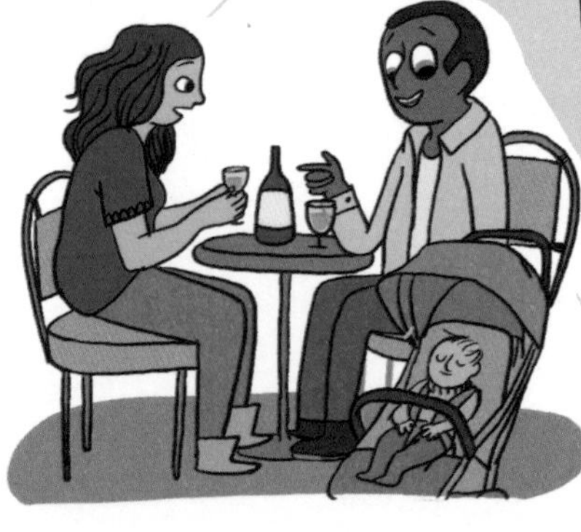

DO YOU REMEMBER SCIENCE CLASS?
WHEN WE DISSECTED THAT FISH! GROSS!
YEAH, BUT MOSTLY, THEY MADE US WATCH THAT BIRTH, DURING SEX-ED CLASS. REMEMBER? THE ENTIRE CLASS WAS TRAUMATIZED. THE GIRLS SAID THEY'D NEVER HAVE KIDS, AND THE BOYS SAID THEY'D NEVER HAVE SEX!
LOOKS LIKE IT DIDN'T AFFECT YOU, THOUGH.

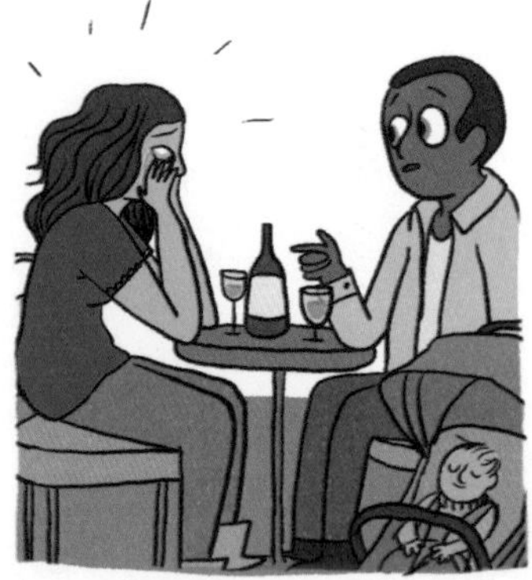

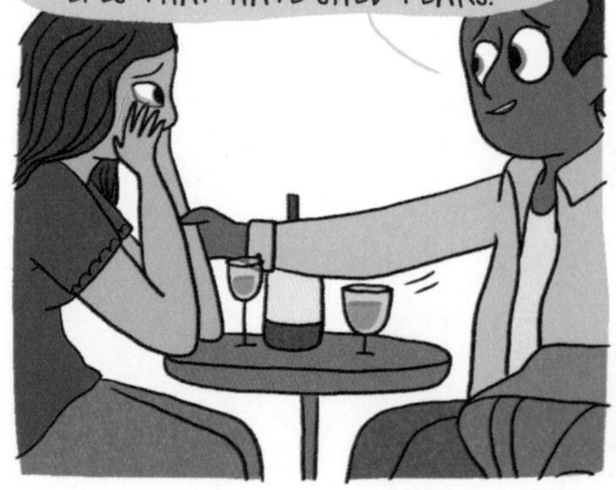

YOU KNOW WHAT WE SAY IN CÔTE D'IVOIRE? THAT SOME THINGS ARE SEEN MORE CLEARLY THROUGH EYES THAT HAVE SHED TEARS.

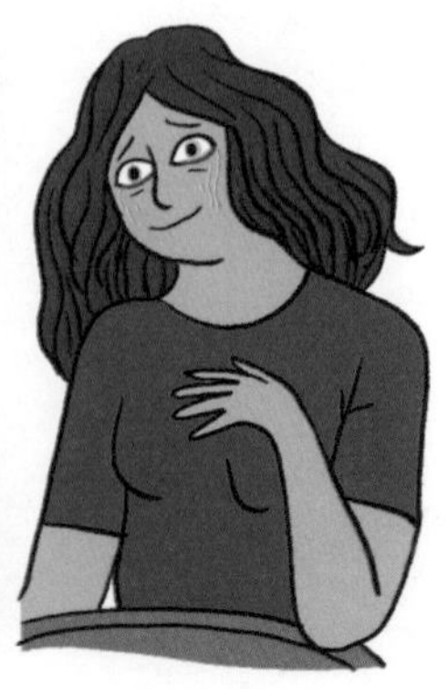

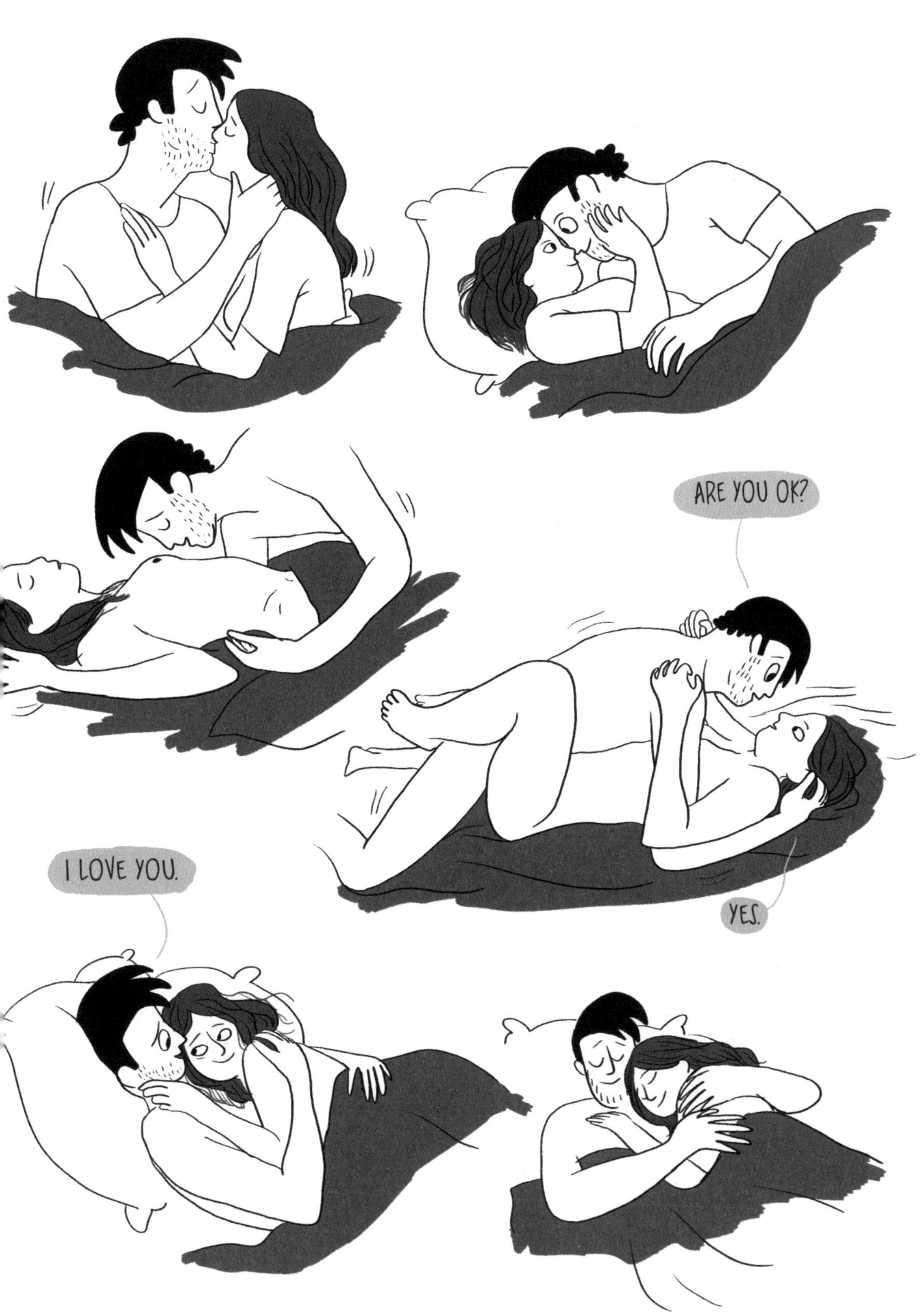
ARE YOU OK?
YES.
I LOVE YOU.

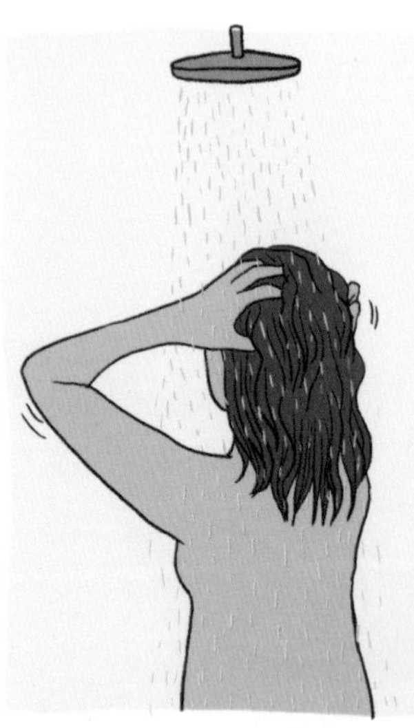

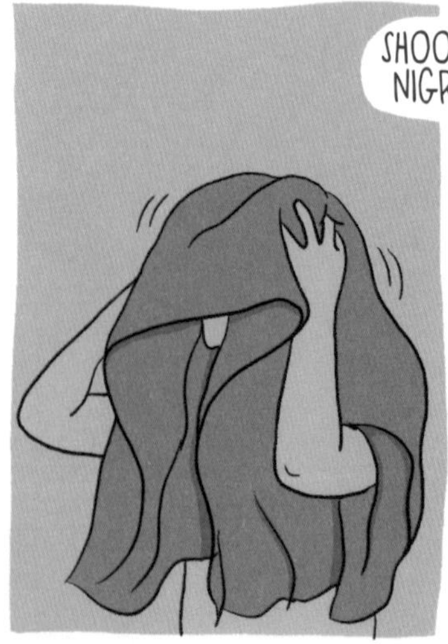

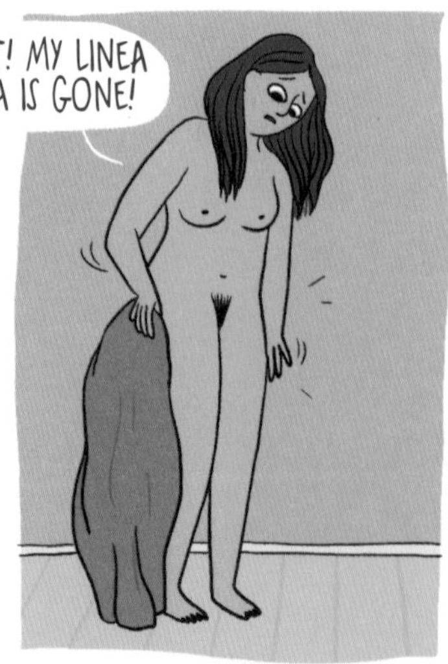
SHOOT! MY LINEA NIGRA IS GONE!

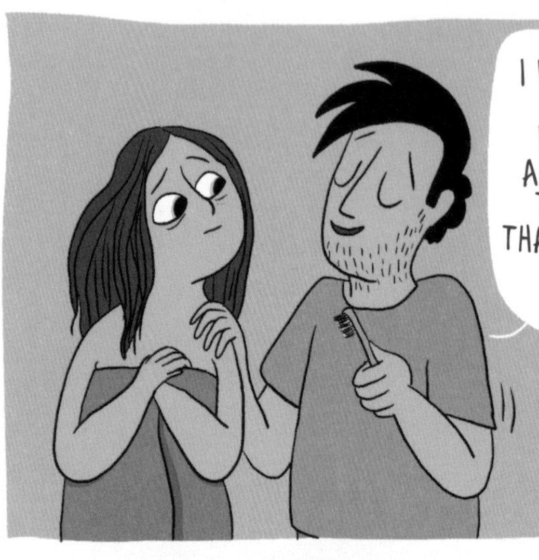
I DON'T THINK IT'S GONE. I THINK IT'S ALWAYS BEEN THERE, AND THAT IT'S HIDING, JUST IN CASE.

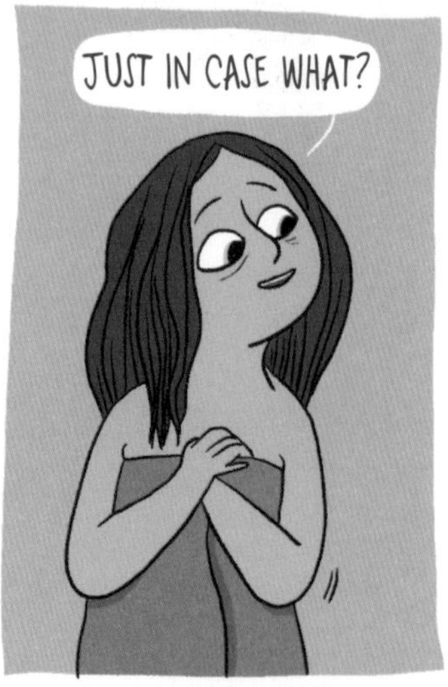
JUST IN CASE WHAT?

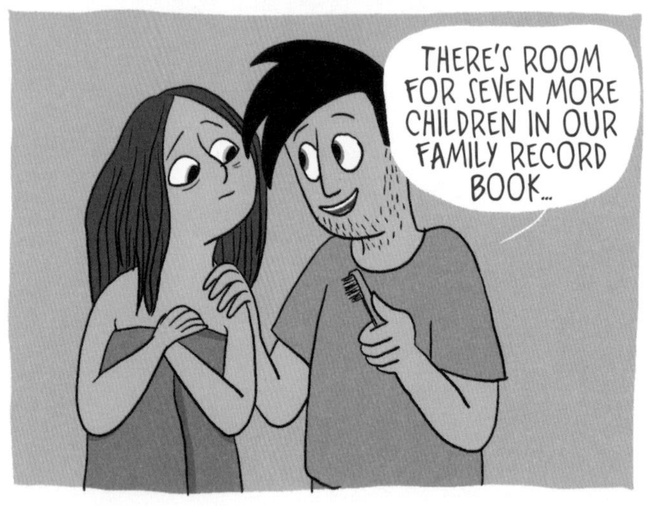
THERE'S ROOM FOR SEVEN MORE CHILDREN IN OUR FAMILY RECORD BOOK...

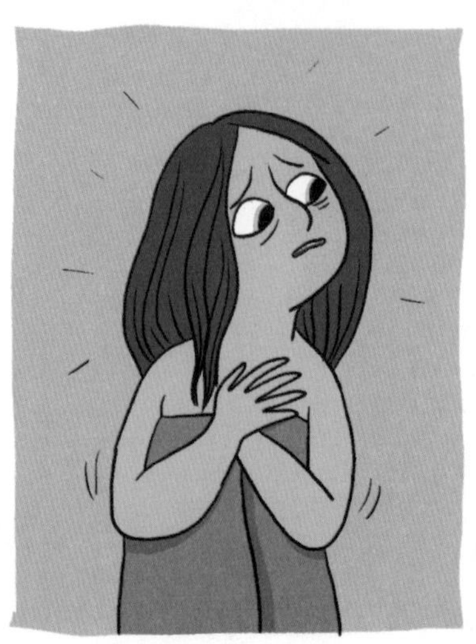

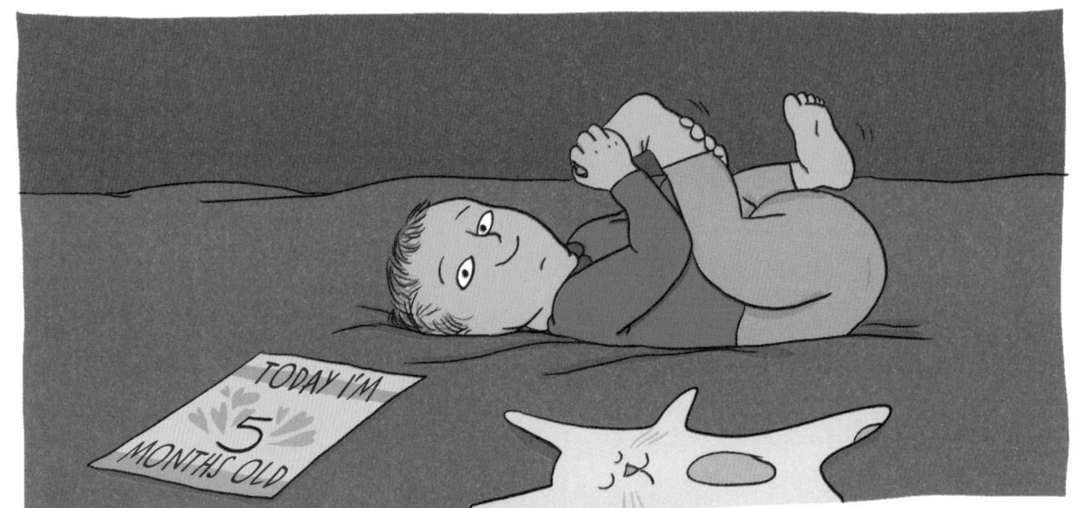
TODAY I'M
5
MONTHS OLD

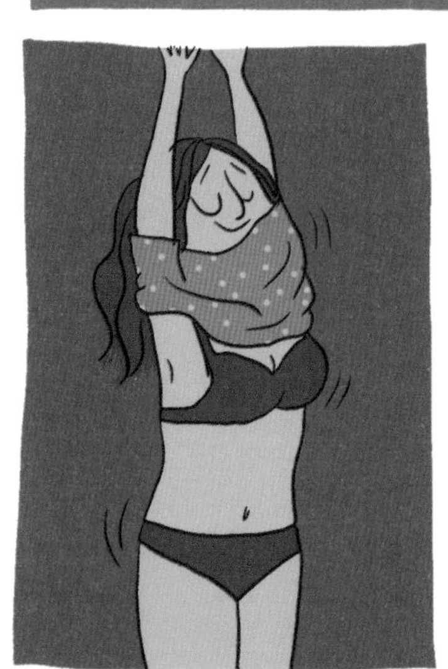

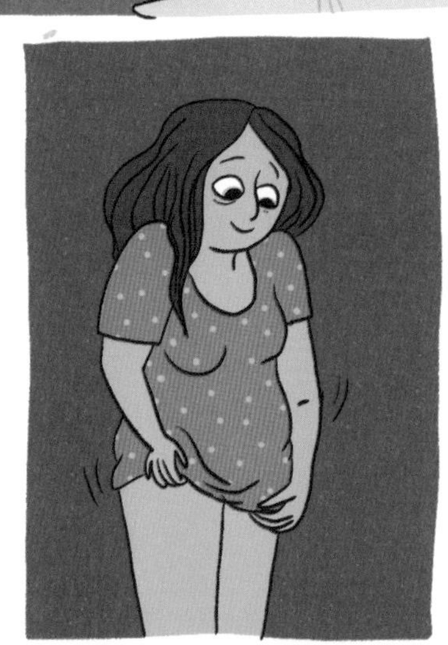

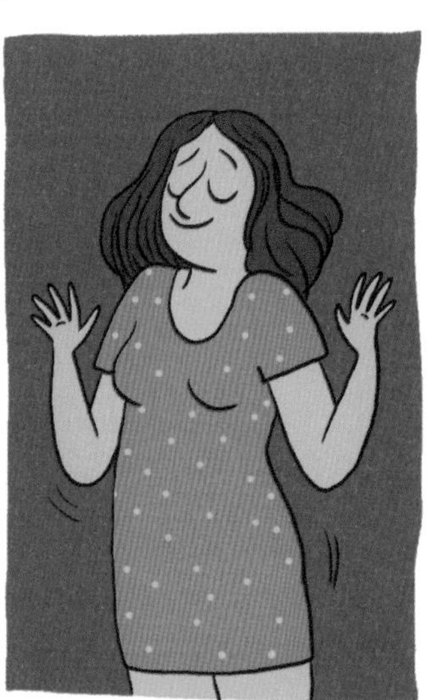

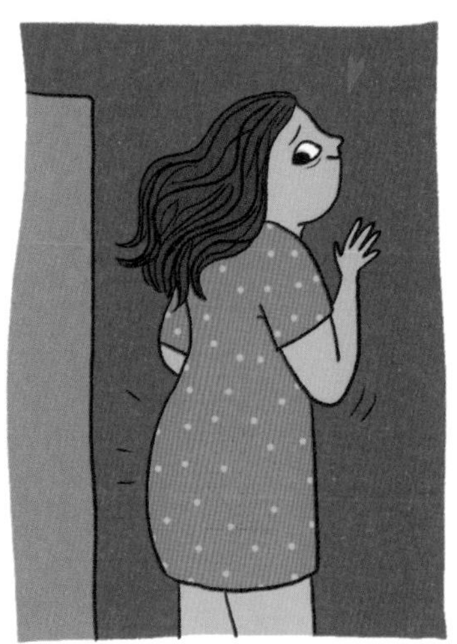

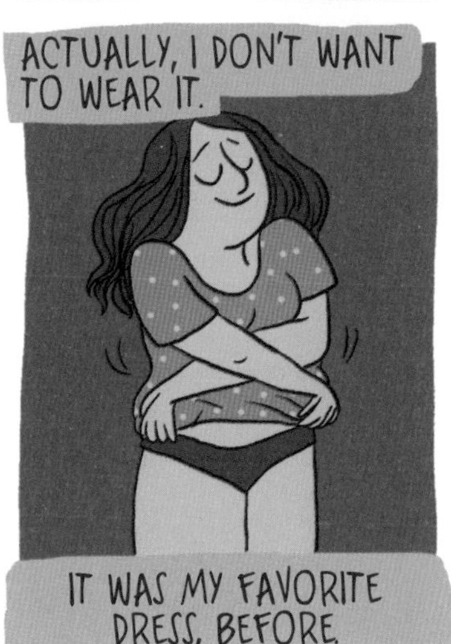
ACTUALLY, I DON'T WANT TO WEAR IT.
IT WAS MY FAVORITE DRESS, BEFORE.

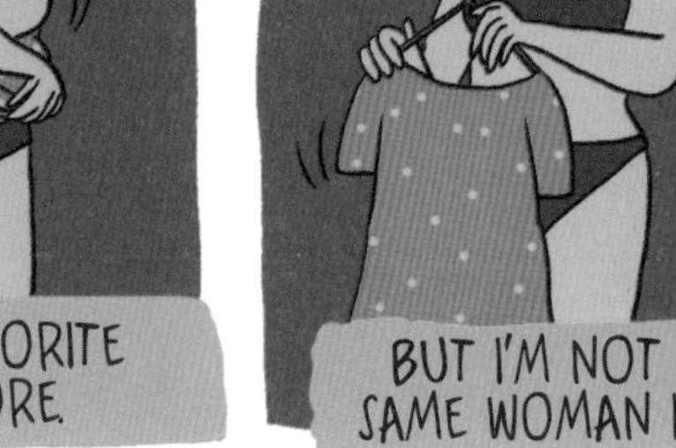
BUT I'M NOT THE SAME WOMAN I WAS.

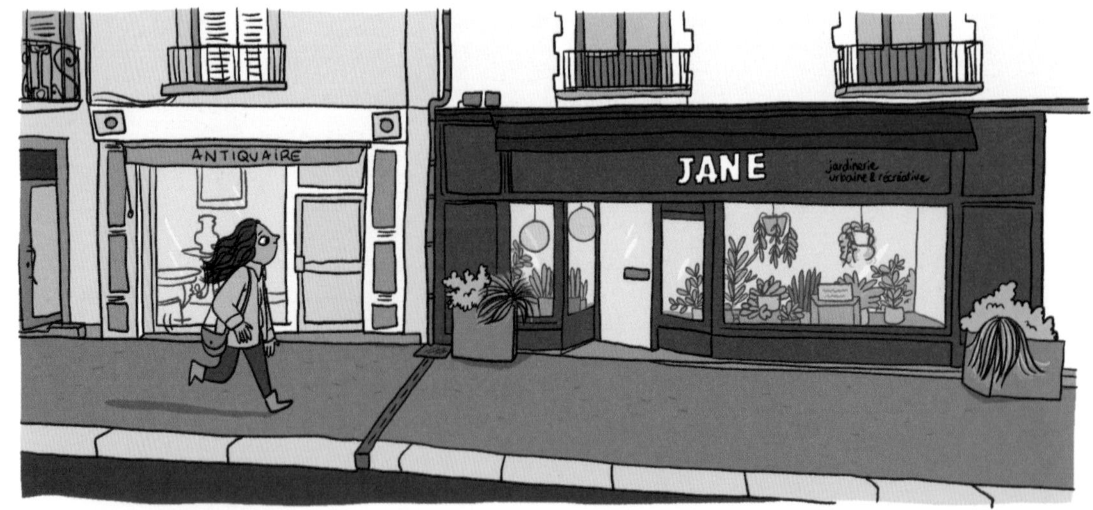
ANTIQUAIRE
JANE
jardinerie urbaine & récréative

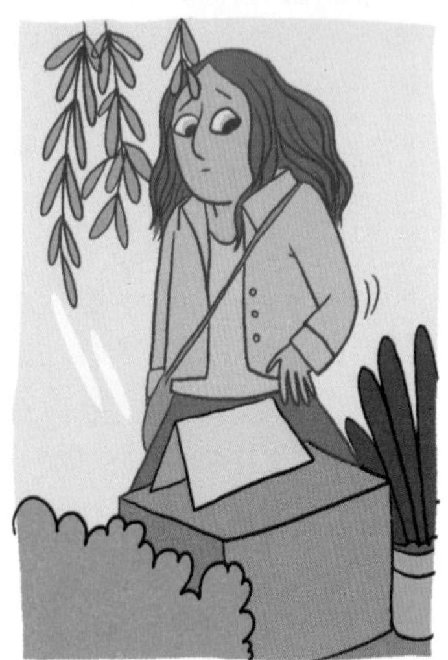

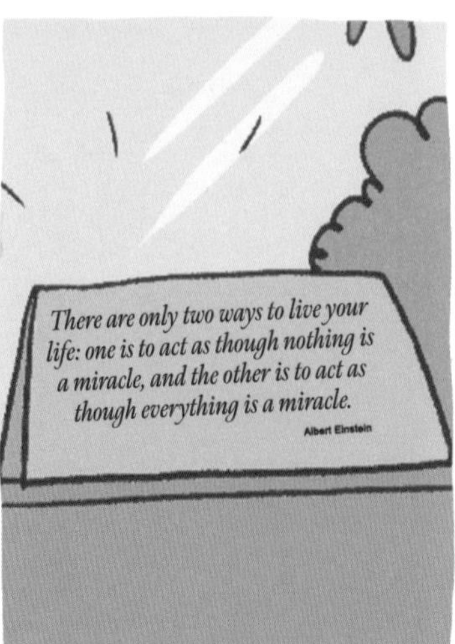
There are only two ways to live your life: one is to act as though nothing is a miracle, and the other is to act as though everything is a miracle.
Albert Einstein

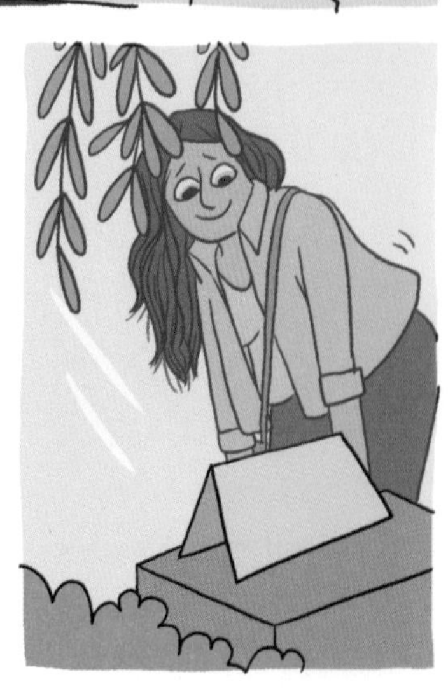

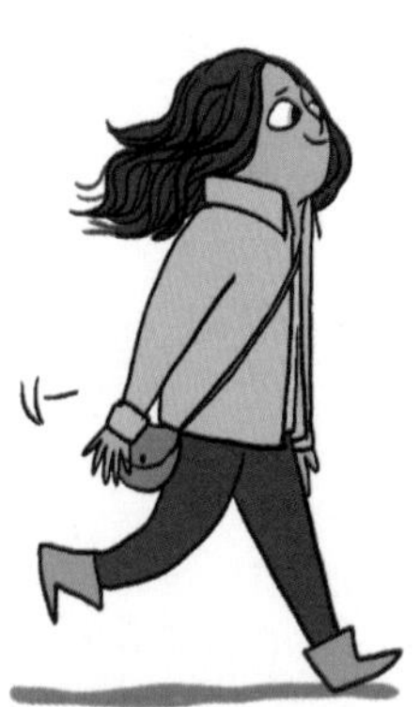

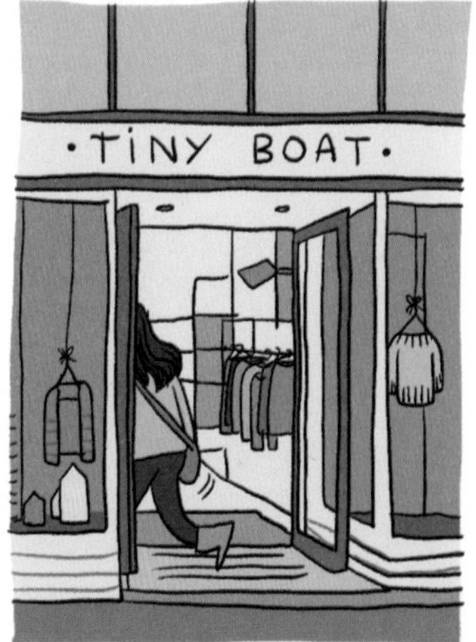
·TINY BOAT·

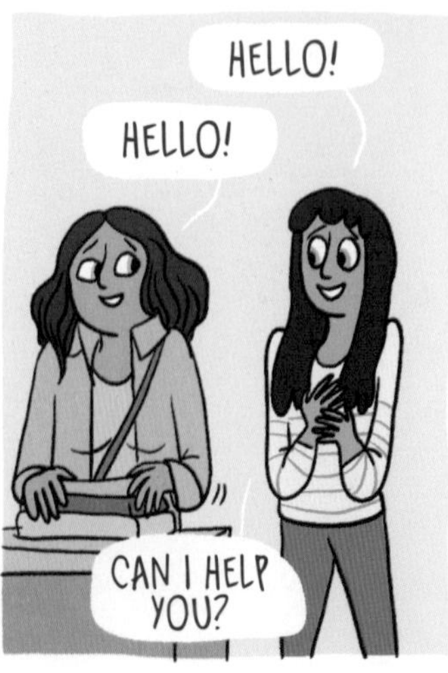
HELLO!
HELLO!
CAN I HELP YOU?

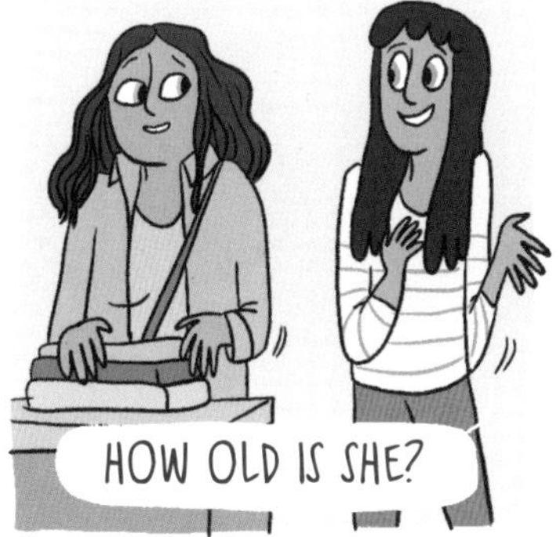
I'M LOOKING FOR ONE-SIES FOR MY DAUGHTER
SURE.
HOW OLD IS SHE?

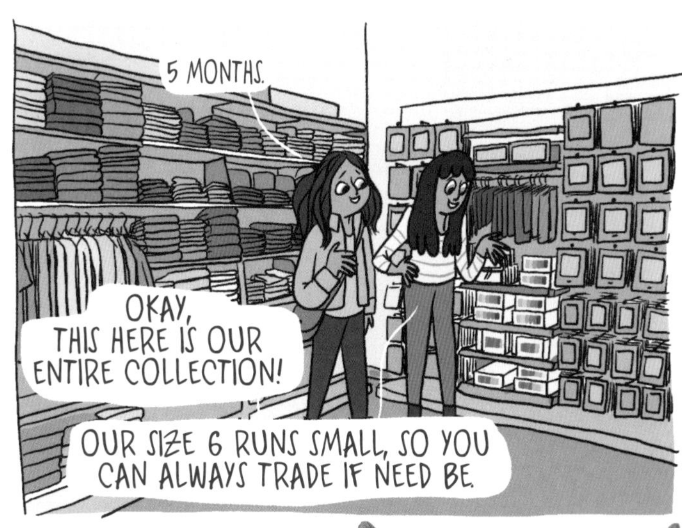
5 MONTHS.
OKAY, THIS HERE IS OUR ENTIRE COLLECTION!
OUR SIZE 6 RUNS SMALL, SO YOU CAN ALWAYS TRADE IF NEED BE.

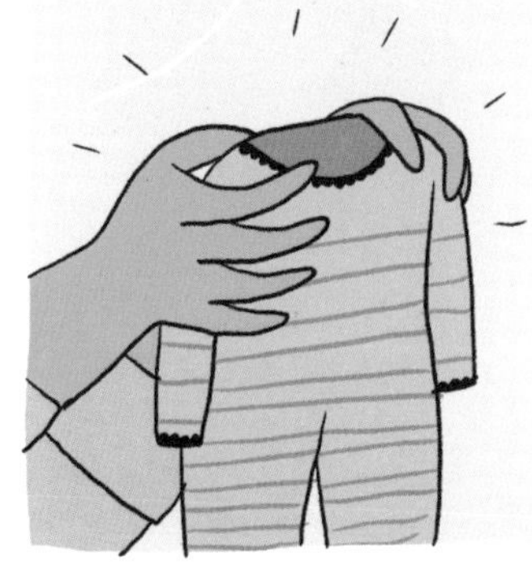
GREAT. I'LL TAKE THIS ONE, AND THE YELLOW ONE TOO.

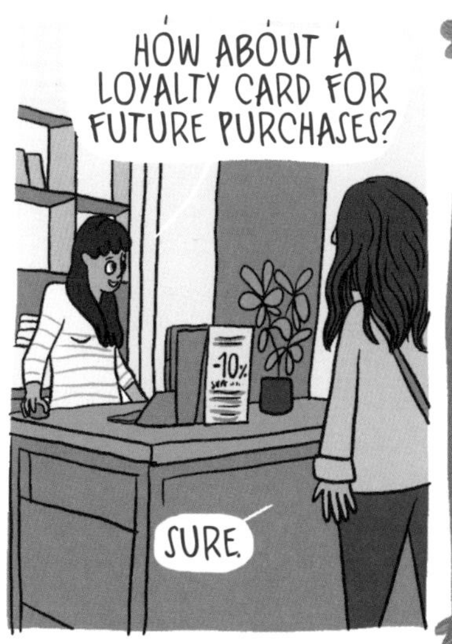
HOW ABOUT A LOYALTY CARD FOR FUTURE PURCHASES?
-10%
SURE.

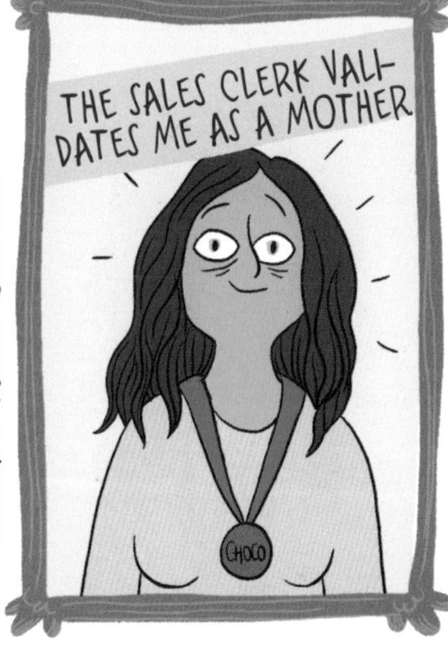
THE SALES CLERK VALI-DATES ME AS A MOTHER.
CHOCO

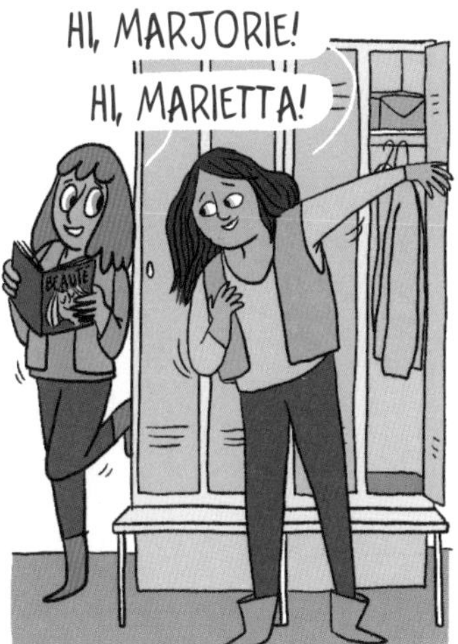
HI, MARJORIE!
HI, MARIETTA!
BEAUTE

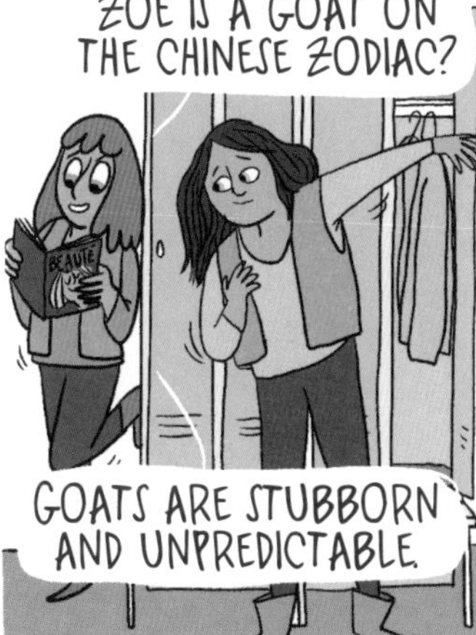
DID YOU KNOW THAT ZOE IS A GOAT ON THE CHINESE ZODIAC?
BEAUTE
GOATS ARE STUBBORN AND UNPREDICTABLE.

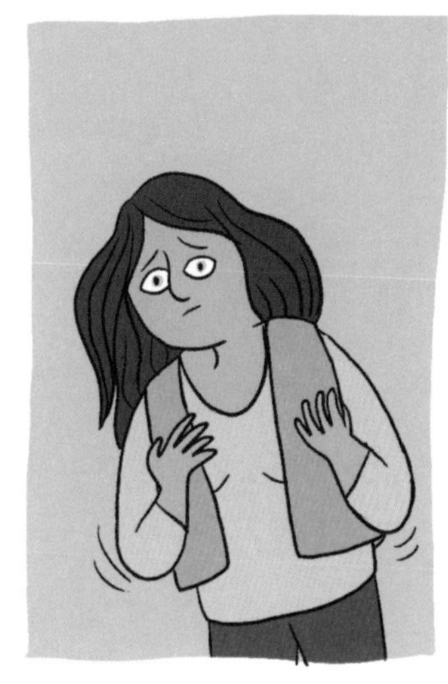

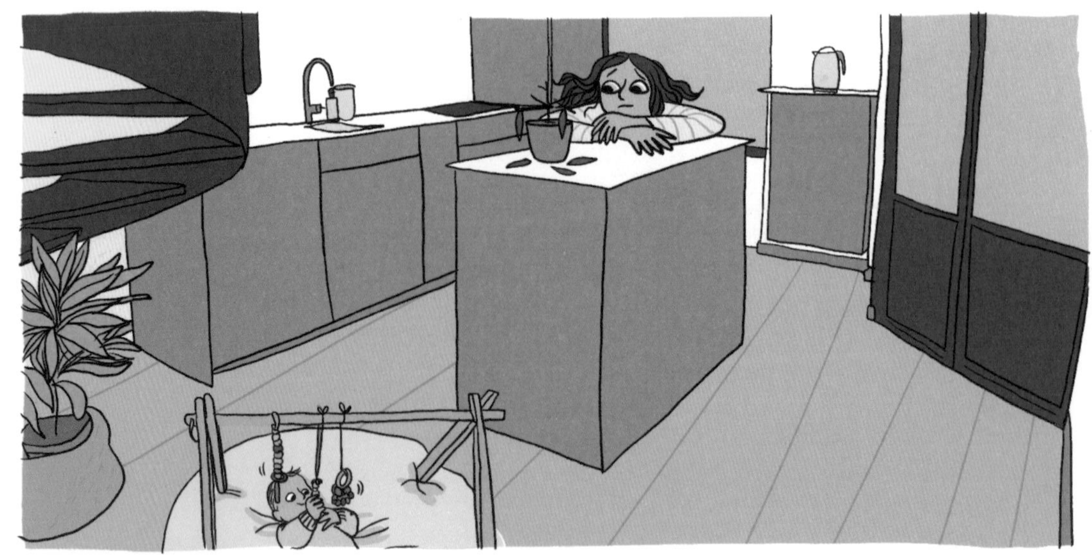

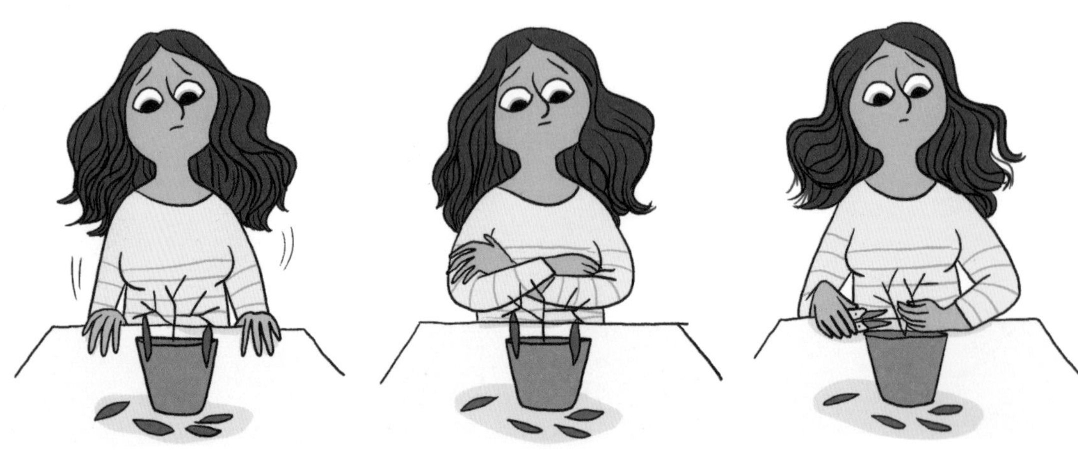

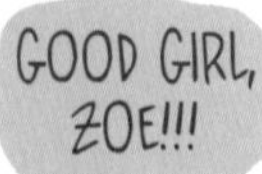
GOOD GIRL,
ZOE!!!

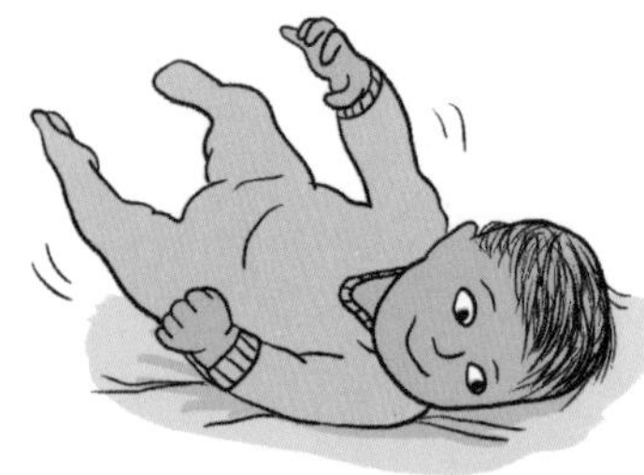

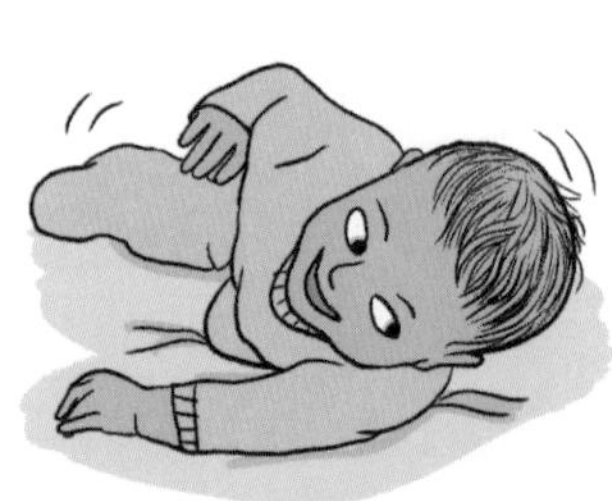

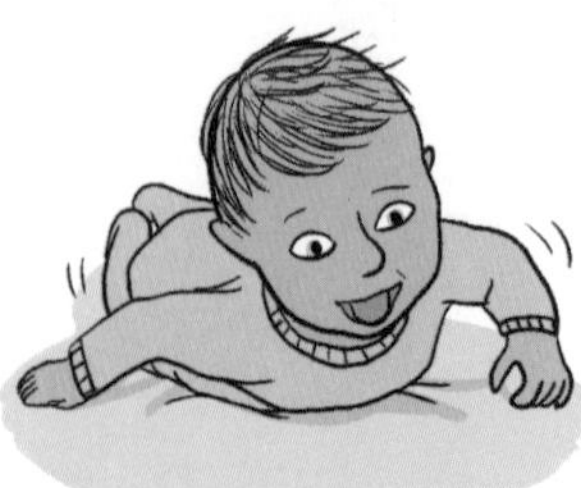

NICE WORK!!
WHO'S A BIG GIRL?

ARE YOU HUNGRY?

LOOK, YOUR FIRST MASHED VEGGIES. CARROTS, YUM!

READY?

WELL? DO YOU LIKE IT?!

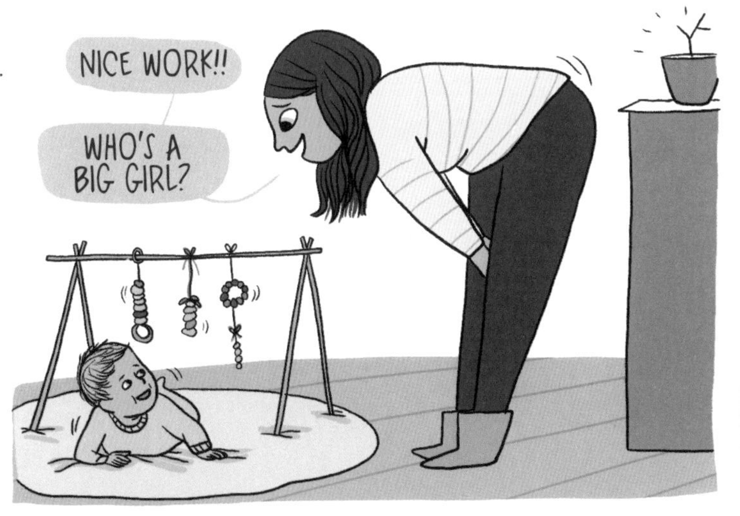

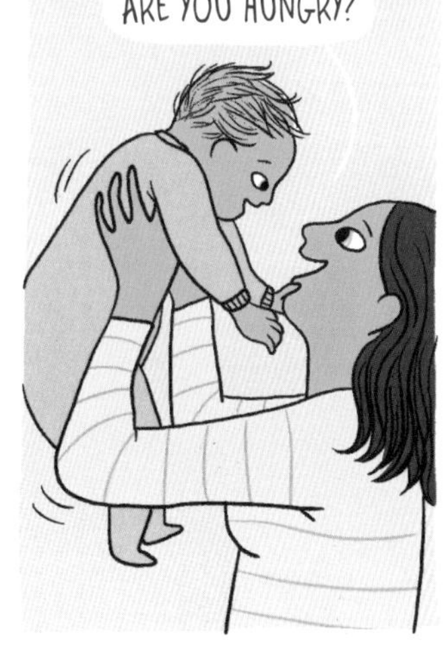

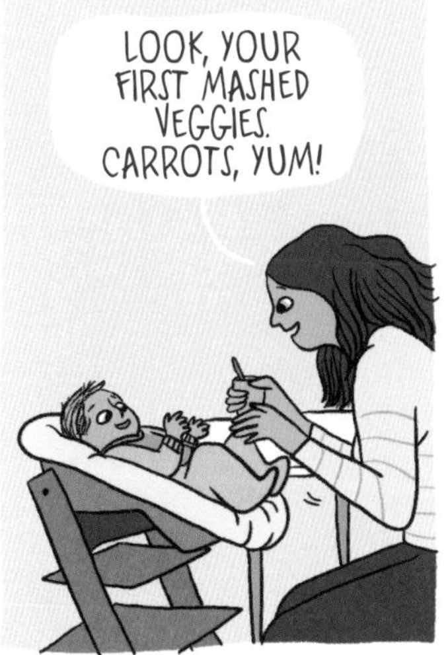

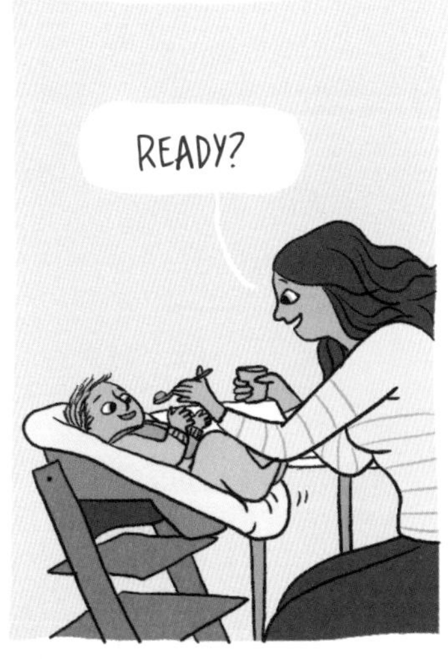

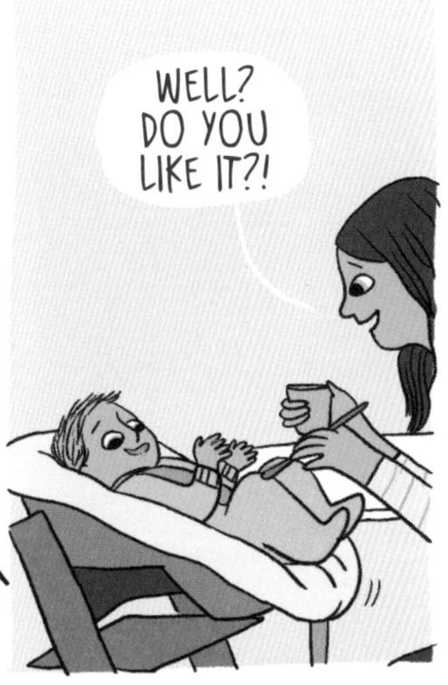

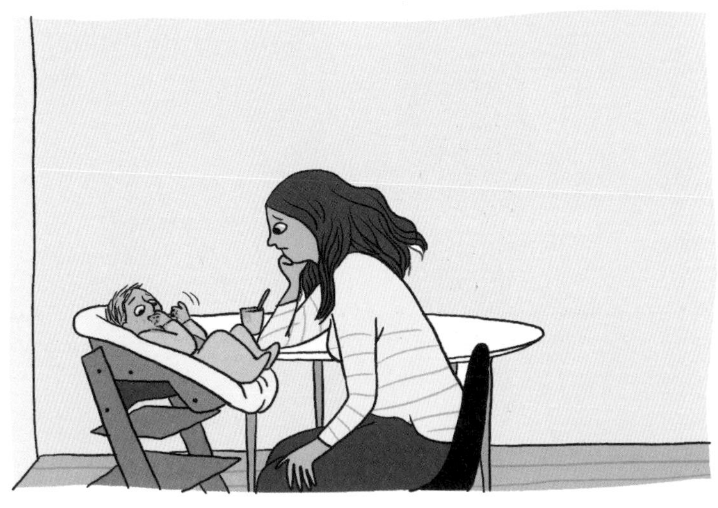

WHAT IF ZOE HAS A CONDITION?

A DISEASE YOU CAN'T DETECT?

A WHOLE BUNCH OF ALLERGIES?

12 CHOCOLATE MEDALS.

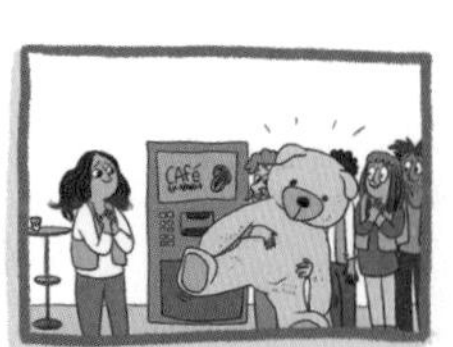
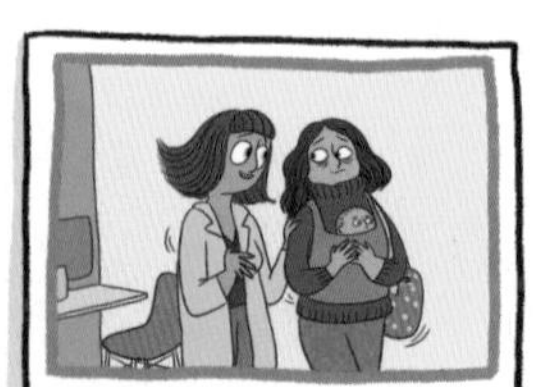
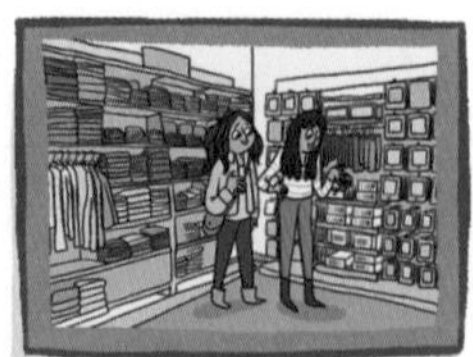
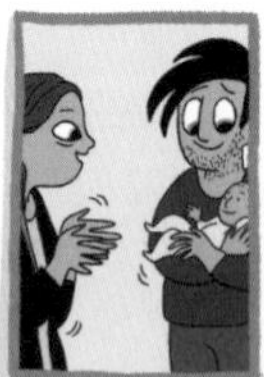
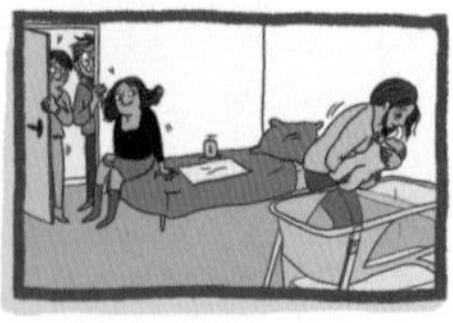
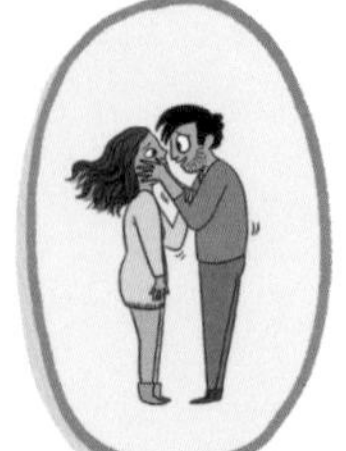
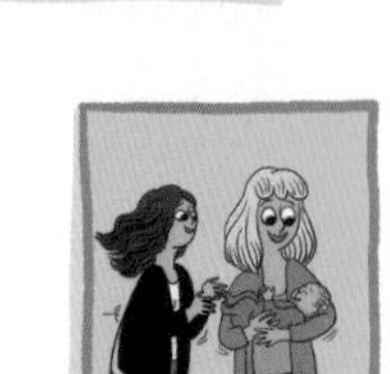
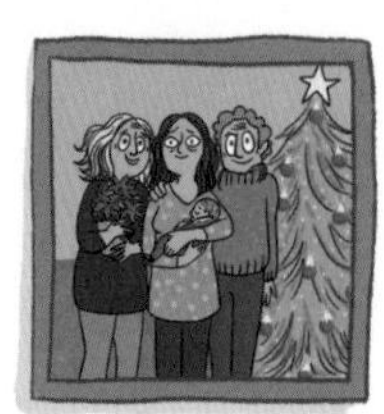
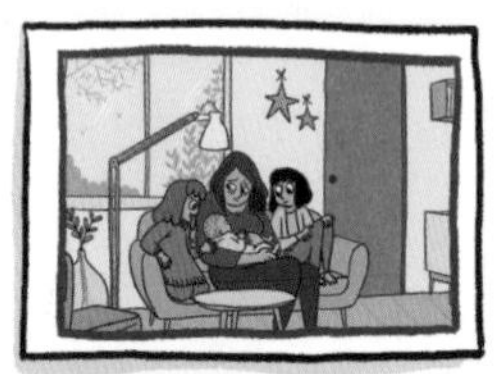
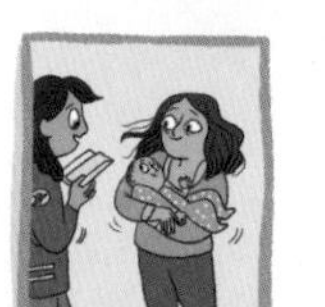
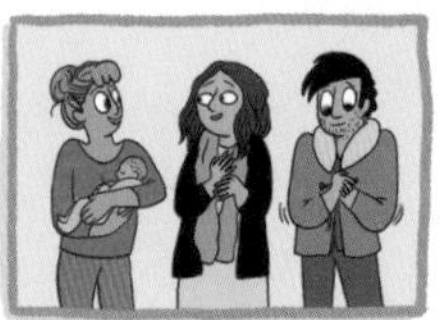
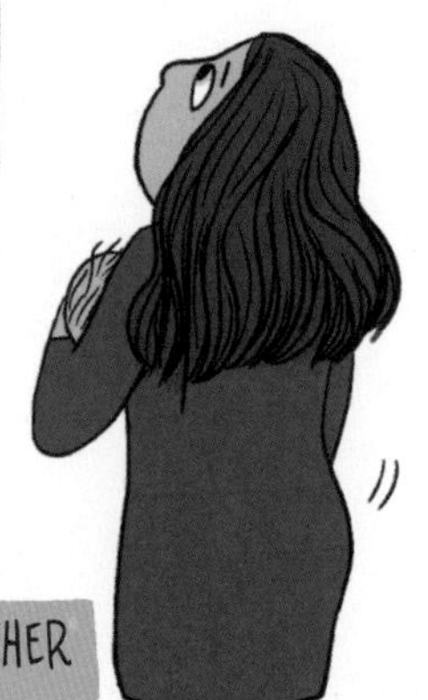

12 PEOPLE WHO VALIDATE ME AS A MOTHER

BUT I STILL DON'T KNOW WHAT THAT MEANS.

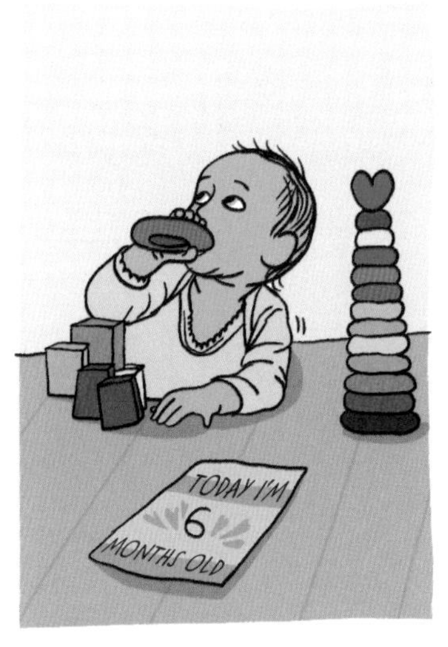
TODAY I'M
6
MONTHS OLD

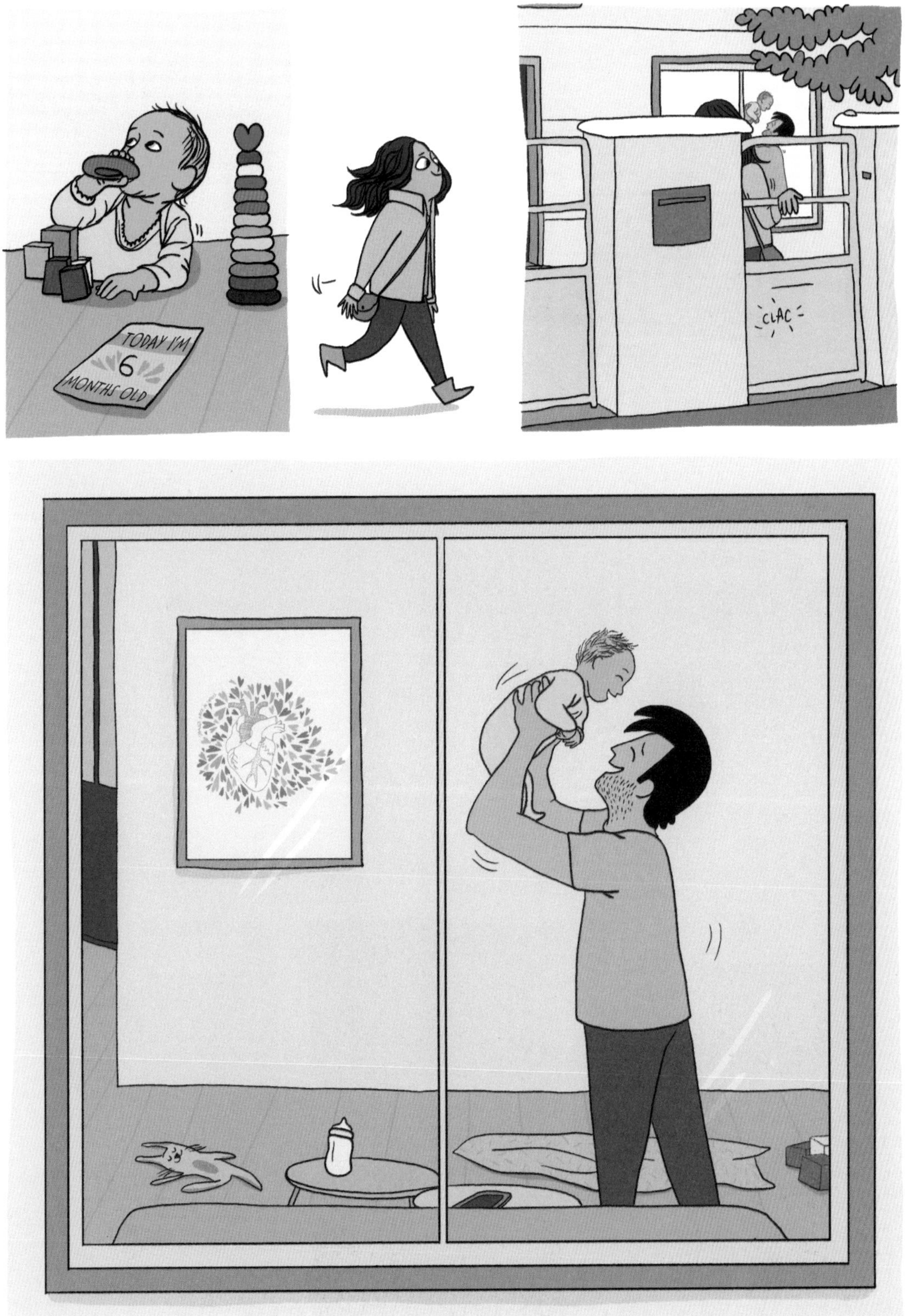

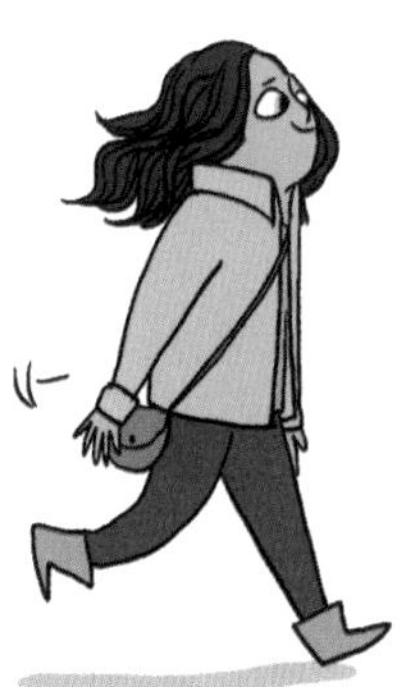

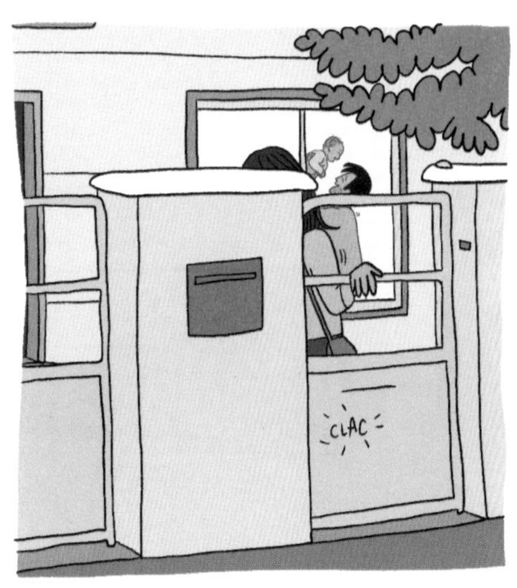
CLAC

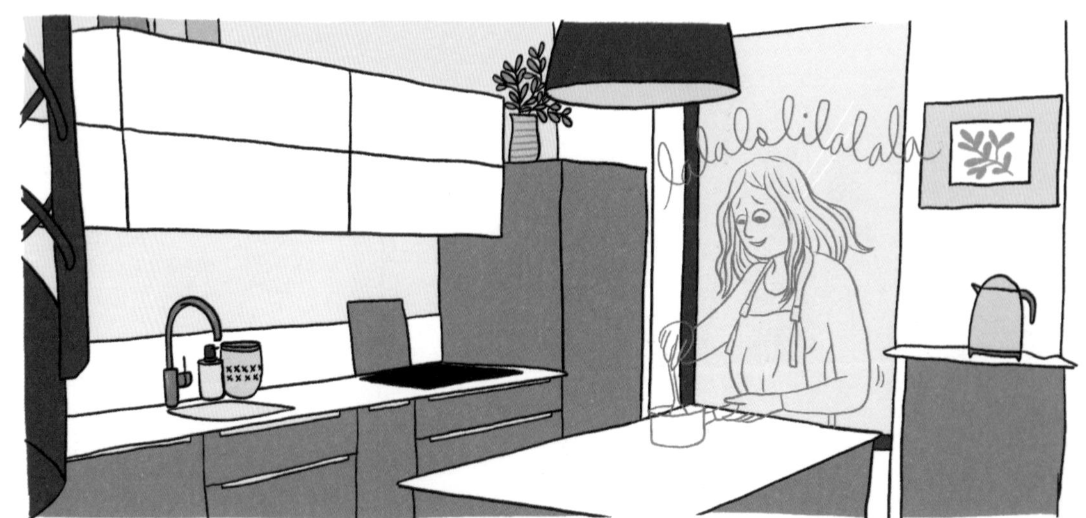
lalalolilalala

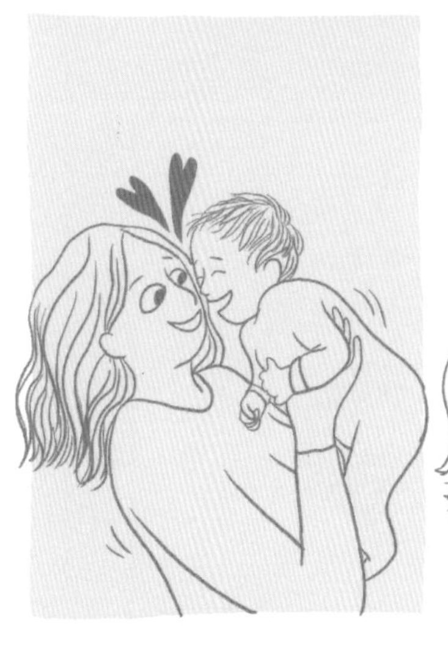

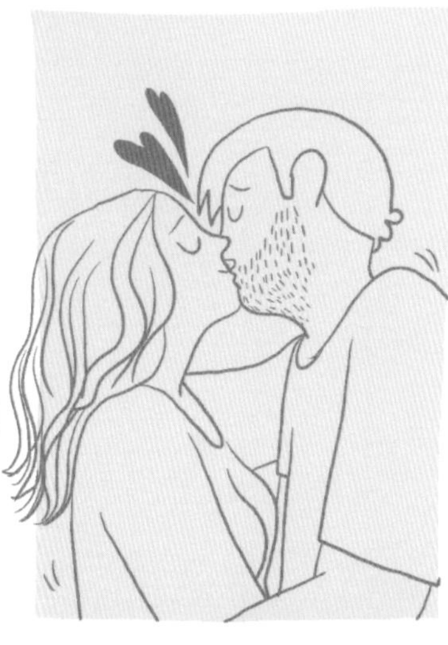

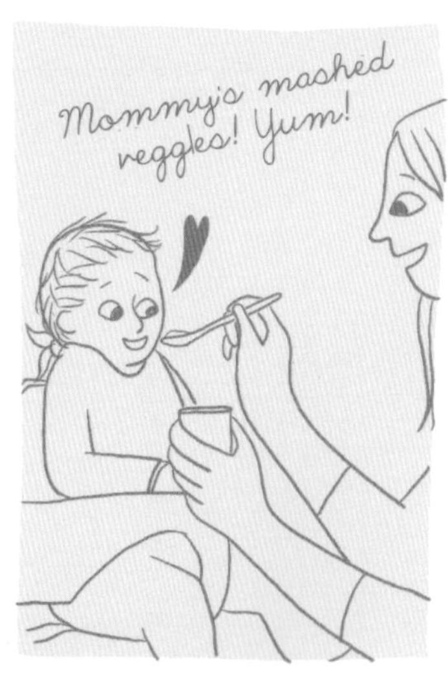
Mommy's mashed veggies! Yum!

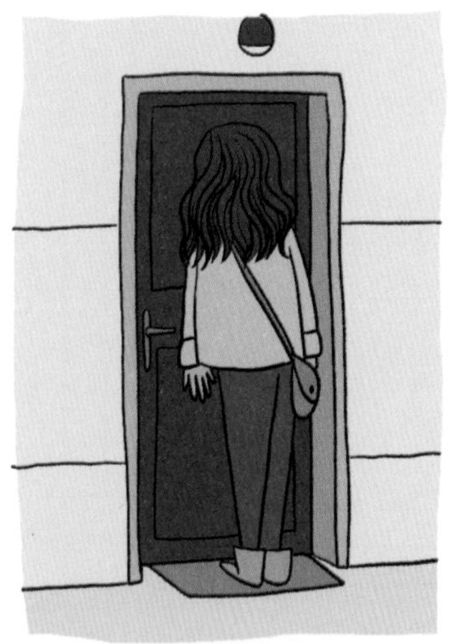

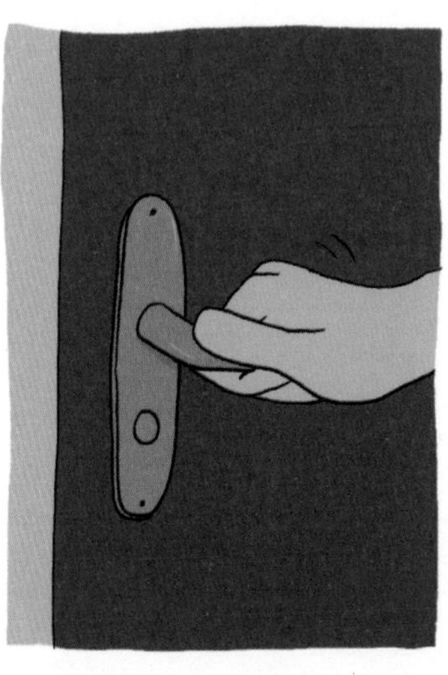

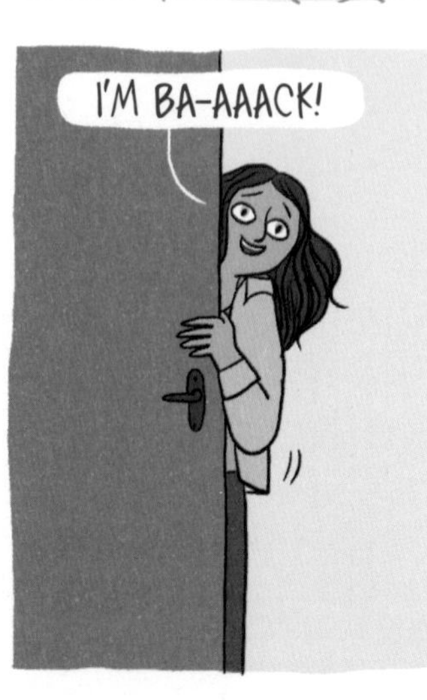
I'M BA-AAACK!

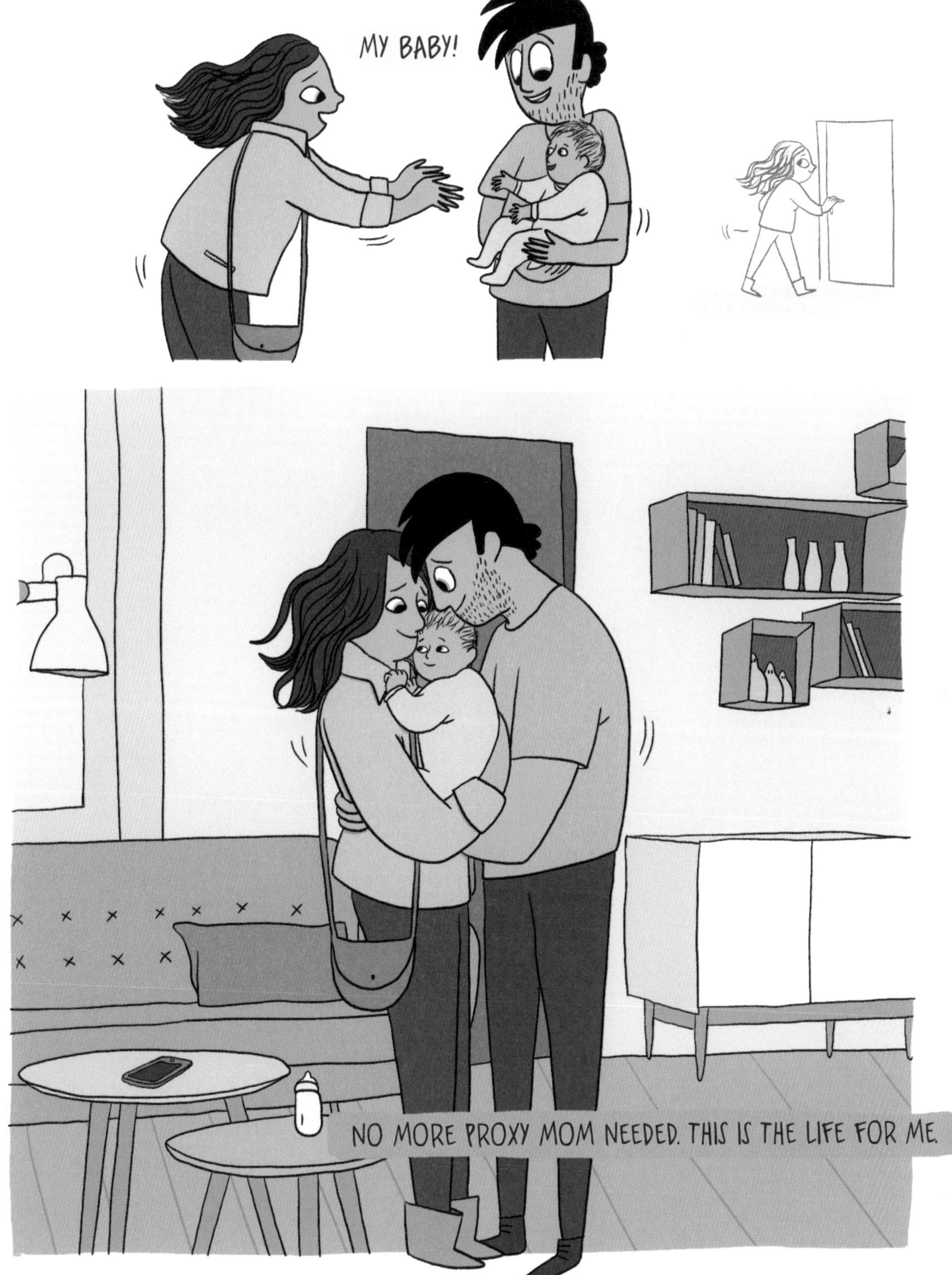
LOOK, ZOE, IT'S MOMMY!
MY BABY!
NO MORE PROXY MOM NEEDED. THIS IS THE LIFE FOR ME.

WHICH IS WHY I'M GOING TO GO FOR IT, JUST DIVE IN ONCE AND FOR ALL. REGARDLESS IF MY BABY IS SIX MONTHS, SIX DAYS, OR SIX MINUTES OLD: MY BIRTH AS A MOTHER FINALLY HAPPENED.
IT'S NEVER TOO LATE.

THERE IS NO DIPLOMA FOR MOTHERHOOD.
WE ALL JUST DO THE BEST WE CAN.

I DID MY BEST.

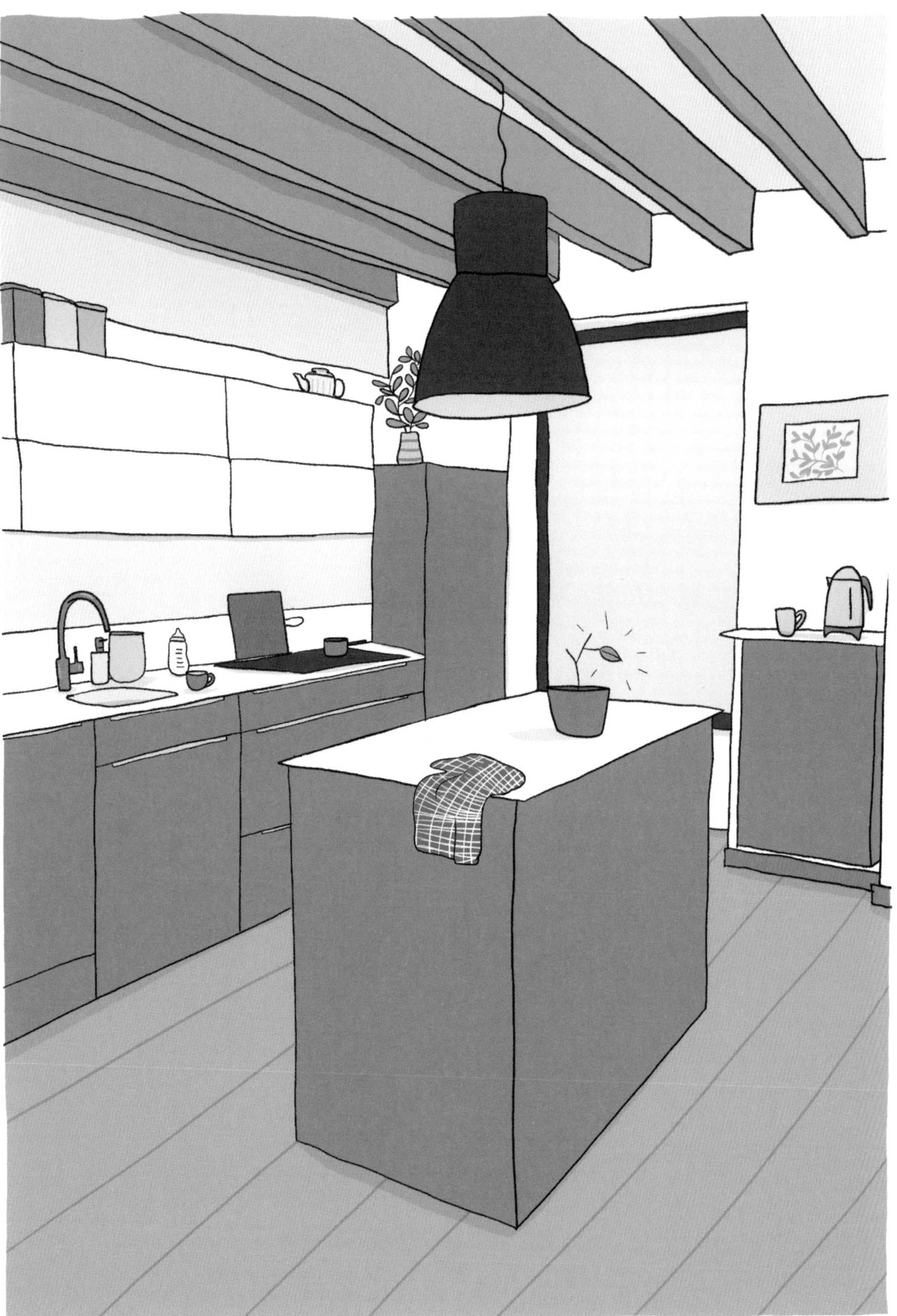

SOPHIE ADRIANSEN & MATHOU

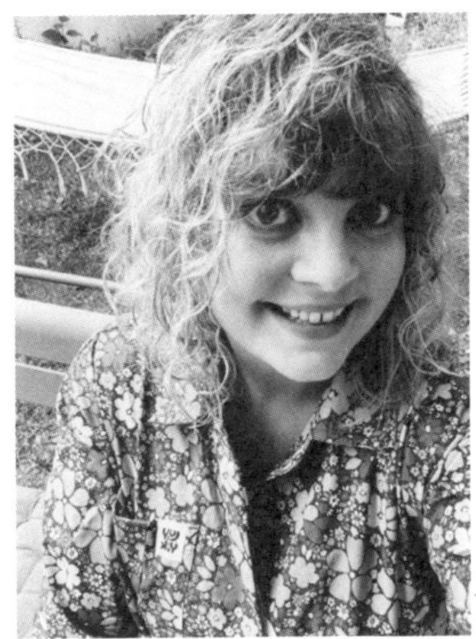

Mathou

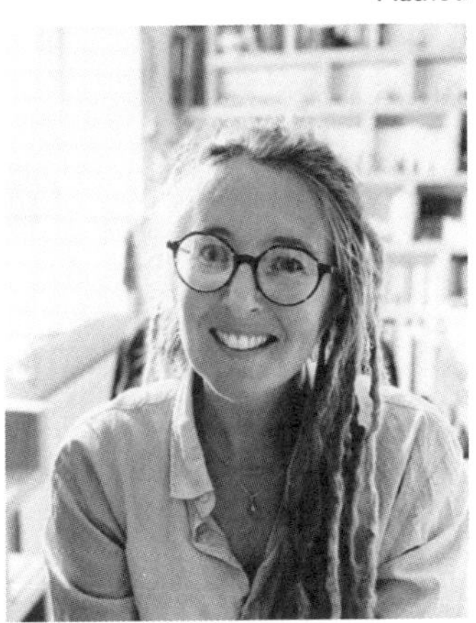

Sophie Adriansen

TWO GIRLS FROM WEST FRANCE

Sophie and Mathou met at a 2016 book fair in western France, where they both live. They immediately clicked thanks to their common interests, and it wasn't long before they read each other's work. This further increased their sense of connection, and the two women kept in touch. As their friendship deepened, so did their mutual admiration.

TWO ARTISTS EMBARKING ON A NEW CHAPTER IN LIFE

École Supérieure de Commerce (Graduate Business School), Sciences Po (Graduate School of Political Science), Faculté d'Économie (Graduate School of Economics): between the two of them, Mathou (pron. Matoo) and Sophie boast twelve years of higher education at some of France's most prestigious institutions. In 2011, they embark on new lives as artists. Hello, impostor syndrome! But they bravely overcame the feelings of self-doubt with a lot of hard work: more than fifty publications for Sophie since then, while Mathou has worked on six comics, a popular series of illustrated diaries, appointment books and wall calendars, and countless projects with other artists.

MOTHERS X 2

Sophie and Mathou were born only a few months apart and are both mothers. They both had children with men who were already fathers and who "knew what they were doing," while the women both struggled with a maternal instinct that was anything but instinctive. Impostor syndrome rearing its ugly head again!

A PROJECT DESTINED TO BRING THEM TOGETHER

The challenges of becoming a mother turned each woman's life upside down, led to some deep soul-searching, had a pivotal effect on their artistic journey, and inspired them to share their experience publicly. When you add it all up, it almost looks as though Fate conspired to lead them to *Proxy Mom!*

ACKNOWLEDGEMENTS

The idea for The Proxy Mom first came to me when I was in the maternity ward, shortly after giving birth to my second child. As I walked past a young mother in the hallway, I flasbacked to three years earlier and saw myself looking the exact same way: dazed and confused after the birth of my first child. I went through a long period of postpartum depression the first time. Right then, in that hallway, I decided it would be different this time around. Some time later, at home, the story began to take shape.

My heartfelt thank you to Mathou for her generosity, her emotional honesty and her friendship, and for helping this endeavor feel like the right thing to do.

A big thank you to Marie-Anne Jost-Kotik for the royal treatment, and to Aline Sibony for helping to bring this project to fruition.

Thank you to the women who started #MonPostPartum for liberating the words and putting them out there.

Thank you to Marc Zaffran/Martin Winckler and Michel Odent for their advocacy on behalf of women, in the medical context and through words—thank you, thank you for the words.

I would also like to thank Dr. N. Alassas and the entire team at the Redon-Carentoir maternity ward, thanks to whom I went through a second period of postpartum without attaching the word depression to it.

Thank you to my men for learning about motherhood. Love, ♥

Sophie

"We will not change the world until we change the way we are born."
Michel Odent

Sophie, thank you for sending me that email during the lockdown of spring 2020; it brought a ray of light into such a dark period. I am very happy that you chose me to illustrate this wonderful story of rebirth, love and resilience. For this story is a bit like your own story, as well as my story and the story of all mothers. And it finally talks openly about all the things that can go wrong, after centuries of hearing nothing but "you'll see, it's absolutely wonderful!"

I am very proud and touched to have been part of this amazing adventure. Thank you for listening, thank you for all those endless conversations we had, and thank you for the champagne, of course!

A big thank you to the amazing team at First Éditions, Aline, Marie-Anne and the whole team of women who work with them; I'm really lucky to have come across people as supportive and attentive as you all were.

My Loulou, these drawings are also for you, in a way, because even though nine years ago, it wasn't exactly love at first sight and I didn't exactly experience the most beautiful day of my life, with a little hindsight, I'm sure of one thing: in the baby store, I would have chosen you, and even though, at first, I debated on whether or not to return you for a refund (I was told it wasn't an option, which I find outrageous), you are the best person in the whole wide world and I am unbelievably proud to be your mom.

I would also like to thank Salomé, who taught me that you could also be a parent, even a "half-parent," without losing part of your perineum and with fewer sleepless nights.

A big thank you to Yohann for taking on (almost) without flinching both shares of the mental parental load while I was busy drawing my pages.

Happy reading, and I hope the story of this woman—who's a tad broken, a bit different, slightly confused, but a badass nonetheless—a real woman from real life, will touch you as much as it made me shed tears of both sadness and of joy.

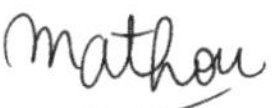

Also by Sophie Adriansen:
NINA SIMONE IN COMICS

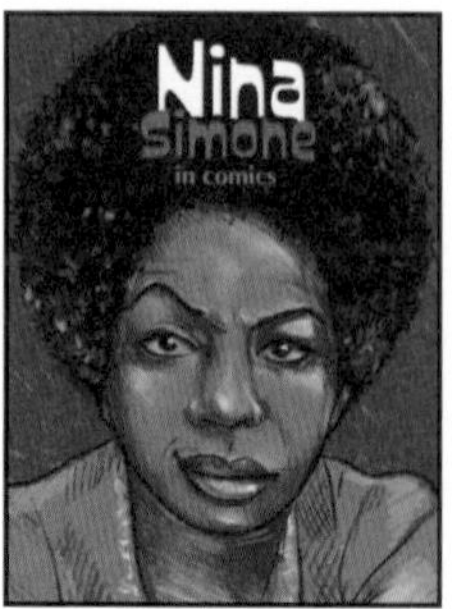

Also available from NBM Graphic Novels:
WOMEN DISCOVERERS
Top Women In Science
"RECOMMENDED. Educators, librarians, and readers will be motivated to further research and share the stories of these heroic minds."
-School Library Connection

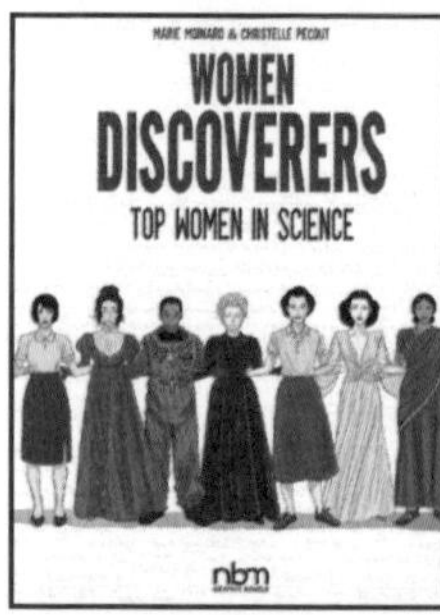

PHOOLAN DEVI
Rebel Queen
"STARRED REVIEW. A woman operating with an eye-for-an-eye attitude is a rare and powerful thing, and this heroic tale of Phoolan's journey from despair and abuse to justice and renown, is intoxicating."
-Library Journal

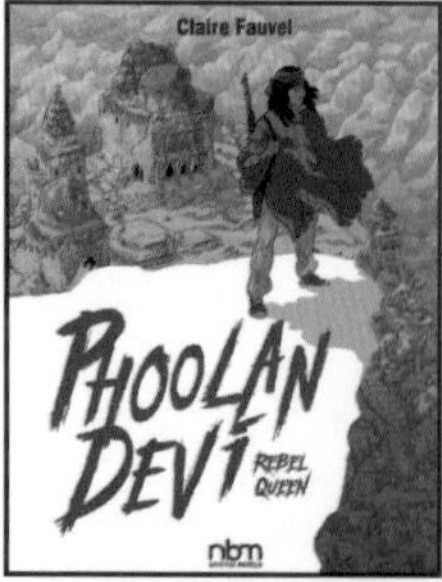

FISTS RAISED
10 Stories of Sports Star Activists
Rich in authentic anecdotes, this book tells the fate of women and men who have written the political, social or cultural history of sport by taking a stand.

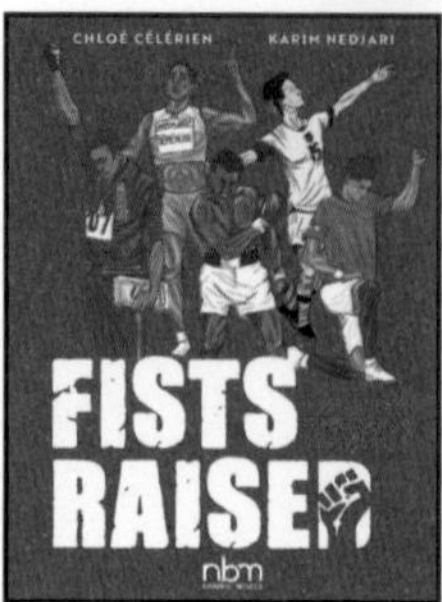

See previews, get exclusives
and order from:
NBMPUB.COM
We have hundreds of graphic novels available.
Subscribe to our monthly newsletter
Follow us on Facebook & Instagram (nbmgraphicnovels), Bluesky (@nbmpub.bsky.social), X (Twitter, @nbmpub).